INFORMED
IS BEST

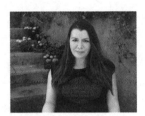

About the author

Professor Amy Brown is based in the Department of Public Health, Policy and Social Sciences at Swansea University in the UK where she leads the MSc in Child Public Health. With a background in psychology, she first became interested in the many barriers women face when breastfeeding after having her first baby. Three babies and a PhD later she has spent the last twelve years exploring psychological, cultural and societal barriers to breastfeeding, with an emphasis on understanding how we can better support women to breastfeed and subsequently raise breastfeeding rates. Her primary focus is how we can shift our perception of breastfeeding as an individual mothering issue, to a wider public health responsibility, with consideration to how we can make societal changes to protect and encourage breastfeeding.

Professor Brown has published over 100 papers exploring the barriers women face in feeding their baby during the first year. In 2016 she published her first book *Breastfeeding Uncovered*, followed by *Why Starting Solids Matters* (2017), *The Positive Breastfeeding Book* (2018) and *Informed is Best* (2019). She is a regular Huffington Post blogger, aiming to change the way we think about breastfeeding, mothering and caring for our babies.

INFORMED IS BEST

How to spot fake news about your pregnancy, birth and baby

AMY BROWN

Informed is Best: How to spot fake news about your pregnancy, birth and baby
First published in the UK by Pinter & Martin Ltd 2019

ISBN 978-1-78066-490-3
Also available as an ebook

Edited by Susan Last
Index by Helen Bilton

British Library Cataloguing-in-Publication Data
A catalogue record for this book is available from the British Library

Cover image: Shutterstock

Printed in the EU by Hussar

This book has been printed on paper that is sourced and harvested from sustainable forests and is FSC accredited

Pinter & Martin Ltd
6 Effra Parade
London SW2 1PS

pinterandmartin.com

CONTENTS

For #girlyswots and those who love them

INTRODUCTION

You should breastfeed. No wait, he'd sleep better if you formula fed. He looks like he needs a bit of cereal in his bottle… No, don't give them anything till at least six months. They need spoon-feeding. Let them feed themselves. Co-sleep. Put him in his own room. Soothe her to sleep. Let her cry to sleep. He's manipulating you. Dummies are a must. Dummy? He'll go off to university with one! Vaccinate. Don't vaccinate. You're spoiling that baby. Eat soft cheese. Whatever you do, don't eat soft cheese! Water birth. Home birth. Hospital birth. Give birth in a stream birth. Rod for your own back. Get induced. Don't get induced! A glass of wine won't hurt you. Don't touch wine again until they've left home! And whatever you do don't get stressed…

Is it any wonder that pregnant and new mums are so exhausted all the time? I mean, I guess growing and birthing and caring for that new baby is going to take it out of you a bit, but maybe the barrage of unsolicited 'advice' is the real reason mums are so frazzled.

In the age of digital media we are inundated by information seemingly every moment of the day telling us what to think, do and buy. This seems to get even worse as soon as you're pregnant. Everyone has an opinion on what you should think and do, with the underlying suggestion that every decision you make is of vital importance and will affect your child's entire future. Suddenly you are public property and your every move is scrutinised, even by those with no experience of babies. And that's before increasing numbers of experts, self-proclaimed or otherwise, pop up telling you what the right thing to do is, based on their own experiences or interpretation of 'evidence'.

In the sea of voices, how do you know who to trust? How do you know if the headline screaming at you has even a hint of truth in it? And how can you confidently rebut the latest 'wisdom' imparted to you over a family dinner?

The answer is by being your own judge of what is important and relevant to you and your family. By understanding the tricks the media play, and learning how to separate facts from conspiracy-style theories and make judgements about the research evidence yourself.

If you're looking for '*the one most definitely right answer*' when it comes to growing, birthing and caring for babies, unfortunately this book won't give it to you. No single book can do that. No one individual can be an expert in *all* the research around caring for babies. And – spoiler alert – there is no one right answer when it comes to the majority of baby care decisions anyway. People are complicated. Lives are complicated. Babies, despite their deceptive smallness, are remarkably complicated.

What this book will do is help you cut through the media spin and nonsense online and give you the skills to understand the research, what it means (and also what it doesn't mean), so that you can make your own evidence-informed decisions about what is best for you and your family. It will help you think about what research evidence really means on an individual level, and it will expose the gaps in our understanding, particularly when it comes to the health and wellbeing of mothers and babies.

It will cover topics like thinking about who is giving you information, and why. It will help you explore the research that information is based on, and how it applies to your own day-to-day life. It will get you thinking about context and individual risk and how different options might protect you and your baby. It will help you see the bigger picture and feel more confident in making decisions.

What do I mean by 'informed is best'?

Information can be empowering. It can help you make the decisions that are right for you. But what it can't do is change biology. Or often circumstance. You can have all the information in the world, and things still might not go the way you'd like them to. I am not suggesting that if you just have a bit more information and knowledge, things will be different. Information doesn't mean that you don't still need support from others, either – support from professionals and others is a vital part of enabling you to put your informed decision into action.

However, whatever situation you find yourself in, *being as informed as possible will help*. It won't solve everything, but it will help. If a caesarean section ends up the right decision for you, then knowing all about it will help, even if you'd have preferred not to have one.

Ideally, you would always be at the heart of any discussion about your body and health with the professionals supporting you. There is increasing recognition that 'shared decision making in healthcare' – actually involving the person things are happening to – is important.[1] It is recognised as benefitting physical health outcomes, satisfaction with care and general wellbeing, including in maternity services.[2] You should be presented with the different options available, their risks and benefits, and be able to make a shared decision with your healthcare professionals.

This may sound simple and obvious, but it is not. Even with the most supportive health professionals in the world it involves having a full picture of what might be right for you in your individual circumstances, and there are plenty of people out there trying to drag you in one direction or another. And professionals are not always supportive. Research has shown that obstetricians tend to focus on the potential risks of labour and birth, and in a discussion on birth options may be thinking about the potential for complications. You can understand their bias – most obstetricians will deal with mainly complex cases, increasing their perception that birth is a risky process. However, research has shown that sometimes this means they only explain the risks of one option, without fully explaining the risks of surgical procedures.[3]

So knowing what is right for you, and feeling confident in your decision, makes any discussion much simpler. It will give you a much better handle on:

1. Whether you are being given the whole picture and what the real risk is to you (i.e. what is your *individual* risk? Suggestions that something is 'double' or 'triple' the risk don't help – double the risk of what?)
2. What wider factors in your life might affect this decision and why you think those are important
3. Being an informed player in the discussion

The aim of this book is therefore to help increase your understanding of how to make informed judgements when it comes to you, your body and your baby.

'Science' should only be part of your decision

This book is going to talk about how understanding science and research can be important when it comes to growing, birthing and caring for your baby. Science helps us to understand more about the world. It gives us an evidence base that we can use to shape our decision-making, at an individual and policy level. And it's really useful when it comes to thinking about growing and caring for babies. For example, bioscience can help us understand the mechanisms of how infant feeding, birth or care might affect a baby's health and development. Epidemiology can help us spot patterns in behaviour and outcomes in large populations. Social sciences can help us understand the complex social, cultural and psychological factors that shape and influence health outcomes. Health economics can model the costs of different behaviours and interventions for us. Philosophy can help us think more deeply about if, how and why these things matter.

Conducting research into pregnancy, birth and babies is vitally important because we live in a society that relies on an evidence base to produce health guidelines and secure investment in services that support women. If there is a 'lack of evidence', women miss out on care and support that they need. And we're already fighting to catch up, because the majority of well-funded scientific research is conducted by rich White men, who tend to do research that they believe matters... to other rich White men. Research into the female body, and especially perinatal health, is sparse in comparison and this absence of 'evidence' is used to keep women down.

Nonetheless, this book is not going to insist that science and data should always be the main or only tool that you use to make decisions that are right for your family. Your circumstances and preferences, alongside things that are important to you such as your family and your culture matter. Research, data and external expertise can play an important and useful role in your decision, but are by no means the top or only priority. And you certainly don't need 'permission from science' to make decisions. You don't have to justify your decisions, and certainly not to people who haven't been involved in creating and caring for your baby.

You have a right to expect your body to work, and to use it in the way that was intended, without needing science to support your view. It is your right to want to breastfeed your baby, for example, not because study X says this and study Y shows that... but simply because it's a biological norm and you want to use your body in that way. This isn't to be mixed up with biological imperatives (e.g. you must use your body in a certain way because you can) but rather a desire and right to be able to mother that way, just like we expect and hope to be able to hear or smell. And if you can't breastfeed, it's okay to feel angry or mourn the loss of it.

11

One final note: a lack of research evidence is not proof that something is not important. Just because science hasn't caught up with what women have 'known' for generations, doesn't mean those behaviours and rituals should be dismissed. Women know what is important. Cultures know what is important. And they get to define what is important, or indeed, not see it as important at all – rather a case of just being. The burden of proof should fall on any intervention to prove its safety and benefit. Benefits of breathing, anyone? Exactly.

So, use this book wisely. Use it to gain skills to explore what the science says when it comes to you and your baby. Use it to push for more investment and care for women. Use it to overthrow the science patriarchy. And remember science is not the be all and end all. Your instincts and desires matter too. You do not need to present a complex systematic review for every parenting decision you make.

Reflecting on my own bias in research

It wouldn't be right to write a book criticising (some) research without reflecting on my own inherent bias and place in all of this. We are all biased in one way or another. Every single one of us, including researchers and policy makers. Recognising this and reflecting on it is a really important step in trying to reduce or mitigate bias. I'd like to think that given the right tools, an open mind and an understanding of just how natural bias is, we're all capable of spotting our bias and reflecting on what things really mean.

As an academic and researcher I have trained for many years (15 to be precise, although I did squeeze in – or should that be out? – three babies during that time) in different forms of science, research and analysis. I've worked across psychology, business studies, early childhood and now public health. I've worked on intervention studies, trials, survey data and many a qualitative interview and focus group. I've published over 100 research papers and books and am now a professor of public health.

This has given me an understanding of how things should work in research, and the natural pitfalls and limitations that apply to absolutely every piece of research out there. And that very much includes my own research, done to the best of my ability at the time, which has its flaws just like any other work. However, science is not built upon any individual study. It's how individual research fits into a bigger picture that counts. No single study can give a full answer.

Through all my research, reading literally thousands of research papers, I have formed scientific opinions based on the evidence of those papers on the optimal outcomes we should be striving to promote and protect across pregnancy, birth and babies. But I'm also a mum of three, and therefore affected by my own experiences of growing, birthing and feeding my children. It is only natural (as we will cover in more detail later) to like it when a piece of information supports what you want or do. But it's also important to stay abreast (pun intended) of other research that competes with or challenges your views.

I am hugely fortunate in that my preferred 'choices' about having babies were possible through a combination of my biology, experiences, a bit of luck and relative privilege. I wanted to give breastfeeding a go – and it all turned out pretty fine for me (minus the mastitis). I wanted to avoid a caesarean if possible – and that worked out too (just). I wanted to be able to keep my babies close day and night – and that mainly worked out, although I had to go back to work sooner than I wanted. But I also had things I would have preferred not to happen – three rounds of hyperemesis (oh, how I'd planned to eat healthily!), hideous experiences in labour, and some horrible times postnatally.

So if I combine my science background, and my life as a mum, what do I get? Here is my 'stance' on the major things to do with birth and babies, stated openly:

- I have my own personal preferences, but I believe in informed choice – giving women the information they need, and supporting them in making and following through with their own decisions.
- I believe in a 'public health' approach rather than an 'individual focused' approach – that means I think we should create environments in which the options that data suggest are the 'healthiest' are more easily supported.
- I believe in the importance of recognising individual context. What is shown to be 'best' on a population level, may not be 'best' for any individual. I believe that culture, history and family traditions play a huge role in decision-making.
- I believe most of all that women should be given accurate information and not terrified or moralised into making decisions by someone else. A big part of this is opening up the discussion about research and how it is conducted so we can understand risk more clearly.
- I believe in supporting the 'biologically normal' where it is beneficial – for example by keeping mum and baby close, not leaving women to die in childbirth! I believe we need to value new parents and their connection with their baby more.

Most of all, I believe that families should have access to the best evidence, and be given the tools to understand, critique and judge how research affects them – free from judgement, justification or guilt. And that is what this book is about.

1

WHAT DO YOU WANT TO BELIEVE?

Imagine you're scrolling though social media. First up is the acquaintance with the very carefully selected (and likely Photoshopped) pictures of her holiday. Next, the guy who really likes posting photos of his 'babies' (they're actually cats). Then that one person you think is absolutely crazy but you keep for amusement purposes. And then... something catches your eye. Someone has shared the latest study suggesting that something you do in pregnancy *definitely really absolutely strongly* affects your baby's life chances. What do you do?

Be honest. Do you jump for joy because you happened to do that very thing (without actually meaning to, as you had no idea it was important)? Does your stomach start churning because you did the exact opposite and now you're worried you've screwed up? Do you get angry because you feel judged? Do you roll your eyes at yet another study about a 'miracle' thing? Do you share it?

If you share it, do you add a comment proclaiming it to be a marvellous/awful study? What do other people do in response? Do they react? Does a fight break out? Do you wish you'd just stuck to looking at Snookey the cat?

Most of us think we are logical when it comes to new

information. We may pride ourselves on our ability to be critical thinkers. We hope that in this situation we would have the sense to at least check what the research was actually about before sharing it, rather than relying on the emotive, barely-grasping-the-facts news summary of the study. And let's face it, given the current political climate, we really ought to check that we haven't accidentally shared a spoof *Daily Mash* article thinking it was real. However, it takes real effort to genuinely approach each new piece of information from an unbiased perspective. And who has time for that?

The biggest problem we have when faced with new information is our own brain. We are pre-programmed to seek out information that reinforces how we already think, in the fastest possible way. This is known as 'confirmation bias'. Thinking is tiring and our brain will do whatever it can to sneakily skim read and ignore things we don't like, even if we consciously try to stop it doing so. Worse, the brain's top five blind spots are religion, money, health, relationships and family.[1] So you can see where anything to do with growing, birthing and raising babies fits in.

Why does confirmation bias exist? Well, stability and continuity feel comforting and reassuring. And anything to do with babies can feel stressful and uncertain, especially if we are really concerned about a particular area. So anything that helps make us feel comforted and reassured helps.

The bad news is that we are all prone to confirmation bias. Even when we think we're not doing it, we are. Humans are made that way. Researchers do it. Health professionals do it. Politicians definitely do it. The good news is that with a bit of understanding and reflection, and, importantly, recognition of how we are led to do it, we can minimise its occurrence.

1. Is confirmation bias persuading you to think a certain way?

Confirmation bias, as we've seen, is the tendency to seek out and pay attention to information that fits with how we already think.[2] Confirmatory information makes us feel like our decisions are the 'right' ones. It's comforting. It tells us we're doing a really good job of this 'adulting' thing, even if our top is on back to front and we've got baby sick down our arm.

Most of us worry at some point about whether our decisions about caring for our babies are the right ones. Confirmation bias dampens this worry right down. No need to worry, brain, some random person on the internet has confirmed that we're okay! Research has even suggested that when we find information – or 'new proof' – that our ideas are right, we get a rush of dopamine to the brain. This is one of the reward hormones that makes us feel happy and exhilarated. Confirmatory information literally stimulates the reward pathways in our brain, making us feel great. It's no wonder we like it.[3]

Our brains also love it when we find information that fits into what we already think. Although our brains are pretty complex and clever, actually all they really want to do is get things done in the quickest and simplest way and then go back to watching cats on the internet or singing a mindless tune. A relevant term here is 'sense-making'. People want order in their world, so they look for information that reduces uncertainty and helps them make sense of the world as a rational place. Avoiding conflicting information is part of that.[4]

Conversely, our brains don't like to admit they were wrong. On an evolutionary level, our bodies still think that decisions can be life or death. Long ago, doing the wrong thing – for example, trying to stroke a man-eating tiger because it looked cute – could have extreme consequences. Nowadays, when we mostly worry about things that are less important, our brains still freak out if we receive information that suggests we are wrong. This is where that paranoia that you've done something to irreversibly harm your baby comes from.

So we seek out – consciously or otherwise – information that confirms what we already think. This can be as simple as surrounding ourselves with only one type of information or voice, for example relying only on particular websites, groups or newspapers, or it can be as blatant as refusing to listen to or read any information that goes against our beliefs. The more you surround yourself with people who confirm your beliefs, the more entrenched you get as you hear fewer diverse views (more on this later).

This means that once we have developed a belief about ourselves or the world, it can be difficult to change it. In one study, participants were given data that showed that how happy someone was to take risks in life correlated with their skills as a firefighter. Two groups were used, with one group being told that low risk-taking was associated with being a skilled firefighter and the second being told that high risk-taking was associated with being a skilled firefighter. Half the participants were then told that the information they had just been given was complete nonsense and that there was no association at all between risk-taking and firefighting skill. Participants then went on to judge whether they felt certain individuals would be good firefighters based on a bio including details about their background and risk-taking. In all groups (whether they had been told the information on the link between risk and firefighting was nonsense or not), participants believed that the information they had initially been given was true and rated the firefighters according to their risk-taking.[5] The information, once in their brains, just seemed to stick.

You can see how this plays out in family conversations around birth and babies. Guidelines change over time. When we do more research, and understand more about a topic, we know more, so we change the guidelines. I could write a whole book about things that have changed in the last few decades of parenting. When to introduce solid foods to babies. How long women 'should' stay in a hospital after giving birth (and where is best to give birth in the first place). Whether you can eat peanuts in pregnancy (yes, no, who knows?). Whether drinking Guinness is good or harmful during pregnancy. And so on.

Anyone who has had a baby in the last 10 years or so will almost certainly have been told by someone who had a baby in a previous generation that 'things were different' when they were having babies. And you can see why this is an issue. At the time they were told that what they were doing was best according to the evidence available. And it was! So it is very difficult for them to understand that there are now new guidelines based on new evidence, and it's very difficult to change a view that you have held for a long time (and have been told was right). Even if you can see the logic, your brain will fight you every step of the way.

2. Are you trying overly hard to create an explanation for something you want to believe is true?

Our brains also like patterns. It helps us believe that the world is organised, structured and logical. Being able to predict things helps us feel secure and safe as we believe that we can control the future through our actions. If we can construct a theory for ourselves about why two things are connected, then all the better. Look at us being all in control (rather than tiny creatures on a spinning planet in the depths of space).

In the study about firefighters and risk-taking,[5] some of the participants were asked to write down an explanation for why they thought risk-taking would be linked to firefighting skill. The researchers found that in those who wrote a detailed explanation of why they thought the two were linked, the tendency to not change their opinion after hearing that the information was false was particularly strong.

So if we believe that there is an explanation for why something happens, rather than just being told two things are linked, our beliefs are particularly hard to shift. Again, once we have convinced ourselves that the relationship exists, our brain pretty much refuses to think otherwise. This is particularly true if we have made a decision with the hope of a particular outcome. Our brains will fight to link to a positive outcome and create an explanation for why it happened. And if there's one thing our brains do not like it is coincidence or random occurrence. It's no wonder that the gif of Sherlock Holmes stating 'there is no such thing as coincidence' is so popular.

A great example is the idea that giving young babies solid food earlier than is recommended (or more of it, or before bedtime) will help them to suddenly become brilliant sleepers. Research comparing sleep outcomes has pretty much shown that this isn't true.[6,7,8] But that doesn't stop countless people telling you otherwise. Often they say that they gave their baby solid food and soon after their baby started sleeping more. Great. Everyone loves a bit more sleep. But just because two things happened close together, doesn't mean there is any reason whatsoever that they are linked. Because we do not have access to parallel existences (where we could compare and contrast ourselves in universe A, with ourselves in universe B or C), we can never know what would have happened if they hadn't given that baby solid food.

But our brains love to think that things that happen close together are connected to each other. Research can help uncover the truth – and we will look more closely at how we can be more confident that two things are actually linked later on. With regard to solids and sleep, not only does research tell us that there is no link between solid foods and sleep, but there is also no rational explanation for why the two would be linked. Why would a different energy source (particularly one often lower in calories) affect sleep? Why would eating more help? As adults, if we went to sleep just after a big meal we would likely be more fitful and unsettled, not sleep better. Further, babies do not only wake up at night because they are hungry. (Again, think about the reasons adults wake up at night – is it because they are hungry?)

The real nail in the coffin for the idea that introducing

solids can improve sleep, however, is the research that tracked babies' sleep, showing that they often wake more frequently at certain ages before settling down again. A really common time to start waking up more is at around four months old.[9] Parents will try anything to cut down on these wakings and some will introduce solid foods. Often these babies then start sleeping better. But actually, babies also start sleeping better again in the coming weeks if they *haven't* been introduced to solid foods. They most likely wake up more because of a big growth spurt and developmental leap, rather than because of anything to do with food.

One reason that people often want to link food and sleep is because they (consciously or subconsciously) prefer the idea that their baby's sleep is controllable and predictable. Thus this 'fact' gets passed on as misinformation to the next generation of parents, and so on and so on, strengthening the belief as it rolls on.

3. Are you doing something because everyone else is? (Even if you left high school quite some time ago?)

Another thing that we get a lot of comfort from is thinking that our choices are also made by other people. If we feel that everyone around us is acting differently, it can make us feel anxious about the decisions we have made, even if we spent a lot of time making them, or had no real choice. So if lots of other people share particular information, or state that they believe it is right, we are more likely to go along with it if we can. And if we can't – we may feel pretty unsettled.

Things that are common or 'usual' in our wider social group are known as *social norms*. We are influenced by the social norms around us, both consciously and subconsciously. There can be a lot of pressure to fit in – and acceptance when we do – which can lead us to doing things even if, really, we would prefer to do something else. There are many different types of social norms, but two key variants are 'descriptive norms', which are perceptions of what other people typically do, and 'injunctive norms', which are perceptions of what behaviours are approved or disapproved of.[10]

There are some really interesting studies in the wider psychology literature into how highlighting unwanted social norms to people can increase unwanted behaviours. If you tell people that *'most people are doing X'* even if 'X' is something undesirable, and you say that it is undesirable, then people are still more likely to do it. For example, in his book *Nudge* David Halpern[11] gives the example of how an advert attempting to prevent littering actually increased it, because although it said littering was wrong, it also said that lots of people did it. More people therefore thought it was socially acceptable to litter, as everyone else was at it too.

Similarly, another study highlighted how an attempt to stop people taking petrified wood from a national park in Arizona backfired. In a series of experiments the team showed that if a sign was put up saying *'Many past visitors have removed petrified wood, please don't remove it from the Park'*, almost 8% of people picked up a carefully placed piece of wood just past the sign. However, when the sign read *'Please don't remove the petrified wood from the Park, in order to preserve the natural state of the Petrified Forest'*, only 1.6% picked up the obvious piece of wood.[12]

The importance of fitting in and doing what everyone else is doing can be seen in many aspects of baby care. Although we joke about different 'types' of parents with distinct parenting styles –'routine queens' and 'crunchy mamas' – and the tendency of certain behaviours to become popular within communities (having a certain pram, driving a certain car, children all wearing the same things), there is a real phenomenon behind it. Many of our choices are 'contagious': we copy those around us because it is reassuring, and it makes us feel like we fit in. Known as *'behavioural or social contagion'*, it can be seen across human behaviour – we look to those around us when deciding what to do. Rioting, stockpiling, daft toy crazes sweeping the internet – these are all examples of social contagion,[13] which can even be seen when it comes to pregnancy and birth. Examples of behaviours that have been shown to be 'socially caught' are teenage pregnancy,[14] pregnancy rates in offices[15] (it's not your imagination – they double in the year after someone else has a baby) and postnatal depression.[16]

Perceptions and feelings of pressure around infant feeding are another good example. Where you live can determine whether you feel pressurised to feed your baby in a certain way. Particularly in some low income communities, low breastfeeding rates have become the norm, meaning that many mothers feel pressure *not* to breastfeed because hardly anyone around them is doing so. Mothers are encouraged to bottle-feed and reprimanded socially for breastfeeding publicly or in front of others.[17] Conversely, mothers living in communities where breastfeeding rates are very high report that they feel pressured *into* breastfeeding, or guilty if they can't, because everyone around them is doing it.[18]

Feeling part of a group, particularly one that you identify with and feel connected to, can be wonderfully protective for your mental health.[19] We will look at this in more detail when we consider the role of social media in our decision-making, but you only have to look at the many thousands of social media groups and their popularity to see how comforting being part of a group with similar interests and ways of thinking can be. But at the same time it can also feed into confirmation bias and a belief that there is one 'right' way to feel, increasing feelings of inadequacy and anxiety.[20]

4. Are you thinking too quickly?

You might have heard of the concept of 'fast versus slow thinking' – or to give it more scientific terminology, 'reflexive versus reflective thinking'.[21] Again, this goes back to our brain's desire for everything to be simple and easy, as thinking rationally is complicated and exhausting. Over millennia we have developed all sorts of brain tricks to help us make the quickest possible judgement. The problem is that a lot of our quick-fix brain solutions developed in different contexts that are less helpful now.

Very simply (very, very, simply!) our brains are made up of two parts. The first, more basic part is what we share with many mammals. This primitive part allows us to make very quick decisions, often based on a sense of danger or other strong emotions. Central to this part of the brain is the amygdala, which is responsible for many of our basic emotions.[22]

However, our brains have developed over millennia and humans pride themselves on having a more complex part of the brain – the prefrontal cortex. This is responsible for our developed skills, such as thinking, critical analysis and reasoning. Our amygdala may yell at us that something is very, very scary indeed, but our prefrontal cortex can hopefully tell us that it's just a *Daily Mail* headline. The prefrontal cortex matures during our teen years.[23]

The problem is that sometimes it's just too much like hard work to properly engage the prefrontal cortex. It takes energy. And our brain prefers to use shortcuts if it can, which is not surprising when you think that humans make up to 35,000 decisions every single day.[24] From the big things to the tiny. Which socks. Which piece of dinner to eat next. Which seat to take on the bus. Coat on or coat off? People who experience significant anxiety and struggle with smaller decisions will tell you how time-consuming and exhausting it is to think deeply about this stuff.

Our brains have evolved to make the decision-making process a whole lot simpler. We have a whole system of stored information, knowledge and shortcuts in our minds that lets us 'just do stuff' without thinking too much, called heuristics. Heuristics are shortcuts to thinking. Our brain collects information in a 'usually good enough' way so we can respond. When we are presented with new information, we use these existing heuristics to decide what to do. Heuristics are great. They let us make all sorts of small decisions all day long without stopping to think and dwell and reflect on them.[25]

There are many specific types of heuristic that we use:

Anchoring

We are more likely to stick with the first piece of information we hear, even if subsequent information tells us otherwise. Between my first and second pregnancies the guidance on peanuts changed. In pregnancy one I was told not to eat peanuts and worried dreadfully if I did. By pregnancy two the guidance was to eat peanuts, but I still had a niggling fear when doing so, despite having access to the research in front of me telling me it was a good idea. My brain kept anchoring to the initial information and nagging me about whether eating peanuts was a good idea.

Representative heuristic

This is to do with how probable we think it is that two things will be linked to each other. We use our prior experiences of individuals and their behaviour to make assumptions about new people. We are especially likely to do this when we are busy and faced with lots of decisions at once. The problem is that we are often wrong and we can end up displaying discriminatory or unpleasant behaviours.

This heuristic is one of the explanations for why people end up stereotyping others. You might find, for example, that because you are a younger mother, everyone assumes you aren't going to breastfeed your baby. This is because overall, on a population level, younger mums are less likely to breastfeed, but of course many individual mothers who are younger breastfeed, often for many months or years.[26] So rather than being helpful, this stereotyping can be a significant issue, as research has shown that when health professionals do not expect a certain group of mothers to breastfeed, they provide less breastfeeding support. Research with Black mothers in the US for example has consistently found that they receive less breastfeeding support because their health professionals expect them not to breastfeed.[27] This can lead to a vicious circle: if professionals assume that Black women are less likely to breastfeed, and so offer less information and support, women are then even less likely to be able to breastfeed, and the heuristic is reinforced in the professionals.

Conversely, growing evidence is accumulating that although on a population level in the UK Black mothers have higher breastfeeding rates than White women, this can lead to health professionals believing they know what they are doing, and again give less support, increasing the chances that women encounter difficulties and feel unsupported.[28] So generally, this heuristic is at the heart of many problems when it comes to women receiving the support they need.

Familiarity heuristic

This is when we use our prior experiences to predict what will happen in the future. We assume that because two events appear similar, that all the different circumstances surrounding them will be the same too. A great example of this is when a grandparent says 'W*ell you were introduced to solids at six weeks old and you're fine*'. They have taken a similarity – you as a baby and their grandchild as a baby – decided you're 'fine' (still alive) and assumed that the two situations are essentially the same and therefore your baby can have solids at six weeks too. Of course, this completely disregards all the other circumstances that are part of you 'being fine', like genetics, your other early life experiences and even good old chance. And that's without addressing the deeper question of whether you are actually 'fine'.

Availability heuristic

This is based on how easily we can think or worry about something happening, which depends on how much we hear about it, particularly from news stories. So if we hear lots of scare stories in the news about sharing a bed with a baby being dangerous, we're more likely to agree, because of our perception that the risk is more common than it is.[29] The problem is that some things are more publicised than others. For example, we hear far more about the small number of people killed by terrorists each year than we do about the much greater number who die falling down the stairs. We think our chances of one are greater than the other, when in fact we should be being far more cautious on the stairs.[30] More on this later.

Escalation of commitment

This is a bit like the 'sunk cost fallacy'. If we have already invested money (or our time) in something, we are more likely to keep throwing money (or time) at it, even though we realise it may be even more expensive overall. If we buy a second-hand car, and something on it breaks, we pay to fix it, even though it might not actually be worth it.

The more effort we spend making a decision, the more time we have taken, the more committed we are to it… the more difficult it is to change our minds. Imagine you spend three months decorating your baby's nursery, buying a really expensive swinging crib and ensuring the blinds don't let a single ray of 5am sunshine in. Your baby then flat out refuses to sleep anywhere other than on top of you. But you keep trying, every night, over and over… until they eventually grow out of the swinging crib and you sell it on eBay (to another parent full of false hope).

In my own case, I was determined that baby number two was going to take a bottle of expressed milk. Therefore I bought practically every bottle and teat on the market. I should have stopped after she refused three, or perhaps five, different teats. But no, I carried on (spending hundreds of pounds in the process). And she never took that bottle.

All of this means that despite our potential for higher brain function, we don't always act logically. Far from it. Any good book on behavioural economics, such as Richard Thaler's *Misbehaving*, will give you countless examples of how we often make very strange decisions indeed.[31]

5. Are you deciding with your head or your heart (or your sympathetic nervous system)?

As we have seen, our behaviour (or at least our first instinct) is strongly driven by our emotional reactions, whether we like it or not. We end up making decisions based on how something (a headline, a story on social media) makes us feel in that initial moment, over and above the logic of what we know to be true or the actual risk.

Emotions actually have many benefits on a subconscious, evolutionary level.[32] Think about it: fear, anger, disgust, empathy, happiness – they all bring rewards in the right context and our ancestors who experienced and reacted to emotions probably lived longer to reproduce and pass on those traits compared to those who didn't. For example:

- Those without fear would have ignored the rustling in the trees, and been eaten by the tiger.
- Those who had no feelings of disgust would not have had reduced contact with those showing signs of infection.
- Those incapable of smiling and getting along would have been ostracised by the group.
- Those who displayed no anger would not have helped shape behaviours that would help the group thrive.
- Without empathy members of the group who needed support to survive and thrive would have been abandoned.

So emotions have been part of our evolutionary survival.

The problem is that modern-day society doesn't need us to have the same type of emotional reactions. If you feel threatened by someone in a meeting, it's now less acceptable to try and slingshot a rock at them, set your mates on them or run away and hide behind a tree no matter how tempting that feels.

There is also some evidence that emotion and decision-making are linked in our brains. People who have brain damage in the part of their brain where you experience emotion often find it difficult to arrive at even simple decisions, suggesting that both processes originate from the same areas.[33] And it also appears that emotion can often override logic – we see this all the time in political campaigns and court cases. Support is about hearts and minds, not facts.[34]

Emotions – and stories – therefore often win out over evidence. And the press, social media, and certain organisations know this – consider the tacky but true phrase 'if it bleeds it leads', used to justify lurid headlines.[35] If someone has a heartbreaking, emotional story about damage that has been done to their life, then logic, other rational explanations or influencing factors and the actual risk of the same thing happening to others often fly out of the window, and our natural first instinct is to panic.

It can therefore be extremely difficult for 'science people' to discuss things with 'emotion people', because the science people are easily portrayed as heartless villains. Few researchers or scientists want to make an individual feel 'bad' by discussing the actual research evidence if they can clearly see someone is grieving in front of them. If you have a mother in front of you whose baby died during a home birth, you're going to react kindly, not suddenly start spouting about the (very small) actual risk of that happening. It happened to her and no statistic will ever change that for her.

The issue is further complicated now that, thanks to technology, our discussions take place on a broader stage. If something terrible has happened to an individual, and they highlight that on a social media site with thousands of people watching, it becomes exceedingly difficult to both respect them as an individual, and also share accurate information about what happened to them. And some individuals or organisations manipulate this by effectively shutting down any debate. Paul Ofitt, a vaccine scientist, is quoted as stating that he will not appear with a parent who believes her child has a vaccine disability because *'Every story has a hero, a victim, and villain'* and the scientist often ends up the villain.[36]

We are also selective about which emotions we choose to prioritise. Evidence from psychological experiments shows that we focus on negative emotions much more strongly than on positive ones. We love positive emotion – they give us a great buzz – but negative ones can have a much stronger and lasting impact. Brain imaging even shows that the response to a negative emotion is stronger than for happier ones.[37] This makes sense historically: fear, anger and uncertainty all had much more dangerous implications for us, and our brains therefore pay serious attention to them. This was fine when we were dodging sabre-toothed tigers, but can now lead to us overreacting to social media headlines.

Language also plays an important part in emotions.[38] Anything that contains words that are scary makes people afraid. *'Imagine'* is a particularly powerful word. It encourages people to bypass any sort of reality and critical thinking and imagine a future filled with horror. Unfortunately, our imaginations are often far scarier than reality, so if invited to imagine, we inflate risks.

Getting people to think about the 'future' is another powerful tactic, which is used by a certain follow-on formula milk brand aimed at toddlers. Adverts ask you to imagine 'your baby's future'... implying that it will be all the better for buying their product. There is no evidence that buying a certain brand of follow-on formula milk will affect your baby's future in any way. Indeed, there is little evidence that follow-on formula for toddlers is of *any benefit at all* (first-stage milks have a slightly higher nutrient content and are suitable for the whole time your baby has milk, and you can give cows' milk after 12 months).[39]

Descriptive language is another particular persuader. One fascinating study asked two groups of people to rate how tasty they found certain foods. In both groups the food and presentation was exactly the same, but the description differed. One group was given a descriptive name for what they were eating, e.g. 'succulent Italian seafood fillet'. The other group was given a boring name, e.g. 'seafood fillet'. Those in the descriptive group not only rated the food as tasting better, but also rated it as more appealing to the eye and believed it to contain more calories – despite having eaten exactly the same food, with the same presentation, as the other group.[40]

Formula manufacturers are particularly good at targeting words and descriptions to appeal to their different markets. We know that there is very little difference between first-stage formula milks. The ingredients are determined by law, and if new ingredients are found to be necessary, they are added to all formulas.[39] However, the manufacturers work hard to convince parents that there are differences between them, through adverts, promotions and marketing on the packaging that is tailored to appeal to specific groups.

Another example is the names given to baby foods. First Steps Nutrition Trust examined the content of 191 different baby food products, comparing the name of the product to the actual content. It was surprisingly common for:

a. the order of ingredients in the name not to match the % volume in the ingredients, and

b. for other ingredients not listed in the name to make up a considerable portion of the product.

Often more 'exotic' or 'nutritious' ingredients that parents might be keen for their babies to try are listed at the start of the name, but there is very little of that ingredient in the product, which will be mostly made up of a more mundane fruit such as apple or pear. Sometimes, a seemingly bizarre combination of ingredients is used in the name to appeal to parents who want their baby to have a variety foods, when in fact once it's all mushed in together it tastes more like the main ingredient of apple or pear than anything else.[41] Here are some examples:

Product	Ingredients
Aldi Mamia 'Sweet potatoes, pumpkins, apples and blueberries'	Organic apple purée (52%), organic sweet potato purée (23%), organic pumpkin purée (20%), organic blueberry purée (5%), lemon juice
Little Freddie 'Tender spinach, peas and apples'	Apple (82%), spinach (12%), peas (6%), lemon juice concentrate (0.1%)
Ella's Kitchen 'Broccoli, pears and peas'	Pears (79%), peas (14%), broccoli (7%), lemon juice concentrate (a dash)
Heinz by Nature 'Strawberry, banana, raspberry and apple'	Apple (79%), strawberry (8%), banana (8%), raspberries (5%), antioxidant ascorbic acid

Returning to the example of the seafood fillet labels, the marketing of baby foods reflects our tendency to value 'descriptive' labels, whether they are accurate or not. For example, Ella's Kitchen produces a 'Mighty Grains' range, which sounds very wholesome and far more appealing than just saying that it has added flour in it. Each of the products in the range is based on fruit purée plus around 3–5% of different flours including quinoa, buckwheat, amaranth and wholemeal spelt.[42]

HOW TO KEEP INFORMED:

Your brain won't initially thank you for it, but when you're reading information or research, stop and think. Read it more than once. Take your time.

Own up to your own bias. We all do it. It's natural. It's fine. But we certainly don't all admit it or recognise it. And we certainly don't all challenge ourselves about it.

Try to 'consider the opposite'. If it fits with what you know you want to hear, read it through again with a critical hat on. Ask yourself if you would be thinking that the way the study was conducted was so great if the findings were the opposite.

Try to take the emotion out of it. Avoid getting 'facts' from stories that are trying to play on your emotions. Where possible find the actual research paper. They tend to be less melodramatic.

Always check the actual ingredients!

2

HOW THE NEWS MEDIA
SHAPES OUR VIEWS

Picture the scene. It's holiday season and you're at home with the extended family. Maybe you're pregnant. Or have just had a baby. Or have an older child who isn't sleeping through the night yet (whatever that means).

Distant relative one: *'Ooooh you don't want to be doing that, them experts say pregnant women mustn't do that.'*

Distant relative two: *'It's true, my television programme just the other night said you mustn't!'*

Random family friend: *(nodding head vigorously)* *'It's true, it's all over my newspaper.'*

Every day the media manipulates and twists scientific research into sensational headlines in order to sell papers and advertising space and make money. And every day these ideas are touted on social media and in discussions around the dinner table as 'true'. Yet 'fake news' and a distrust of science and experts has become a sign of our times. Conversely, well-conducted research is dismissed with anecdotes rather than data, and the well-known claim that *'My Granny lived till 96 and she smoked and drank a bottle of whisky a day'*.

Unfortunately, these attitudes are increasingly common

in the world of pregnancy, birth and babies. With a whole industry pushing parents to make choices that make money or fit in with certain beliefs about women and the family, the headlines and discussion presented are often very far from the truth. Newspapers do not neutrally present facts – they use emotions and fear to make a profit, and they allow those with power (think money and politics) to shape the news. Using all the underlying theories presented in the previous chapter they design headlines to cause as much discussion and chaos as possible. Spotting this is a vital part of judging what is news or just nonsense.

Although sales of hard copies of newspapers are down, online web traffic to the main news websites is phenomenal. The BBC has roughly 39 million novel viewers each month (a novel viewer is considered a device, not necessarily an individual) and the *Sun* and *Daily Mail* battle it out for second and third place with around 29 million novel viewers each per month.[1]

We used to think that we could receive our news fairly neutrally, with it being a place for facts and information (although in reality it was always screened and politically motivated). But now there is increasing recognition of just how manipulative news headlines can be, especially in the tabloid press. Fuelled in part by technological and digital revolutions that mean that news can be far more immediate and 'breaking', fear-based headlines, warning people of increasingly rare or unlikely events, are now an everyday occurrence. Simply put, fear sells. Fear-based headlines grab your attention and then try to make the story relevant to the reader (using tactics such as headlines that state '*What YOU need to know about...*' or '*Happening in YOUR country*').[2] Unsurprisingly, the more people are exposed to these types of headlines, the more they become anxious and worried about themselves and the world they live in.[3]

This fearmongering leads a significant proportion of the population to believe that things that they feel are 'scary' are far more common than they really are. Bobby Duffy, managing director of the Ipsos MORI social research institute, highlights in his book *The Perils of Perception* just how much we over or underestimate what is happening around us.[4] One example he gives is our guesstimates of the proportion of the population that is aged over 65 (and therefore, in the eyes of a tabloid commentator, presumably all sick, bed-blocking and using our taxes). All countries surveyed overestimated the proportion of the population aged over 65. In the UK the average guess was 37% when in fact it is just 17%. In the US the average guess was 36% compared to an actual 14%. In Australia it was 37% compared to an actual 14%.

Why do we overestimate this? Well, for a start it's difficult to look at the news without seeing a story about ageing populations, strain on health services, increasing retirement ages and so on and so on. You'd forgive anyone for thinking that a large percentage of the population is dependent on pensions. Interestingly, although it still had a gap between reality and estimate of 14%, Sweden came bottom of the overestimation rankings. Sweden is known for having a very good social security system. Taxes are high, but public health and social care services are some of the best in the world.[5] This again suggests that fear plays an important role in our estimates.

Ageing populations are not the only thing we overestimate. We seem to overestimate anything that we perceive as a problem. Terrorism, teenage pregnancies... we overestimate them. One Ipsos MORI survey on the top misperceptions of the UK public found:[6]

Issue	Perception	Reality
What is the teenage pregnancy rate?	15% of girls under 16 pregnant each year.	Just 0.6% – that's a misperception of 25 times as many.
Are crime levels falling?	58% say no.	Crime rates are falling every year.
Do we spend more on pensions or Jobseeker's Allowance?	29% more on Jobseeker's Allowance.	We spend 15 times as much on pensions.
How much does benefit fraud cost us?	£24 in every £100 spent.	70p in every £100 spent
Is foreign aid one of our top three expenses?	26% say yes.	It makes up just 1.1% of expenditure. Pensions cost ten times as much.
What proportion of the population are immigrants?	31%	15%
Is capping benefits the way to save the most money?	33% say yes.	Capping benefits to £26K per household saves £290 million. Raising the pension age to 66 saves £5 billion.

You can see this play out across the news headlines every day when it comes to pregnancy, birth and babies. My own research has been over-dramatised by newspapers many a time. Key messages are misconstrued, and findings are twisted to draw in readers, despite our efforts to word our press releases cautiously and positively.

One example that will forever haunt me came when we did some research exploring whether there was any difference in weight between babies who were baby-led weaned (allowed to feed themselves) or spoon-fed. The article that the *Telegraph* newspaper printed was fine and fairly balanced. But the accompanying picture was a photo of a morbidly obese baby on a hospital bed covered in wires.[7]

Who owns the press?

A report in 2015 found that in the UK:[8]

- 71% of national newspapers are owned by just three companies. If you include online content this rises to five companies for an 80% share.
- 80% of local newspapers are owned by six companies, who take 85% of newspaper revenue. The other 20% of titles are owned across 50 companies.
- The top three biggest selling newspapers are the *Sun*, *Daily Mail* and *Daily Mirror*. Together the *Sun* and *Daily Mail* account for over 50% of sales.
- Two companies – News Corp UK and Ireland, and Associated Newspapers (now *Daily Mail* Group Media) account for over 50% of turnover.
- News Corp is owned by Rupert Murdoch. Lord Rothermere owns the *Daily Mail* group. Together they control 60% of national newspaper circulation.

So pretty much 60% of our newspapers come through two people – Rupert Murdoch and Lord Rothermere. But who are they and why does this matter?

A quick glance at Wikipedia shows that Murdoch has been close to a number of prime ministers, was seen as sympathetic to Thatcher, was very close to Tony Blair and then supported David Cameron, apparently meeting him at least 26 times during his 14-month tenure as prime minister (including flying him by private jet to have a chat on his yacht). He bought the then-failing *Sun* newspaper and appointed Larry Lamb as editor, stating '*I want a tearaway paper with lots of tits in it*'. He recommended that Cameron hire former *News of the World* (owned by Murdoch) editor Andy Coulson as a communications director. Coulson was later jailed for 18 months for his role in the phone hacking scandals. Murdoch thinks the Brexit result was 'wonderful'.[9]

Lord Rothermere was also supportive of David Cameron and claims non-dom status in order to avoid paying taxes on his stately home. He runs his businesses though offshore holdings and trusts and has an estimated wealth of over £1 billion. Just your average bloke then.[10]

Generally, these men have a lot of money, a lot of connections and a lot of power. Nonetheless, we (or at least some of us) are buying and reading their newspapers (and not just in a horrified 'what are they doing now' way). The strange thing is that we know our news is biased. A survey by Reuters[11] found that two-thirds of us recognise that the media is influenced by politics, and three-quarters of us recognise it is affected by commercial influence. We also don't particularly trust journalists: just 29% of us said that we trusted journalists most of the time. Those who are right wing or centrist, in political terms, are more likely to trust the news that is presented than those on the left. This is probably because the majority of news published has a right-wing leaning (more on this later).

Different newspaper audiences

So you don't have to be a conspiracy theorist to know that what is presented in certain newspapers is biased towards certain views. Newspapers know that they have a 'type' of reader who will buy their paper, and they target their content, language and ideology accordingly. For example, the target age range differs. While the *Mirror* is aimed at those under 30, *Daily Mail* and *Telegraph* readers are mainly over 60. The *Guardian* and *Independent* are read by a wider range of readers. *Telegraph* readers tend to want serious, detailed stories appropriate to their age, while *Mirror* readers want emotion and stories.[12]

Handily, YouGov has compiled some additional characteristics of typical readers:[13]

Newspaper	Favourite pet	Favourite foods	Favourite sports
Guardian	Cat	Antipasti, aubergine parmigiana, braised endive	Cricket, cycling
Daily Star	Dog	Neapolitan ice-cream, chips, curry sauce	Boxing, darts
Daily Express	Dog	Meat pie, ham salad	Long jump, golf
Daily Mirror	Bird	Chips, curry sauce, ham and eggs	Football, boxing
Daily Mail	Dog	Cheese and tomato sandwich, lobster, sweet and sour prawns	Golf, tennis
Daily Telegraph	Cat	Vichyssoise soup, Stinking Bishop cheese, tournedos Rossini	Cricket, rugby union
The Sun	Dog	Pork chops, chips	Darts, horse racing
The Independent	Cat	Antipasti, braised endive, gambas al ajillo	Cycling, cricket
The Times	Cat	Tarte au citron, baklava, pommes Lyonnaise	Rugby union cricket

There are clear educational/income-based splits (and differences in the size of the bill when eating out). But what really matters are the political leanings of the newspapers and their readers. *The Times*, *Telegraph*, *Daily Express*, *Daily Mail* and *Sun* are Conservative, while the *Daily Mirror* and *Guardian* are Labour. The *Independent* is somewhere in the centre, although leaning more towards the left.[13]

Given that the *Sun* and *Daily Mail* make up over 50% of all newspaper sales, and that eight out of ten of the bestselling newspapers in the UK are considered right wing (The *Mirror* makes the top ten, as does the *Daily Star*, which is politely described as not having any political leaning), is it any surprise that the majority of the messages that are given out to the public via the newspapers are right wing?[8]

Ignoring your own political preferences for a moment, it's important to think about how a predominantly right-wing news media has the power to shape the messages we are given about parenting and caring for babies. Broadly speaking, because of course you can't (and shouldn't) group everyone's beliefs and preferences based simply on the political party that they vote for or the newspaper that they read, research has shown that left or right-wing tendencies are associated with a number of attitudes that could affect the type of content that could appear in newspapers in relation to mothers and babies.

1. A link between right-wing beliefs and sexism towards women

Numerous studies show that there is a link between right-wing beliefs and sexism towards women (both from men and women, because women can be sexist towards their own sex too). Not all sexism looks the same, however. Broadly speaking there are two types – benevolent and hostile sexism. It is possible to exhibit both types at once.

Benevolent sexism

Research shows that those with right-wing leanings are more likely to be high in benevolent sexism. Benevolent sexism is the view that women should be cared for and looked after. On the surface that doesn't sound too bad. I fully believe in 'mothering the mother' after birth, caring for her and looking after her. But that's not where individuals high in benevolent sexism are coming from. People high in benevolent sexism feel that women need looking after because they are weak, childlike and overly emotional. Particularly if they are pregnant.

Those who are high in benevolent sexism tend to believe that women should be in traditional roles: in the home, looking pretty, not being too challenging. The issue with benevolent sexism is that the benevolent bit goes straight out the window if a woman won't sit on her pedestal. If she is seen to be challenging the belief that she is weak, or be overly powerful and have an opinion of her own… the benevolent sexists can get a little angry. Some men use benevolent sexism and its restrictions on women to try to keep them in place: the message is 'conform and you will be cherished and supported, break the rules and you will be punished'.[14] You can easily see how women who end up in weak positions, reliant on men for money and housing, can be very badly treated by 'benevolent' sexists.

A good example of the impact of benevolent sexism is in research looking at the link with attitudes towards breastfeeding. One study found that men who scored highly for benevolent sexism loved the idea of women breastfeeding (feminine, pure, nourishing a baby)… as long as it was in private.[15] They were hugely supportive of it as long as they met the traditional 'woman at home' criteria, alongside the private, self-conscious behaviour of only breastfeeding in the house. However, when they were asked how they felt about women breastfeeding outside the home, they were horrified. She was jumping right down off that pedestal and showing the world her breasts. Men who did not score highly for benevolent sexism were pretty much happy for women to breastfeed whenever and wherever they want. Thank goodness.

Those high in benevolent sexism also like rules being applied to women, particularly rules that restrict their movement, freedom or ability to speak out. They really, really like it when these rules can be imposed as a way of 'protecting' women, usually giving the reason that 'it's for their own good'. On the one hand this could be seen as protective, but usually what she is supposedly being protected against is nonsensical.[16]

One study looked at a whole host of behaviours a pregnant woman could engage in, and a man's measure of benevolent sexism. The higher a man's benevolent sexism score, the more highly he rated the following as risky for pregnant women: using a microwave, travelling abroad, having house plants (!), eating starchy foods, eating fatty foods, eating sweeteners, eating ready meals, sleeping on your back, having oral sex, having any sex (but this was less risky than oral for some reason), exercising, having her hair dyed... and oddly, given the list of restrictions, being stressed.[17]

Although some of these things are on recommended advice lists – for example, don't sleep on your back once you are heavily pregnant (mainly because you might get stuck there forever!) – the majority are plain nonsense. This didn't stop the men high in benevolent sexism from thinking they were supposedly risky. And there was a strong link between sexism and how willing a man was to step in and stop pregnant women from doing outrageous things like owning a house plant. This all suggests that 'benevolent sexism' is more about controlling women than any real risks to them.

It is probably unsurprising that men high in benevolent sexism really hate abortion. One study found that men high in this trait hate abortion when it is a choice, and they also still hate it even when a woman's life is endangered by the pregnancy.[18] This says a lot. Benevolent sexism is not about protecting women, but about protecting men's control of women, alongside their ability to get a woman pregnant and pass on their genes.

Hostile sexism

Hostile sexism is also closely tied to right-wing views.[19] This is your common or garden variety sexism: generally thinking women are lesser than men, disliking and distrusting them and scorning anything about them that is symbolic of being overtly feminine (for example being pregnant, giving birth and breastfeeding). There is a whole academic literature out there describing it. How some men have come to the conclusion that women are weak is beyond me. Growing whole new human beings, without which our species wouldn't exist, giving birth with all that entails, and then keeping our children alive with our breasts is a display of immense power and strength. Perhaps the real reason some men are so keen to believe that women are weak is that we, and our power, scare them.

Hostile sexism is closely tied to concepts of masculine ideology in which men are seen to be superior and all-round wonderful. Men who score highly on this trait base their identity on appearing 'tough', dislike emotional intimacy between men and women and believe men should be the breadwinners. They measure their success typically in terms of how successful they are at work, and how successful they are with women (in terms of how many they have slept with). Women are typically viewed in terms of their sexual worth.[20]

The press exploits this tendency – such as in the *Sun*, which features women in various poses, and in the sidebar of shame on the *Daily Mail* website – encouraging others to judge women according to their appearance, and either lifting women up or putting them down depending on whether they're acting within the 'rules'. We absorb these messages. Men high in sexism are invited to judge, and women are judged, whether they want to be or not.

Research supports this too: the more men view media that objectifies women, the more strongly men believe in gendered roles. Of course, this could work either way, and men who strongly believe in gendered roles may be more likely to seek out media.[21] However, one study back in the 1990s showed one group of male undergraduates objectifying adverts and another more neutral adverts before they made judgements about a hypothetical female job applicant. Those exposed to the objectifying adverts recalled more about her appearance than her qualifications and viewed her as less competent than the group who had seen the neutral adverts.[22]

You don't need a PhD to guess that men who strongly hold these sexist views are less likely to respect birth and feeding babies as important. When a woman becomes pregnant, gives birth, and continues to use her body to feed her baby, she is not 'prioritising' being a sexual being for these men, and (if she is not their own partner) she is in fact a symbol of another man's 'conquest'. Men high in hostile sexism and masculine ideology get very annoyed about that. When they see a woman breastfeeding in public they see someone daring not to submit themselves to him, along with a mix-up of images of motherhood and sexuality that they find really uncomfortable.[23] The poor things.

Men high in masculine ideology are more likely to view childbirth as something disgusting that they would not want to see their partner doing. They are also more likely to think breastfeeding is disgusting and should be done in private, as for them breasts are first and foremost sexual and breastfeeding gets in the way of sex.[24] Seriously, dating apps should give you the option to screen men for this stuff.

Women are affected by a dominant society view that breasts are primarily sexual. A core reason for women not wanting to breastfeed is a fear of whether breastfeeding will affect the appearance of their breasts or make them less attractive to their partner.[25] Women worry about doing a 'sexual' thing in public, and if I had a pound for every time I've heard or read a story in the right-wing press judging women for breastfeeding in public (and the predictable comments that follow), I'd be writing this from my superyacht in the Caribbean.

Men high in hostile sexism also become angry when women break the supposed 'rules' around pregnancy. They really like the idea of there being rules controlling what women can and can't do during pregnancy and believe that women should be punished if they break them. In one study those high in this trait strongly believed women should not drink alcohol, eat deli foods, eat seafood or do strenuous exercise during pregnancy. They also believed women should be punished (how?!) if they broke these rules and dared to eat a Scotch egg. What is telling is that how strongly men believed women should be punished was not linked to how risky they felt the behaviours were. It was simply about punishing naughty, out of control women.[26]

2. A link between right-wing beliefs and the personality trait right-wing authoritarianism

There is an association between the tendency to hold right-wing beliefs, and a personality trait known as 'right-wing authoritarianism'.[27] Those who are high in authoritarian beliefs tend to hold strong views about the power of authority and tend to be quite rigid in their beliefs, as opposed to believing people should be able to think what they want. This trait is typically associated with right-wing views. Three common aspects of right-wing authoritarianism are:

a. Acceptance of and submissiveness towards perceived legitimate authorities such as government, the police and medical authorities.
b. Aggression against those perceived to be an outgroup or deviant against authority (or 'our way of doing things').
c. Strong adherence to established norms and traditions, particularly with regard to traditional family values.

Research has shown that those high in right-wing authoritarianism (RWA) have low tolerance for ambiguity and do not like change. They are more likely to be pro-capitalist, support conservative economic policies and be anti-abortion. They also are more likely to be generally prejudiced towards women, particularly lesbians. Finally, those high in authoritarianism are more likely to score highly on traits of self-righteousness, feeling themselves to be morally superior with the right to point out to others when they feel they are beneath them and acting accordingly. They also score highly on social dominance orientation: the belief that the group one feels you belong to should be superior to those groups you see as 'other'.[27]

Surely it's unfair to say only the right can be dominant and rigid? Yes it is. Emerging research shows that those on the left can also hold authoritarian stances. However, the views they generally hold determine what they will be authoritarian about. Those on the left are more likely to be authoritarian about equality and support for all – so they are more likely to be rigid about liberal beliefs and allowing people to have their freedoms.[28]

So how does this all fit in with pregnancy and babies? Well, just by reading that description you can pretty much guess what someone high in RWA is going to feel. Although I cannot find any direct research, I can make an evidence-based guess that your average RWA is not going to like the concept of women a) having the option to make decisions around where they give birth and b) as a consequence of that making the choice to give birth at home. At home! Outside of the hospital building! Making her own decisions! Not bowing to senior (male) medical staff! Quick – get them some smelling salts (the right-wingers, not the woman calmly giving birth in her living room).

What all this goes to show is that there is a body of evidence that you can piece together to explain the bias of the right-wing press, leading to the following conclusions:

- Women's reproductive rights are more likely to be limited in countries with high levels of right-wing authoritarianism.[29]
- Individuals who are high in RWA are more likely to believe that women shouldn't work, or if they do, then they should not take on significant roles in the workplace (presumably leaving them for the men). You can see why newspapers that have right-wing tendencies despise working mothers.[30]
- This isn't limited to men's views. *Women* who are high in RWA are more likely to believe in traditional gender roles, and women not pursuing their careers once they have a family. This explains why women columnists write some pretty nasty things about other women – women defying their status quo are threatening.[31]
- There is an association between RWA views and the medical profession. Of course, not all medics will hold these views and many will feel the complete opposite. But it

does seem that those with RWA views are perhaps drawn to become medics. One study looked at how strongly groups of students held RWA views, finding that medical students held the strongest views compared to all other subjects.[32]

- RWAs are angered (terrified?) by change, particularly when it is instigated by those who they feel are not at the top of the hierarchy – for example, pregnant women. When RWAs perceive something to be threatening their lives, they get much more angry when it is seen to come from others in society rather than their close-knit circle.[33]

What is the impact of all this?

This brief look at the background serves to explain the headlines we see every day. They are anti women making their own decisions, blame women for negative outcomes and try to scare and shame women into acting in a certain way. Here are a few examples of classic right-wing news headlines from the last few years:

Headline	Translation
Pregnant women reveal why they REFUSE to ditch alcohol (Daily Mail, *03/04/18*)	We're using capitals to really make you angry about the fact that women have minds of their own and are not doing what they're told.
Deaths during pregnancy are on the rise again due to obesity rates and increasing age of expectant mothers (Daily Mail, *01/11/18*)	Terrible things are happening and we're angry that people we think are too old and fat get to have lots of sex.
Mumsnet is driving women to request caesarean sections, a leading midwife has warned (Telegraph, *12/08/18*)	Somehow, women talking to each other and sharing facts and experiences is leading them to feel they have the right to be involved in what happens to their bodies, and this is the end of the world as we know it.

Generally, the right-wing press like to blame women, whatever they do. On googling 'Daily Mail working mothers child obesity' to find an article I had recently seen that was particularly awful I got the following search results:

Scientists blame working mothers for Britain's childhood obesity crisis (09/03/19)	See, it's not us, it's those mysterious judgemental scientists.
Rise in obesity is blamed on women going out to work (27/06/16)	Those pesky women again, leaving the house.

If this seems like conclusive evidence that working mothers are the problem, consider this:

Working mothers LESS LIKELY to have obese children (26/10/17)	This one had the handy clarification 'but only if they are in the office for under 24 hours a week'. Presumably if you work a few hours in the local coffee shop or something, you're okay.

And next, something else that is now women's responsibility:

Women can help prevent their children from becoming obese by exercising during pregnancy (07/04/19)	Next sentence – 'US researchers tested the theory on mice and discovered youngsters were less likely to gain weight throughout adolescence if their mother regularly exercised during pregnancy'. They're even trying to give female mice a complex now.

Who else can we blame? Here we go...

Single mothers are more likely to have obese children (12/02/19)	But don't you go working, as it will make your children obese. Stay at home instead! Oh no, we forgot we don't like this either. Why did you magically conceive a baby entirely on your own? Why do you exist?
Parenting classes could reverse UK's obesity crisis (30/04/19)	Be a good girl and run along to this eight-week class. It will distract you from your repeated attempts to try and overthrow the patriarchy.

And then we're back to the original article...

Children with working mothers 6 times more likely to be fat (04/02/11)	Apparently their 'survey found that working mothers have less time to prepare more nutritious meals'. I had forgotten that men are genetically incapable of cooking dinner.

HOW TO KEEP INFORMED:

Always consider where the story was published – and what the underlying motivations may be. If a story appears across the press, compare how different newspapers present the issue. If only for the simultaneous amusement and horror.

It is always worth trying to track down the original research article a piece is based on. Often the press article will be vague (as they know they have stretched the meaning of the research) and sometimes only give the researcher's name or the journal the paper was published in rather than a direct link. If you go to Google Scholar, set the dates to reflect only recent research and search for the topic, you should be able to find it.

Do yoga or something for the rage.

3

THE ROLE OF THE INTERNET

High speed, accessible internet, and the affordable devices we view it on, has led to a world of social media that few of us 25 years ago would have even dreamt was possible. I clearly remember the internet becoming more mainstream when I was a teenager. But it involved signing up to a specific company, getting sent their installation CD in the post, and using dial-up. Some people used the internet to join chat groups, which became increasingly popular. But few of us imagined we'd soon be carrying the internet around in our pockets, able to search for whatever information we wanted at any given time.

The change has had a huge impact on our lives. What did we do before the internet, both in terms of finding out information and wasting time on it? Now most of us use it. The most recent research in the UK shows that over 99% of those aged 16–44 years had used the internet recently, with large increases in older populations which used to be less-frequent users. In 2011 just 20% of those aged over 75 used the internet, but this has now risen to 47%. Among the slightly younger group of 65–74-year-olds, in 2011 just 52% used the internet, rising to 83% now. So most parents and grandparents and even some great-grandparents are now connected. The

UK is now the third most prolific internet user in the EU (after Denmark and Luxembourg).[1]

This has been fuelled by the increase in the number of smartphones and the ability to access the internet wherever we are. Statistics show that 95% of individuals aged 16–34 now own a smartphone, 91% of those aged 35–54, and 51% of those aged 54–65.[2] And yes, we are mainly using it to look at videos on YouTube and get into fights on Twitter.

This technological advance has revolutionised how we get our information. In 2016, the internet officially overtook television as our main news source. And as the population has started to use the internet instead, printed newspaper sales have fallen. An age difference is seen – among those aged 45 and under, the internet is clearly their favourite source of news, with 84% of 18–24-year-olds, 62% of 25–34-year-olds and 53% of 35–44-year-olds stating it is their main source. Television remains the main source for 45–54 and 55+ year-olds. However, 31% and 21% respectively of these groups use the internet as their main source.[2]

In terms of direct news stories, there does seem to be a possible benefit of using the internet instead of television or print sources for primary news. Research conducted by Reuters found that those who use search engines end up viewing an average of 3.61 online news sources, compared to 1.97 for those who don't search for news in this way.[3] However, the study didn't check whether these sources represented a spread of different viewpoints.

Seeking health information online

We're not only using the internet to get our news. We're increasingly using it to find information about our health. A survey done a few years ago in the US by the Pew Foundation found that almost three-quarters of adult internet users regularly search online for health information.[4] In the UK, NHS Choices gets over 15 million hits per month. There's even a new term for hypochondriacs who spend excessive amounts of time trying to diagnose themselves with rare illnesses online: 'cyberchondriacs'.[5]

Globally, people are using the internet to seek out health information more than ever before, using it to make decisions, and, in a considerable number of cases, believing it is more reliable than the information they get from health professionals. A recent study of 1,194 patients attending hospital clinics in Hong Kong found that among those who had access to the internet, 87% had used it to find health information, with 66% regularly doing so.[6] In another study, again in Hong Kong, the internet was the first place patients sought information, regardless of the severity of their issue. What individuals clicked on then had a significant influence on whether they decided to make a medical appointment or not.[7] Indeed, a study of US adults found that a third believed they could essentially diagnose themselves based on online information.[8] Others use it if they are unhappy with what their doctor has told them.[9]

The internet is a major source of information for many pregnant women and new mothers. In the UK, a 2017 report by OFCOM found that 24% of pregnant women were accessing the internet for health information every week.[10] Likewise, a study in Ireland found that 70% of women were using the internet to answer questions about their pregnancy, with 67% using social media sites for this purpose.[11]

It's not difficult to see that this could be problematic. Absolutely anyone can write whatever they like and publish it on the internet. Some information may be high-quality factual information from health-based websites. Which is good. Research suggests that having the ability to access high-quality, accurate, evidence-based health information, and having the confidence to share it with your healthcare provider (who also has the confidence and humility to be interested in what you are saying), is a good thing. Patients can feel empowered, motivated and like they are actually playing an active role in managing their health.[12] So far so good.

Unfortunately, this doesn't apply to everyone who is accessing the internet, and there is a huge amount of bad information out there. Even information from reputable sources is not always accurate. The NHS Choices website, for example, states that '*For babies aged 6 months to a year, night feeds may no longer be necessary*'[13] when research tell us that in fact babies who do not need night feeds at this age are in the minority.[14]

If we ignore things like science, facts and actual evidence, we can convince ourselves that pretty much whatever we like is good for our health. An article from Health Online, for example, states that chocolate is '*very nutritious*',[15] and according to that well-known source of accurate heath advice Business Insider, gin '*can even help you achieve younger, healthier looking skin as well as keeping your waistline trim*'.[16] My latest favourite is that you can drink up to 25 cups of coffee a day before it has a damaging effect on your heart.[17]

All jokes aside, things can go drastically wrong if people are not able to judge the information that is in front of them. It can lead to self-diagnosis (which can be wrong), ignoring medical advice and a whole load of anxiety.[18] In the Pew report, 58% of participants said their search results affected their decision on how to treat their illness or condition, 55% said it changed their overall approach to maintaining their health and 35% said it informed their decision on whether to seek medical advice.[4] No details were given as to whether that led to positive or negative outcomes, but it shows the power of online information.

Using the internet to check information about health and development during pregnancy is increasingly common. In one study the majority of women said they checked it more than once a month for information about their health during their pregnancy. Pregnancy complications and foetal development were the main searches and almost two-thirds of respondents stated that the information that they accessed affected decisions they were making about how pregnancy and birth should be managed.[11]

However, although most women in the study rated themselves as 'intermediate' or 'expert' in terms of having the knowledge and ability to seek out accurate and reliable information online, when this was explored, few did. Most checked who hosted the website, but few checked the accuracy of the research that was being presented, or when it was written. Overall just 11% could list ways in which you could check the quality of the information being presented, over and above who hosted the website.

Of particular concern in the Pew report was how infrequently people checked the source of the information they were reading. Over three-quarters of individuals who used the internet to seek health information stated that they checked the source and date of the information 'only sometimes, hardly ever, or rarely'. The report equates this to over 85 million Americans not checking the source of the information they are using to guide their health decisions every year. Worryingly, compared to the previous version of the report, far fewer were now bothering to check the source.

Notably, while 69% stated they had visited websites where information was wrong or misleading, and few believed that the majority of information found on the internet was high quality, at the same time 83% believed that the information *they* had found was good or excellent. This pattern was found in another study, this time of parents with a baby in neonatal intensive care. Around half used the internet to search for information while their baby was in hospital. However, just 10% stated that they believed information on the internet was reliable. Yet 49% believed it could answer their questions.[19] Clearly people are (correctly or incorrectly) deciding that the information they have found and decided to believe is the correct information – as opposed to all the other stuff out there. They may well be right, or their brains may be bathing in a sea of confirmation bias.

Another study looked at how accurate online information about pregnancy weight gain was. They reviewed search engine results for 181 different web pages that came up in the first 10 pages of their search for accuracy and depth of information. Of these pages, just 22% contained information that was both accurate and gave sufficient detail. Most pages were accurate but scant on detail (27%), completely inaccurate (12%) or gave very little information at all (34%).[20]

Inaccurate information is a concern, especially when it can affect the health of mother or baby, and/or the mother's wellbeing (if she changes her behaviour unnecessarily). Another study asked callers who contacted a helpline about exposure to teratogens (things that can potentially harm a baby during pregnancy) whether they had searched for information online and what they had found. Overall, half of respondents had searched for information online. Of those, thankfully, 59% had found accurate information. However, among the remaining mothers, 18% had been informed that their exposure was dangerous when this was untrue (likely causing unnecessary concern), 4% were wrongly reassured when they were actually at risk (potentially causing increased exposure) and the remaining women couldn't work out what the website was trying to say.[21]

Thinking back to what we know about confirmation bias, there is a risk that, consciously or otherwise, some people are searching for the information that they want to find. And you can find support for almost anything on the internet. This isn't helped by misleading adverts trying to sell things that will supposedly improve your baby's health, development or behaviour, such as suggesting your baby will sleep better if they have a certain brand of formula (they won't),[22] or that you should buy a music-playing device to place inside your vagina so your baby can listen to music because apparently that a) helps babies' development and b) that's how babies in the womb hear best. Um... no.[23]

Where are people getting their online information from?

In the study that looked at the information pregnant women seek out online, the top place they looked was general search engines such as Google.[11] The good news is that the most popular websites for health advice do appear to be reliable. A compilation of the most popular global sites that people use includes the National Institutes of Health, WebMD.com, and Mayo Clinic – all sites which generally at least give good health information.[24] In the UK, the NHS website gets over 18 million visits per month.[25]

Unfortunately, just because information is linked to government, medical or academic sources, that doesn't automatically mean that it is high quality. One study in the US looked at the websites of crisis pregnancy centres referenced in state resource directories for pregnant women seeking an abortion. These were essentially government-approved websites. Researchers assessed the information given to check whether it was accurate. In total, 80% of the websites carried at least one misleading or false piece of information. The most common false links given were a link between abortion and mental health risks, preterm birth in later pregnancies, breast cancer and future infertility.[26] A similar issue has occurred recently in the UK, where a seemingly professional-looking website claiming to support women through abortion has been accused of stringing women along to delay their decision until it was too late.[27]

Some web pages *look* very professional and formal. Take the Nestlé Nutrition Institute for example.[28] The site carries many scientific articles and features experts talking about infant nutrition, including breastfeeding. However, the organisation is funded by a formula manufacturer to promote

Nestlé products (and the site carries many adverts, both obvious and dressed up as infographics). Without getting into people's individual decisions about infant feeding, it is obviously not in the interests of a company selling formula milk to give breastfeeding advice. So we cannot be sure that the information given is in the best interests of women.

Another popular way to get health information is via a 'symptom-checker' where you input your symptoms and get a result. These can be the perfect way for a hypochondriac to pass a few hours, but in some cases they may be useful. One study looked at whether symptom-checkers gave accurate diagnoses. Researchers compiled a list of illnesses and their general symptoms and ran them through symptom-checkers online. They found that the symptom-checker got the right answer the first time in just 34% of attempts. Worryingly, the more urgent the illness, the less accurate the checkers were, with just 24% of urgent care situations being recognised as such. In contrast, real-life medics got the diagnosis right first time 72% of the time, even though in the study they could only work with the information they were given and weren't allowed to do any tests, such as blood tests, which would presumably increase their accuracy in real life.[29]

Symptom-checkers usually make a number of suggestions based on your symptoms. When researchers widened the criteria, 51% of checkers got the right answer in their top three results, and 58% got it in the top 20(!). Again, the more urgent the problem, the less likely the symptom-checkers were to get it right. The researchers also found huge differences between symptom-checkers, with some doing pretty well and others where you might as well have asked your cat what was wrong with you.

I couldn't find a study looking at pregnancy symptom-checkers, but by entering fake symptoms of 'stomach pain' into one, and pretending that I am pregnant, gives me a choice of pulmonary embolism, blood clot in the legs, pre-eclampsia, melasma (skin discolouration?!) or 'pregnancy'. On balance consulting a real-life doctor is probably better if you are actually pregnant and experiencing stomach pain.

What about good old Wikipedia? We all use it, but we should exercise caution – especially if we are doctors using it to look up health information. Every year we tell our new students not to cite Wikipedia articles, as you can't guarantee the accuracy of the information. But apparently it's a common source of information for medics. A review article considering its accuracy on the subject included findings that in one study 50% of physicians surveyed used it to answer health questions,[30] along with 70% of junior doctors graduating from a London medical school[31] and over a quarter of pharmacists, predominantly to check the safety and interactions of medications prescribed.[32]

No matter what we try to tell our students, Wikipedia is a go-to source that is frequently in the top 10 most-visited websites and the top 10 of health-related searches. Unfortunately, on pretty much every evaluation of its health information it falls short. Often it is technically accurate (but not always). But it lacks depth and fails to include relevant information such as drug interactions or contraindications to taking certain medications.[33]

Another growing source of health advice is YouTube. Where we used to go for videos of cats, is now a resource for making judgements about your health. Research has shown how dangerous YouTube can be when it comes to health information in pregnancy. Although there are useful videos, misinformation is rife. One study evaluated 651 different videos on YouTube talking about the safety of medications in pregnancy. Over two-thirds of videos were made by law firms presumably trying to persuade people to make some kind of claim. Of the different medications discussed, the majority were antidepressants (72%), which in general, dependent on the medication and individual circumstances of the woman, are safe for women to take during pregnancy. However, 88% of the videos about them stated that they were unsafe. When the researchers looked up the safety of the individual medications discussed in the videos, the vast majority were rated as unlikely or minimal risk.[34] If women see these videos and believe them, they are at risk of potentially catastrophic consequences if they stop their medication abruptly as a result.

Another example is information about abortion. Pro-life activists have ensured that some awful, inaccurate videos are within the top search results returned.[35] These too could have serious consequences for women's health.

Then there are the vloggers and bloggers, and many high-profile cases have shown how misinformation can be spread. A few years ago in Australia, blogger Belle Gibson claimed that she had cured her brain cancer with whole foods. She went on to write a book and app and supposedly made at least 430,000 Australian dollars. However, she didn't have brain cancer (or any other kind of cancer) at all.[36] Gwyneth Paltrow's Goop brand has famously published advice including getting a coffee enema (priced at $135 – and you thought your morning latte was expensive!) and putting jade eggs in your vagina to help spice up your sex life. The eggs were a step too far and the California Food, Drug and Medical Device Task Force fined her $145,000 in civil penalties.[37]

Some bloggers receive money to advertise baby-related products, or are sent 'gifts' that they then talk about. Some are sponsored by brands to produce content. Some 'Mummy bloggers' have been criticised for having moved from leading an anti 'perfect mother' discussion on formats such as Instagram to being salespeople, effectively promoting brands for companies through their extensive followers.[38]

Recent examples include Mrs Hinch (2.6 million Instagram followers, famous for cleaning) being sent a Tommee Tippee Perfect Prep machine, which she then shared photos of. Of course it is her choice how she feeds her baby, but there are valid safety concerns about the machines that make up formula for you, which focus on how hot the shot of water is when it hits the formula. Contrary to popular belief, making up formula bottles with water that is at least 70 degrees C is recommended because it can kill any potential pathogens in the *formula powder* (which is not sterile) rather than the *water*. It is not clear that the 'hot shot' of water in the Perfect Prep machine is big enough or hot enough to do this effectively.[39]

Danone, which makes Aptamil formula milk, appears to be significantly investing in promoting its products through mummy bloggers. In 2018 the watchdog OFCOM ruled that Ferne McCann's reality TV show breached guidelines by giving 'undue prominence to a baby formula milk' in the programme (translation: it was clearly visible and was talked about all over the place).[40] Other examples of bloggers who have Instagrammed photos including placement of Aptamil products or hashtags include Amy Childs (590k Instagram followers), Binky Felstead (1.4 million followers) and Candice Brathwaite (39.1k followers). There are a lot of strangely posed Instagram photos of 'celeb' mothers and babies with tins of formula in front of them. I mean, don't we all cuddle up in front of a fire with our baby and our formula tin?

I am not making a judgement about anyone's decision to use formula milk, but rather pointing out that the formula companies are using these platforms to circumnavigate the rules on the advertising of first-stage formula milk.[41] We also know that the costs of marketing formula are passed on to parents – so if you use formula, you are paying the company to pay the bloggers to feature the product.[42] Why not ditch the dodgy promotion and pass the savings on?

Thankfully, there is also a healthy level of scepticism out there. One study exploring how mothers used the internet to find out about their child's health found that the favourite sources of information were academic websites or those of not-for-profit organisations. Many mothers automatically distrusted information that came from commercial websites, and believed that the companies were just trying to sell their products.

The internet and information overload

One of the major problems with getting health information online is that there is simply too much of it. In general in our daily lives we are suffering from information overload. Everywhere we go there is more and more information. There is even a term – 'infobesity' – used to describe it, caused by 'feasting' on all the different types of information available.[43]

Noreena Hertz, in her book *Eyes Wide Open*, gives an example of how much information we are exposed to in this digital era.[44] The amount of information in the *New York Times* weekly edition is more information than the average person in the 17th century came across in their entire lifetime. Our brains change and adapt over time, in response to our environment. But not at that speed. And the amount of information we are exposed to is growing every single day.

Estimates of just how much are pretty jaw-dropping. One study has estimated that we are exposed to the equivalent of 34 gigabytes of information every day *just during our leisure time* – so not even taking into account all the mind-numbing data you might be exposed to during working hours.

Information is being created for us every second. In his book *The Organised Mind* Daniel Levitin describes how television stations around the world create 85,000 hours of new programmes every single day. YouTube gets 6,000 hours of video uploaded to it every hour. Apparently all this adds up to over 300 exabytes of information currently existing in the world. An exabyte is one quintillion bytes. Or 1 billion gigabytes. That's an awful lot of stuff.[45]

It's therefore not surprising that women can end up feeling absolutely overwhelmed by the sheer amount of information given to them when they become pregnant, especially for the first time. Even during antenatal appointments a vast amount of information is presented (often at a superficial level), with no time to discuss or dig deeper. This can increase feelings of anxiety about there being so much information available, but not knowing enough. It can be exacerbated by women not always seeing the same midwife or their appointments only being 10–15 minutes long.[46]

Our brains don't like this information overload. We weren't designed to have information coming at us from so many different sources. We weren't designed to interact with so many people, even if they are in our computers and not our living room. We have seen how thinking and making decisions is physically tough for our brains, and that we are programmed to want to make decisions quickly and easily. Being given lots of competing information can make us very anxious, as it forces us to think and makes decision-making complicated. And when we feel overloaded by information we often end up paying less attention to everything, rather than focusing well on one thing.[47]

The same goes for those who are meant to be helping us in our decision-making. The sheer amount of information published in medical journals (some good, a lot bad – see Chapter 10) is overwhelming medics too. They can't possibly keep up with it all. This has been recognised for a long time, even before technology and the internet took over – back in 1986 it was noted that 20,000 papers in biomedicine were being published each year, and that even if you stuck to a very specialist area it would mean reading a paper almost daily to be able to keep up.[48] Today, if you enter the search term 'pregnancy' in Google Scholar and set the date parameters to just 2019, you get 24,100 results! It is basically impossible to try and read all that evidence.

How does this affect our everyday lives?

Our desire and tendency to make decisions using the minimum amount of effort has a name: Zipf's law, or 'principles of least effort'.[49] We will do whatever we can to minimise the effort involved. With information we take the easiest route and are happy when we find an answer that we deem acceptable enough. But there is just so much information to wade through.

Imagine you have a decision to make. You go to the internet and put in your question: *'Which brand of baby food should I buy?'* Click search and get... 3,490,000,000 results in 0.69 seconds. Okay. That's not a great help. We start scrolling through, but of course we can't scroll through 3.5 billion results, so we end up looking at the first few. Research has shown that we're most likely to click on the first few links – particularly links one and two.[50]

For this search we get lots of web pages showing supposed rankings of baby food according to different online forums and baby magazines. Scanning through the first few, each lists a 'top ten', and each differs from the others. We are not much closer to an answer, are we?

You abandon Google and head to the supermarket instead. But even there you are met with hundreds of different options, all screaming *'Buy me!'* But which is the best? Which will your baby like? Which is the most nutritious? Is it any wonder that once you pick one brand or product and your baby likes it, you are more likely to return to that product again and again?

Another example is when parents make the decision to formula-feed their baby. *'Which is the best formula?'* they often ask. Every formula company out there exists to make a profit, so there are incentives to get you hooked from the very start, as research shows that once a family has settled on a brand of formula, they tend to stick to it. And for subsequent babies. And even across the whole family. Formula companies know this and deploy many tricks to get their customers.

In reality, in the UK all formula milks are pretty much the same. They have to have certain ingredients in them by law. And anything else they throw in as a 'teaser' isn't necessarily for the good of your baby, and is often a marketing gimmick designed to stand out in the deluge of competing information you receive. If that 'special ingredient' was vital, it would have to be in all formula by law. So I can help you out here, with this perennial question: pick whichever formula is sold in your local shop and fits your budget, and that your baby seems to like.[42] If you have more time to read, have a look at the First Steps Nutrition Trust reports that compare formula milks on the market.[42] And there's no need to feel particularly loyal to any brand – they all just want your custom.

We can no longer concentrate

When we do find a really useful document – perhaps a First Steps Nutrition report on formula milk[42] – we also find that all our wading through the sea of information has messed up our ability to concentrate, focus and think straight. How many times have you been reading something online and got distracted? Maybe by an advert. Maybe by a link on the side. Maybe by a social media notification or an email. We are just not concentrating any more, which means we don't read things in a critical or in-depth way. We remember snippets. Which we pass on.

You probably don't recognise you're doing it as much as you do. Research that tracked this with one group of students found that on average they were distracted by social media at least three times an hour.[51]

We are becoming skim-readers

Linked to our exposure to information is the issue of how we actually try and take it all in. And we do it by skim-reading. Writing for the *Guardian* in 2018, Maryanne Wolf raised the issue of how getting our information from the internet is turning us into less critical, unempathetic readers.[52] She noted how reading is not a genetically inherited ability like vision or speech (on the whole). It needs the right environment in which to develop. Whereas babies are born with the ability to communicate verbally, which develops over time from crying to gurgling to words, a child will not learn to read unless they experience words. Research suggests that this happens through something linguists and psychologists call a 'reading circuit', which allows us to decode symbols on a page. This uses our surface reading of what the word says, but brings along with it our experience – of knowledge of the words and their meaning, critical analysis, analogical reasoning and emotions and processes such as empathy.

Reading a story, particularly one that is in depth and complex (not light holiday reading) requires that reading circuit to really kick in. We need to think about what we're reading, remember the information about the different characters, link it to other knowledge that we have, and experience emotions as we move through the book. If it's a great book we feel it and experience it rather than just reading words on a page.

Now think about how many people do the majority of their reading today. Is it books? Or is it emails, or social media feeds, or doom-laden news headlines? Do we stop and read and feel each one in depth, or do we skim it? When scrolling through a Facebook feed do you think nice status… nice status… or really focus on what each status really means?

Our ability to put up with length and depth is seemingly changing. Bloggers and journalists know that if you write too much it won't be read. I've lost track of the number of times an experienced editor has told me that my piece of 1,500 or even 1,200 words is too long for people's attention spans. Really? I mean if you're still reading this, it's likely you are the exception to the rule. Or perhaps this is the 25th time you've picked up the book since buying it. Or the book just fell open on this page. But I remain optimistic.

Using the internet and computers or phones actually changes how our brains process what we read. It means we apply our dominant reading approach – skim-reading, short attention spans – to pieces that really need us to invoke our deeper reading skills – empathy, critical thinking and analysis. Skim-reading and poor attention skills lead to the sort of thinking that believes lies written on the sides of buses. Research has shown that we read in a completely different way when we skim – we read the start of paragraphs (quickly) and then pick out key words. But we don't just spend less time reading, we spend much less time using the deep thinking skills that go alongside it. We are far less likely to annotate or take notes – which helps us think far more deeply around what we are reading.[53]

In an article in the *Atlantic* in 2008 Nicholas Carr asked 'Is Google making us stupid?' reflecting on his own experiences of losing patience with printed books that he once often read.[54] Others around him felt the same. In a research article of the same name published a few years later, Hooper and Herath explored how people read on and offline.[55] They found that when people were reading books they were far more likely to read the information fully than if they were reading it online. In fact, 82% of participants said that they read paper-based texts from beginning to end, while 87% said that they just scanned online pieces for interest. If they wanted to properly read something, 72% said they would print it off as it helped their retention – probably because they actually read it properly. Conversely, participants said they felt more impatient with online sources, reading them quickly and using hyperlinks to jump about.

Indeed, research has shown that hyperlinks have a lot to answer for. Not only are people more likely to click on them and go off on a tangent if they see one, but they actually act as a focal point. Readers are naturally drawn to them, perhaps considering them key points in the article, with the irony that they are then taken away to another page.[56] In a five-year study, researchers examined computer logs for readers of two research sites (operated by the British Library and an educational consortium) which provided access to journals, e-books and other sources of online information. They found that people tended to hop across different sites, starting on one, finding a link, clicking on that, finding another link and so on. They rarely came back to fully finish the original piece.[57]

Unfortunately this means that we do not retain as much of the information we 'read'. It's unsurprising really: if we are only skimming it and not fully absorbed in it (or indeed only reading a small part of it), we're unlikely to retain it. Worse, we may only retain a partial recollection of it. One study also found that alongside lower recall, we show less patience with online pieces, probably because they seem difficult to read, when in fact it is us not reading them properly.[58]

How we read our information matters. Research has shown that if you read something on a screen you recall less information than if it is printed and physically in front of you. In one study half of a group of students read a story on a computer screen and the other half in paper form. Students who read the paper version had greater comprehension of the story.[59] I'm really not surprised by this – I can read a copy of my writing many, many times, and it's not until a print version is in front of me that I spot the typos.

Reading everything on a screen also means that our information is far more homogenised now. Much of what we read looks pretty similar to everything else. Once we would have looked at different sources, say a newspaper, a journal article, a diary entry, a handwritten note... and our brain would consciously or subconsciously tell us whether it was reliable or not. Now these clues are hidden.[45]

HOW TO KEEP INFORMED:

There are a number of steps you can take to judge information you find online. These include:

Think about who is hosting the page. Generally speaking, health institutions (such as the NHS), government, university or medical schools, or not-for-profit organisations are more likely to give accurate information. Looking at the web address can sometimes help – does it include 'NHS', 'gov' or a university (UK universities use 'ac. uk', whereas US universities use 'edu'). Are they perhaps a recognised charity or organisation?

Can you tell who wrote the content? What are their credentials? Remember that personal stories, although appealing and maybe helpful as part of a broader picture, are not evidence.

Does it use scientific references to back up its statements? If you search for those references, are they real? If you read the abstract does it give you a similar story?

Does it tell you how old the information is? Does the website say when it was last updated?

Look around at other websites. What is the overall pattern of the information you are finding? Especially amongst those web pages that are more likely to give accurate information listed in tip one. This is a really important step in getting balanced information. If the majority of these trusted pages are giving the same message, then it is far more likely to be accurate.

Is this actual evidence, or are they trying to sell or promote something? Just because they are trying to sell you something doesn't mean they are automatically inaccurate, but definitely be more cautious.

One great resource for checking out what really happened in a research study is the NHS Choices 'Behind the headlines' web page **www.nhs.uk/news**. They have reviewed thousands of studies that have appeared in the news, and often do so very soon after media headlines hit so check them out.

4

SOCIAL MEDIA TRICKS

The rise of the internet has also brought us social media. Social media sites are now some of the most popular ways in which people use the internet – YouTube, Facebook, Twitter and Instagram are all up in the top ten most accessed websites.

The latest figures show that out of 7.7 billion people in the world, 5.1 billion have a mobile phone, 4.4 billion have access to the internet and 3.5 billion of those are social media users. And it's growing rapidly. That 3.5 billion is up 9% in the last year alone. That's an extra 288 million people who are users compared to a year ago. And overall 45% of the population globally. There is of course a split between regions – whereas 70% of the adult population are social media users in North America and eastern Asia, just 7% of those in mid Africa and 12% of those in West Africa hold accounts. In the UK we have around 53% of adults using social media.[1]

And we're using it a lot. The average social media user is on it for 2 hours and 16 minutes per day. How much, you say?! I'd never do that. Well add up all those 10 minutes here and there. The random videos you end up watching. The dramas you get dragged into. The accounts of strangers you end up clicking on because they've said something completely bonkers in your opinion on an article about Brexit (please tell me that's not just me). It all adds up.

The most popular site is Facebook with 2.3 billion users per year. This has continued to grow with an increase of nearly 10% in user figures since last year, although growth is slowing down. However, there's no need to feel sorry about that given that the platform made over $13 billion in advertising and other fees in 2018. Instagram has one billion active accounts. Internationally there are roughly 261 million Twitter users.

Social media is used for all sorts of reasons. Although the main ones are social connection and staying in touch, social media is now the main form of news for many, particularly those aged under 40. A survey in the US by the American Trends panel in 2015 asked members of the public whether they had received news from different sources in the last week. Among millennials just 37% said they had watched any news on TV, but 61% had read a news story on Facebook. It was pretty much reversed for those in the baby boomer generation, but 39% of this group still read news via Facebook.[2]

Social media and parenting information

Social media is now a major source of parenting information – whether through news articles, specific groups or asking fellow parents. We have always asked our peers questions about caring for our babies. But even ten or twenty years ago this would be a far smaller circle of friends and acquaintances. Now social media is a common method for parents to find reassurance and answers to all sorts of pregnancy and baby-related questions,[3] potentially from billions of people. All with different levels of knowledge, experience and motivation. And craziness.

Ten to fifteen years ago when I was having my babies this interaction was in online groups and message forums. Now, although there are still some major players in terms of forums, such as Mumsnet and Netmums, for many new parents online support is all about Facebook, Twitter and even Instagram.[4]

Positives

Using social media for parenting information and support has both advantages and disadvantages. Let's be positive and look at the advantages first. As there *are* a whole load of them. The internet and social media has really revolutionised the experience of having a baby for many new parents.

First is the social connection and support that social media can bring. Online support isn't just about information. It can play a really important part in reducing feelings of loneliness. It can get people interacting with others, allowing them to be part of a connected online community without ever having to leave the house or physically speak to anyone. This can clearly be advantageous for those who are experiencing social anxiety, feel overwhelmed by life or are in a situation where they are unable to get out and physically meet people for whatever reason – maybe they're a new mother, or a pregnant woman experiencing severe morning sickness, symphysis pubis dysfunction or on bed rest.

Social media can even help reduce people's feelings of depression and anxiety, not only through social contact and connection, but also through normalising asking questions and discussing feelings. Message forums in particular are set up for this. For example, if no one ever asked a question on Mumsnet it would cease to exist. Others also benefit from being able to respond to questions, and seeing others in similar situations.[5]

We know that new mothers are at risk of feeling lonely, isolated and experiencing symptoms of depression and anxiety, from general worries through to clinical diagnoses. We were never designed to have babies alone. Previous generations tended to live near family, or at least have lots of other women in the same situation around them. Loneliness and isolation is a relatively recent phenomenon for new mothers.[6]

Decades of research have shown that social support after birth plays a critical role in protecting mothers from postnatal depression and helping them recover if they are experiencing symptoms. The relationship is bidirectional: mothers who feel unsupported are more likely to develop postnatal depression, but postnatal depression can also make mothers feel isolated and unsupported.[7]

The internet and social media have played a key role in helping with this. It enables anyone who doesn't have a close family, or a close-knit group of new mum friends who know what they're going through, to connect with others, day or night. You can literally pick up your phone at 3am and someone else will be up feeding a baby or trying to get them back to sleep. Many social media groups are multi-continental, meaning that if you have a pressing question at 3am and the UK is asleep, someone will be awake in west coast America or Australia and be able to help. The immediacy of the connection and fast access to like-minded others helps improve maternal confidence and feelings of being connected to other mothers around the world.[8]

It's not just at 3am that the internet is so advantageous. In those early days and weeks, when leaving the house can seem an insurmountable task, social media lets you engage with people without even having to brush your hair or get properly dressed. You can choose a profile photo that was the best one out of the 300 that you took, or even one from five years ago, and engage with the world in a smiley, shiny fashion. On a serious note, those who feel hideously anxious at the idea of walking into a baby group, who generally find the world a bit too 'peopley' or who find stringing sentences together after no sleep last night a challenge, find that social media groups open up a whole new world.[9]

All of this has a fancy term – *social capital* – in other words, the number of people that you have around you who enhance your everyday life. Social capital is really important. Research shows that the more positive social connections you have, the better your health on all sorts of levels.[10] Research is increasingly highlighting the importance of these connections. Facebook groups can be an important way for mothers to feel supported and part of a community of other people who are going through the same thing. Whereas no one else in real life really understands your current angst about whether to go down the baby-led weaning or purée route, or obsession about which sling to buy next, you can find a group online who absolutely get how you are feeling.[11]

The rise of smartphones has made online forums and social media groups even more accessible. Only 10 years ago if you had a question at 3am you had to fire up a laptop or even get out of bed and turn on a computer to connect with the outside world, but now we just pick up our phones. A 2011 survey by BabyCentre found that smartphones were seen as a 'lifeline' for new mothers, as suddenly they had the internet in their hand whenever they needed it. Having a small phone in your hand is also infinitely easier than trying to balance a laptop when feeding a small baby.[12] And you can take it to bed with you far more easily, or look at it in a coffee shop when you're pinned under a sleeping baby when perhaps you couldn't have taken your computer with you.

On social media you can always find a group for your specific needs. Had a caesarean section? There are hundreds of groups around the world for you. Planning one? Loads. Had one before but aiming for a vaginal birth this time? There's more again. Likewise there are groups for home births, hospital births, birth centre births... there is even a group called 'I gave birth in a car'. Only 56 members at the time of searching but still – if you gave birth in a car, there are 56 new friends for you. Knowing that other people have had similar experiences to you can be very reassuring. Research shows how empowering feeling connected to others in this specific way can be.[13]

These groups can also feel valuable if you are making decisions about your baby. If you want to try baby-led weaning, but everyone in your family weaned their babies onto rusks at six weeks old, you can find a group that understands how you feel. Research shows that this can help individuals feel reassured and relieved that they are doing the 'right' thing because others are doing it too. Remember the discussion of social norms in Chapter 1? If we surround ourselves with people who are doing what we're doing, it helps reassure us that our decision is common.[14]

This can be particularly valuable when it comes to decisions that are backed up by science, but the public doesn't generally like to see... like breastfeeding. Breastfeeding is often in the news, with clickbait headlines about mothers getting thrown out of coffee shops for feeding their babies, followed by hundreds of ridiculous comments such as 'I don't urinate in public' or 'I don't flash my penis in public', or 'women who get their tits out in public are just attention-seeking' (all real *Daily Mail* comments). Social media groups aimed at breastfeeding mums can therefore help immensely by providing a 'safe space', where their behaviour is normal and validated, and they are part of a group who are all going through similar experiences. Ultimately these groups can help mothers breastfeed for longer.[15]

Negatives

The social media story is not all positive. Among the reassurance and solidarity, many feel worried that they are not living up to others' experiences of motherhood, feeling that they are failing to meet the standards of other group members. Women see other women's posts about their baby sleeping or feeding well and feel like a failure in comparison, even though we know that much of what is posted on social media is not the full story. Viral trends such as the #motherhoodchallenge, which asked mothers to post saying what made them happy to be a mother, received a backlash for being smug, insensitive to those who are struggling and fetishising motherhood.[16]

And although research shows that positive social media connections can help improve mental health, other studies show that less positive experiences can in fact be associated with an increased risk of depression. Among the general population, very high levels of Facebook use, or less harmonious reasons for using it, have been associated with depression in a number of studies. It is highly likely that this relationship works both ways. Although people with depression may become more withdrawn and therefore spend more time online, the experience of social media can provoke or exacerbate feelings of inadequacy and envy, increasing the risk of depression.[17]

The same is true for mothers using social networks. Mothers who used Facebook more often were more likely to be depressed, but this specifically related to their motivation for using it. Mothers went online specifically (whether consciously or not) to seek validation for how they were mothering, but were left feeling inadequate with increased feelings of depression after using the site.[18]

How does social media affect our decision-making?

The downside of the many, many different support and information groups on social media sites, and the ease of quickly sharing information with wide audiences, is how we are now using them to get our information.

A body of research suggests that, just like with other information sources, we're not really looking for the 'correct' answer when we use social media forums. In fact, we are looking for the answer that validates our behaviour and reassures us we are making the right decision. One study exploring how first-time mothers used social media forums described the relief mothers experienced if they found another member who was doing things the same as them, or whose baby was acting in the same way that their baby was. Having someone else feel the same way, or experience the same thing, normalised their experience and how they felt.[19]

This is potentially a double-edged sword. On the one hand, as we have seen, feeling connected and reassured is vitally important for maternal wellbeing and self-esteem. But it doesn't mean that correct health information is being shared. What it can do is reinforce the message that it is fine to go against established bodies of evidence because lots of other people are doing so too. Remember Chapter 1 and feeling relief if we're doing what others are doing? Well, what do those experts know? People in my Facebook group are saying they ignored their advice and their baby is fine!

If you already belong to a social media group where you feel welcome and like others in the group, this can change your behaviour over time. A feeling of 'homophily' can develop among group members, where you feel connections of similarity and belonging. If some members of the group then start acting in a certain way, and you identify as being part of that group, you are more likely to change your behaviour too. Research has shown that if lots of people in a group start a diet, or stop smoking, other members of that group will too.[20] You can see this play out in 'Due in January' or other birth groups. Members all get together with a shared interest – they are having a baby in January. If lots of those members later decide that they are going to wean their babies at 12 weeks, the likelihood of other group members also doing so is stronger. People trust the group and feel they belong in it, so feel guided by the group's behaviour.

We are also more likely to trust information presented to us by groups we feel part of. As I am writing this, a picture supposedly showing the anatomy of the female chest, complete with milk ducts that look like flowers at the point where the nipples would be is circulating on the internet. It got picked up by numerous websites including the BBC and was shared by social media groups that support breastfeeding. The problem with the picture is that it is inaccurate. Milk ducts do not sit neatly where your nipples are looking like pretty flowers. Fat (which is missing in the picture) means they will be spread out unevenly and stretch further back and all over the place. But the picture was shared by people who trusted what the groups they belonged to were sharing – without knowing whether it was true or not. Posts from those groups got automatic credibility as they were trusted.[21]

Sharing of misinformation and fake news

In 2017 'fake news' was the phrase of the year.[22] Unfortunately, the internet and social media mean that anyone can share anything they like and pretend it's true rather than just their opinion. This isn't helped by increasing political craziness in many countries. I have many friends in the UK who have commented that some days they have absolutely no idea what is truth and what is satire – with satirical publishers such as the *Daily Mash* coming scarily close to the truth at times, particularly during Brexit debates.

It seems that even when we have the best intentions about not sharing fake news, we do so at the same rate as real information gets shared. There is just so much information out there that can seem feasible or comes from trusted sources that we just keep clicking.[23] We even *know* some news stories will be fake: 75% of respondents in one public poll led by Monmouth University in the US believed that the mainstream media reports fake news. Yet we still buy and read (and share) that news.[24]

Fake news has been around since time began. But the internet is its breeding ground because it is so easy to fake being real. It's easy and cheap to set up a website and simple to have numerous social media accounts. You can be whoever you want to be on the internet and share a load of nonsense (harmful or just unhelpful) in an hour or so.

Although most of us would love social media to be the innocent social opportunity that it could be, we are no longer naïve enough to believe that it is. Social media works in a number of ways to expose you to different sorts of information, and in the process affects what you see, think and share, and this process is manipulated by those with vested interests, just like more traditional media. There are two main ways that this happens: through algorithms and bots.

Algorithms

Algorithms are a set of computer-based rules that determine which pages, groups and posts you see, for example on Facebook, which claims it uses them to provide a more tailored experience for the individual. Essentially it looks at what you have previously looked at, and the types of pages you visit most often, and shows you more of them and similar things. This means that what we see becomes more and more filtered each day.

Facebook also sends you targeted ads based on your profile, background and what you view. Companies (and Facebook groups) can target you based on this information and also the likes and interests you tell Facebook you have. There have been some very dubious cases of this happening. For example, recently a formula milk company was found to be deliberately targeting users who had an interest in breastfeeding. Because I am interested in motherhood and breastfeeding, I constantly see related adverts including a series of very irritating ones for a bottle company that apparently makes *the* teat that will help breastfed babies (all the brands claim this too, but apparently don't want to spend so much money advertising to me).

If you're pregnant or a new mum on Facebook, you'll know this because the targeted adverts appear almost as soon as you mention it. Nappies, bottles, weaning products – you can't escape. One day of course these ads will disappear and be replaced with ones for funeral plans instead. But Facebook uses algorithms to look at what other websites you have searched for and things you might have browsed for to buy online. In conjunction with the companies, it will then place adverts for these in your timeline.

Does Facebook use the microphone on your phone to listen to what you say? Mark Zuckerberg denied it in court.[25] Nonetheless, many users report that they have discussed something out loud, and it then appeared in their news feed. One night I watched a film (*This Property is Condemned* – great film). In the film one of the main characters is returning to New Orleans and is trying to convince a woman to go with him. He repeatedly tells her that he is going to New Orleans and asks her to go to New Orleans with him. The next morning I woke up to repeated Facebook adverts offering me plane tickets to... New Orleans.

Other instances are less amusing. Recently a post on Twitter went viral. After Twitter user 'Sam' discussed Instagram listening to her conversations, she yelled 'I'm pregnant' over and over into the microphone. She wasn't pregnant (and hadn't been searching for baby info) but a few days later a large sample of Similac formula turned up in the post via her FedEx account.[26]

All of this means that we end up being more and more exposed to the specific things Facebook thinks we are interested in. And once Facebook thinks you are interested in something, you will never ever escape it. This of course has significant problems for confirmation bias. People get deeper and deeper into their own echo chambers, through no fault of their own.

Bots

The second way in which social media can affect the content of what we see is through the use of bots. Unfortunately, not everything we see on social media is true. Anyone can be anyone they like, and with enough time and effort they can be it multiple times. Sometimes people are not actual people at all.

Bots are social robots designed to be able to interact with humans. They were created with the best intentions: they were meant to be able to talk to you and solve queries on websites, for example. But in the world of social media they can be far more menacing. Designed to be able to produce content and interact seamlessly and realistically with real humans, they are found across social media platforms. Some are great – for example, they can help spread health information in a useful way – but others can be used to try and persuade people to change their behaviour for political reasons. They are also guilty of spreading misinformation.

In the US bots have been used to spread fake news and support or smear candidates in elections. Back in 2013 the Syrian Electronic Army managed to hack the Associated Press Twitter account and post false information about President Obama being injured in a terror attack on the White House. Not only did this cause unnecessary panic, but it also led to a stock market crash.[27]

Bots can affect our parenting decisions too. For example, they have been spotted influencing the vaccination debate.[28] One study used a series of techniques to identify a number of dubious accounts on Twitter, including bots, content polluters (accounts that post random adverts and clickbait) and Russian troll accounts. All three types of malicious account tweeted about vaccines at a much higher rate than your average user. Both bots and polluters tended to tweet anti-vaccine messages, but the Russian troll accounts just disagreed with people posting anything about vaccines, presumably with the aim of causing arguments and chaos.

Bots can make it look like ideas are far more popular than they really are. Get enough bots working on a case and you look like you have a grassroots movement, which can be pretty damaging to evidence-based policies.[29] If you get enough of them working together at the same time, spreading the same information, you have what is known as a 'Twitter bomb'.

One of the main ways in which bots can be used to alter people's thinking is by following accounts, liking and retweeting and interacting. If you set up enough bots to follow you or your organisation and like and retweet whatever you say, it looks as though lots of people agree with you. The bots create the illusion of a large following and audience, which then influences others to change their opinions and behaviour.[30] As we saw with the theory of social norms and wanting to fit in with everyone else, if 'everyone' appears to be adopting a certain behaviour, why wouldn't you follow suit? Bots can also be used for more direct harm. They can be used to attack certain topics or individuals on Twitter and attempt to discredit them.

One study highlighted how active bots are, and how they will do anything to try and increase their followers. The research team created a series of bots, with random Twitter account names, and got them to publish nonsense. No sane person would retweet them, let alone follow the account. But they came... first one bot... then another... then the other bots realised their bot friends were following... and soon these made-up nonsense accounts had a whole heap of fake followers all following each other.[31] Bots can also be programmed to find and follow influential people, in the hope of a like or a retweet.[32]

Bots can seem very convincing. They can be programmed to find key words, e.g. 'caesarean section', and find articles about those online. Once found they are programmed to tweet them, or tweet them at specific people. Combinations of words can be used so they appear to have an 'agenda', e.g. only articles talking about birth using certain words.[33]

We make life easier for bots by our behaviour on social media. Retweeting things that strangers say if you like it is common. How many people have had a celebrity retweet something they have said because they happened to say the right thing at that right time? And on other platforms we end up 'befriending' people who may not be what they seem. One study found that 20% of Facebook users will accept a friend request from anyone. Over half do so if that person has a friend in common. That friendship is apparently a sign we use for deciding whether someone is legitimate or not – but it's easy for a whole group of people to have accepted a request from someone, as one of you is a friend, then two, then ten and so on... and then you're all somehow friends with a bot.[34]

Bots can have friends, or indeed be siblings. One user can have several bots who all have the same purpose. For example, if you were intent on creating media conversation against home birth, but no one was really agreeing with you, if you had sufficient time you could create 100 bots. All these bots would be programmed to tweet awful stuff about home birth. They could all be friends with each other, giving each other some legitimacy. And then of course they'd probably find other bots to befriend and play with.[35]

We also get stuck in a crazy circle. The more followers an individual has, the more likely we are to follow them (and trust what they say). So fake accounts befriend lots of people on the basis that some people will just follow anyone back. They buy followers. And follow other fake accounts and bots. The more followers they get, the more likely complete strangers are to follow them.

One way of spotting a bot is to look at what they share. Often they share the same article over and over – some research suggests up to 100 times or more. They also share articles extremely quickly, within seconds of them being posted, suggesting the article hasn't been read. This is difficult to keep track of.[36] Most people can't tell the difference between a bot and a real person unless they are paying attention and looking critically for the signs (which excludes many regular social media users). In one study students couldn't tell whether a tweet came from a bot or real person. There was no difference in how they rated bots versus humans for credibility, communication or competence.[37]

Thankfully some bots are comically fake. If any bot-makers are reading this, no, we do not want your Facebook friend request from the 'US army vet who owns a boat and puppy' or remarkably similar Twitter profiles from 'man with a big heart looking for a woman to love'. Perhaps try 'man who can cook a great cake, loves housework and has his own gin company' and we might look twice.

Mind games

You don't have to be a bot to deliberately lead people in one direction or another on social media. The set-up of social media – its immediacy, global reach and encouragement of lack of critical thinking – means that it is a perfect hotspot if someone wants to recruit people to a cause without evidence and science behind them. With a few clever tricks and measures they can convince people that they are real, evidence-based and on the ball. Here are some things that can subconsciously persuade people that a group or page is more trustworthy than it actually is:

1. Frequent posts convince people the page is genuine and trustworthy

The more we see information repeated, the more we tend to believe it. Remember back in Chapter 1 when we talked about heuristics – those shortcuts to thinking – and how they affect our perceptions of things? Well the availability heuristic comes into play here. The more we see something, particularly if it is alarming, the more likely we are to believe it. And indeed media richness theory states that if you see a novel piece of information once, you might not believe it. See it again, and again and again... and you become far less sceptical and far more likely to start believing it. After all, it's everywhere isn't it? It must be true.[38]

Based on this, social media groups (or bots) which post frequently, and post long posts, will over time be believed more and more than those who are less vocal about ideas. Organisations know this and use targeted repeated posts to build trust. Facebook allows you to 'boost' posts to be seen by an audience that is not necessarily signed up to your page or even your cause. A lot of amusement can be had once you realise some organisations on Facebook are paying to have their posts promoted to you when you are known to disagree with their behaviours. Thanks but no thanks, I don't want to like your page.

2. A global presence creates a feeling of being in a large group

It used to be that you could only easily communicate with those in your local area. Have a specific issue or complaint? Then finding like-minded others is difficult. Especially if your experience or complaint is unusual. But the internet and social media mean that we can communicate with others easily, all around the world. And you can find a handful of people in your local region more easily... and in your country... and around the world. Now, even though your experience may only occur in 0.1% of cases, suddenly there are thousands of you, all with the same experience! It must be common – look at us all!

The other benefit of the internet and social media being global is the perception it can give you of closeness to people all around the world.[38] Just open up your phone and there are people from lots of different countries, all giving you advice and information. Social presence theory states that the closer we feel to a source of information, the more likely we are to believe it. The internet has brought people together who live many thousands of miles apart. This enables us to feel part of a shared group of large people and also allows us to share information really quickly between those groups.

For example, whereas once the average person in the UK may have known a little about US, Australian or New Zealand politics, now your average person will be far more clued-up (and they all want to be Jacinda Ardern's best friend). This means that social media groups can really gain traction across the world. If, for example, someone had a baby who they felt was negatively affected by postnatal care in one city in America, before the internet very few people outside of that city would likely have heard about it. Now, with a few clicks (and a lot of targeted advertising) the whole world can.

3. Leaders who are present, visible and relatable are very persuasive

People are more likely to join groups on social media that have a visible presence at their helm – a picture of someone and a story behind them, rather than just a topic. For example, a group run by 'Joanna Blogs' with a memorable posed photo, who talks about childbirth being risky, is far more likely to get followers than a group named 'Childbirth is risky'. A similar effect can be seen if the group has a themed name but an individual is clearly leading the show.

Social presence theory is at play again. It states that how close you feel to someone is affected by two main things – intimacy and immediacy. Intimacy is all about how close you feel to someone – do you feel like you know them? Group leaders can create intimacy by sharing details of their stories and work, with occasional posts about family life or their favourite cake. Photos really help. Intimacy is increased if they have a really memorable personal story, particularly one you relate to.

For this reason, on topics related to pregnancy, birth and babies, we tend to believe figureheads who have children more than those who don't, and it's not just due to potential increased experience and expertise – we relate to them. We feel more intimate with them. We also feel a lot closer to people who share our stories and experiences, and who are 'like us'. This of course is natural and part of belonging, but increases the risk of confirmation bias.[40] More on the influence of messengers in Chapter 5.

4. Round the clock posting creates the feeling of being ever-present and important

The second part of social presence theory is immediacy.[39] How quickly does someone react in line with what is happening? If a story breaks, are they there? Or does it take a few weeks? If a social media group is immediately responding to a current topical issue in parenting, we feel closer to them. They are here in real time sharing this issue with us.

This is where having a team behind a social media account works well, particularly if it is a team of people working under the guise of one individual. They will appear very alert and on the ball, when in reality they might be sitting on a sun lounger drinking a cocktail in the Maldives. *Appearing* to have presence is the main thing. This also links in with the volume of social media postings.

5. Discussion and interaction makes people feel like part of a connected group

This again helps create a feeling of social presence.[40] Whereas once you may have read a story in the newspaper and commented to like-minded friends, now, with the internet and social media, you can engage directly with people who have similar experiences. You can go to the social media page of that newspaper and comment and discuss with fellow readers, and get likes and cheers for doing so.

Given the echo chamber that certain groups can create, everyone is likely to be posting similar stories. Or quite possibly, any voices that dissent are being deleted, leaving up only the comments that agree with the page message, to give an illusion of agreement. And given the number of followers of some pages, this can make you feel very much in the majority. These are your people.

Of course, if you are lacking in social media followers, you can always buy yourself some. Yes, this is a real thing. A quick search takes me to a whole host of YouTube clips and articles, such as '10 best sites to buy real Facebook likes, followers and views'. Clicking on the top one, 'Famoid' (with a 4.9 star rating), which is apparently based somewhere in Delaware, US, it has one review from someone saying they easily bought 1,000 likes. As tempted as I am to conduct an experiment and see what happens, I prefer to keep my personal details and credit card to myself, so I won't risk it. However, it costs $44.95 to buy 1,000 Facebook post likes, delivered apparently in a 'drip feed' over 1–5 days to look 'realistic'. Another page, 'ourfollower. com' offers Facebook followers. For $19.99 you can buy 1,000 Facebook followers. Apparently from real Facebook users.

How do you spot this? One way is by looking at the number of followers a page has compared to the active reactions to posts. If a page has hundreds of thousands of followers, but posts get very few reactions and comments, either they attract very quiet social media followers or something is up. Likewise, you might find that some very vocal commentators have very scanty personal details. Of course, lots of people keep their profiles fairly private, but most have a few photos or public posts. Bought or multiple account followers tend to be very, very private.

6. We are misled by professional-looking websites and photos

We trust websites more if they look professional and well put together. We also trust them more if they have an official sounding name.[41] For example, the International Food and Beverage Alliance aims to empower consumers to eat balanced diets and live healthier lives. Sounds good? You might change your mind when you learn that the 'alliance' includes Coca-Cola, Mars, Danone, Nestlé and PepsiCo.[42]

Image costs money. A fancy website costs money. Marketing costs money. Money that many health organisations and voluntary groups do not have – even if the information they are publishing is accurate. Commercial companies have money to spend on looking scientific and fancy – and thus believable

– in a way a local mother support group will probably never be able to do. If a website looks professionally produced and up-to-date, and if social media pages are active and usernames sound credible, we make quick decisions about who and what to trust, without digging deeper.[43]

7. Always check whether qualifications are genuine

It's worth doing this even if the qualifications have nothing to do with the information you're looking at. After all, 'Dr' Gillian McKeith did very well promoting diet and nutrition methods that had no scientific backing whatsoever... although she did get told to stop using her Dr title, given that her PhD in nutrition supposedly came from the American Association of Nutritional Consultants. Investigative scientist Ben Goldacre's cat Henrietta managed to obtain the same qualification a year after her death. (The cat, not McKeith.)[44]

8. Perfect grammar and spelling can convince us that information is true

People who are charming, able to 'talk the talk' and seem convincing and plausible are more likely to be listened to. This is one reason why psychopaths often obtain positions of employment that are far above their skills – they are verbose, use big words on purpose and generally know how to charm with their presentation while distracting from factual questions.[45]

It's easier to hone your language from behind a computer screen. If you know you're not as expert as you might hope to be, try not to appear in public. Instead, do all your communication on the internet, where you can carefully pitch your tone and wording (or have a team to do it for you). Being put on the spot in public might reduce your credibility.[46]

Finally, make sure your grammar and spelling are perfect. We tend to be grammar snobs. Yes, when we aren't sure of a new source, one of the biggest things we look for is how well it is written. Is it spelled correctly? Grammar all in good shape? Great – two ticks on the believability scale.[47]

The overlap between some social media movements and conspiracy theorists

Some social media movements (particularly in health or climate change) have the makings of conspiracy theories.[48] When we think of conspiracy theories we tend to think about fake moon landings, lizard people and chemtrails, but there are some more everyday groups on social media that have conspiracy theory-like traits. Conspiracy theories in health tend to be against public health policy and have some core features:

1. Distrust of government, science and scientific funding, for example dismissing any evidence that suggests a protective element of any aspect of pregnancy, birth or caring for babies.
2. Detailed websites encouraging an anti-public health stance – with a highly rhetorical approach.
3. Emotive appeals, such as having a personal story at their heart, usually a sick child or baby.
4. Ethical allegations such as conspiracy, cover-up and immorality.
5. A clear leader – someone who is recognised as heading the group and held in high esteem.

Do you have experience of groups like this?

A major issue with any type of conspiracy theory-like social media group is the strength of confirmation bias among its members. Research has shown that confirmation bias is strongest in groups that are homogenous and have a clear leader. This fits with many social media movements – large groups of people with a specific goal in mind, with a figurehead at the helm rather than a general coming together of interested parties. Individuals in these groups make decisions more simply, reject information more quickly, and generally feel far more confident in their behaviour than those in more heterogeneous groups without a clear figurehead.[49]

When you think of conspiracy theory followers you

probably have an image of someone wearing a tinfoil hat or colander on their head. But the tendency to believe these theories can affect ordinary people. Those who believe them tend to be in positions in life where they feel powerless, have low self-esteem, feel insecure, voiceless or generally disadvantaged. If they consciously or otherwise feel that they have little social or political power their tendency to believe is even greater.[50] These feelings are common during pregnancy, birth and being a new parent. People can feel vulnerable, and then along comes a group to soothe them and tell them that they are doing the right thing (in a world where public health guidance and evidence is suggesting otherwise).

This means that certain Facebook groups that have the same features as conspiracy theory groups are appealing if you're feeling like this. Groups that claim that policies are wrong and public health organisations are out to get you, and reassure you that you are not alone, can feel very comforting. And women who have been let down may seek this kind of comfort. When we don't receive the information, support and emotional care we need from public health organisations, we turn to those who do offer it. When women aren't listened to and their voices aren't heard, we turn to those who will listen. Unfortunately, those who will listen are not necessarily working with women's best interests at heart.

There is also a suggestion that those who are taken in by potential conspiracies, and are more likely to believe health misinformation, have narrower groups of friends and connections on social media. This means that they are even more likely to see confirmatory information, and a lot less likely to experience anything contradictory. When they do encounter contradictory (typically true) information they are highly sceptical, because everyone around them has been telling them differently.[27]

Look out for trolls, sea lions and strawmen

There are a number of personas and techniques used by individuals online to try and cause chaos and direct debate.

Internet trolls act in a way that is disruptive, deceptive or destructive, or in many cases all three. Their main aim is to cause chaos and try to make others look foolish or to trigger them emotionally in some way. Trolls typically hang out around the 'big issue' topics, or those with lots of followers, expertise or celebrity status. Trolls thrive on someone taking the bait and responding to them – the response, emotional upset, and time wasted is the goal of the troll. Ignoring them, no matter how difficult, is the best thing you can do (both to wind them up and for your own wellbeing).

There are a number of famous trolls in the world of pregnancy, birth and babies online. With a bit of practice you'll spot them a mile off. They typically don't do anything positive themselves, but instead criticise and mock others. They particularly like attacking researchers (even though they don't publish research themselves) and health professionals (even if they are not a health professional, or are no longer a health professional, themselves).

You can spot them by their dialogue and way of communicating. Debate and disagreement is at the heart of academia, research and public engagement. It's normal and enjoyable (most of the time) but it should be respectful and evidence-based. Trolls are neither. They attack individuals, criticising and deliberately misrepresenting their research and making personal attacks. They often have followers who they encourage to do the same. Sometimes trolls work together, using a hashtag to 'call' each other to a thread as back-up, so that they can form some sort of troll army attacking their prey.

Why do they do it? Boredom, desire to destruct and jealousy are the main reasons. Some believe they can find fame by tagging along with those who are famous and successful. Others are angry that others are successful and seek to bring them down.[51] Many score highly on measures of sadism, feeling gleeful when they manage to provoke an individual into responding.[52]

The whole motivation is to derail the conversation, taking the time away from what the targeted individual is successfully doing. It's one way of attacking a certain set of beliefs. Can't do your own research, or be considered an expert in something you want to disprove because you don't like it (let's say something like the success rate of vaginal birth after caesarean)? If you attack those who are conducting research into its benefits, and can distract them or even better dissuade them from engaging in the area, then success! Or not. But that is goal of the troll. #trollgoals.

Sealioning is a more subtle and very irritating form of trolling. Those who engage in sealioning initially appear to be asking polite questions. Someone – typically with considerable expertise on a subject – will post something on social media and the sea lions will turn up with their questions.

The issue is that they are relentless. They keep asking supposedly polite questions, pretend not to understand the responses, and continue to ask questions. The 'failure to understand' is key: they are suggesting that the response is not good enough, or not evidence-based enough. Their style is often over-familiar and casual, but expects the expert to respond professionally at all times.[53]

Sea lions deliberately follow individuals with whom they disagree so that they are alerted whenever they post. Sometimes they work in groups to share the load, often using a shared hashtag. This means they can keep up their relentless pursuit of individuals, asking them for evidence for everything they say, with the aim of wearing them down. Any response is criticised as not being perfect (when no evidence is perfect, as we will see).

Other sea lion tactics include asking questions that are irrelevant, picking at minor points of an argument that cannot be explained fully on social media, and asking questions that could easily be answered elsewhere. They do this over and over, until whoever they are targeting snaps or gets otherwise fed up with them, and thus appears unreasonable to outsiders. They also seek to completely divert the conversation from the focus of the scientific discussion. Essentially they turn up and bark like a sea lion – hence the name.[54]

Something else that crops up in online debate is the strawman. Rather than discussing and debating the idea someone is putting forward, a contributor instead makes up something the original poster has said, or pretends to have heard them say it, then attacks that instead. This is known as a 'strawman argument'. It has many benefits for its creator, because they can:

a. Persuade followers that their opponent really hates, for example, women who decide to use formula or need a caesarean section for any reason (ignoring evidence to the contrary).
b. Completely distract from the actual debate, so there is no longer any need to find any proof for their arguments.
c. Create chaos and arguments, fuelling the concept of the 'mummy wars' and then blame it all on their opponent.

For further effect, these posters may write blog articles or create memes to support their strawmen, declaring that certain experts in the field are evil and hate all other women. They can then publicise these widely and hope people who have never come across the individual, or don't have the energy or will to check out the facts, will agree with them.

Can you change people's opinions on social media?

With great difficulty. If only human beings were rational creatures who worked on the basis of facts! But we know from Chapter 1 that this is simply not (and will never be) true. We all think we know more than we do about subjects, and some of us are unable to understand that our vague knowledge of a topic is less than that of the experts. Unfortunately it seems the less we know, the more we think we know, as we don't realise we don't know! This becomes even worse if we do have a tiny bit of recognised knowledge of something, for example having covered a topic in brief in an undergraduate degree.[55]

Unfortunately, pointing out that someone has made a mistake can actually strengthen their incorrect information. People don't like being told they are wrong, and the arguing and backlash from you correcting them can mean that they become even more entrenched in their view. Others around them might be watching and change their minds – although there is also the possibility that they will take sides with the 'offended' or simply remember the misinformation, not who said what.[56]

In terms of what does work, a key part is acting quickly. If a new piece of 'fake news' comes out, you have more chance of influencing opinion and beliefs if counter-information is given before the fake news becomes ingrained in the public consciousness. For example, it's now extremely challenging to tackle views on the MMR vaccination and autism. Everyone will cite 'that study' that 'proved' that the vaccination caused autism. People remember Andrew Wakefield's name and associate the findings with him. Despite the fact that he and his study were later discredited, it was ingrained in public knowledge as fact.[57]

Confirmation bias plays a large role in this. Once someone has decided they believe something, they are more likely to only listen to information that confirms that belief, rejecting anything else. If you can get to them with facts before mainstream acceptance, you have much more chance of them listening and at least considering your information.[58]

Sometimes, rather than challenging people about why they believe something, ask them to explain more about it. This can be helpful in two ways. Firstly, you can then use counter-evidence, and secondly, it might help them to see what they don't know, breaking the illusion of knowledge. The only issue with this is that people with very strong opinions may simply refuse to give you evidence or explain their thoughts.[59]

Where possible, research suggests that the best means of counteracting misinformation is to be brief, simple and clear, emphasising facts that are supported where possible by further evidence. The person who was stating the information may not agree with you, but the wider 'audience' watching may decide to consider or follow up your information.[60] Unfortunately, this seems to work best when everyone is having a fairly mundane conversation. When emotions are at play, or anxiety is running high (the whole of parenting, then), it is far more difficult to fight misinformation with facts.[61]

Nonetheless, there is some evidence that if people have fallen for highly emotive misinformation, or conspiracy-like theories, you can persuade them to think differently by creating a plausible alternative rather than by debunking their knowledge.[62] For example, as mentioned above, Andrew Wakefield's MMR and autism research is still cited despite the work being discredited and him being struck off the medical register. Research suggests that stating those facts does not work to change people's opinions, but creating a narrative about how he had alternate motivations, such as the money he made from the scandal, can help people to think more clearly about the facts and evidence.[63]

Most of all, try to remain respectful, calm and kind. This is far more likely to have an effect than becoming angry, especially if you are a woman. Copious research has shown that we think angry people are not logical, and women in particular are 'overly emotional' and nonsensical. Of concern is that once a woman is perceived like this, her whole character is written off, while men are forgiven for 'having a bad day'.[64]

Consider whether you are benefitting from social media

It's important to regularly re-examine whether social media is positive for you. It can be a great tool for reading about evidence and other people's experiences around having babies, but as we've seen it can be a complicated arena.

Social media is increasingly implicated in negatively affecting mental health, and you can see why. Katherine Ormerod, in her book *Why Social Media is Ruining Your Life*, discusses findings from a survey by Mush – an app that connects mothers – that revealed that 80% felt that social media was making them feel under greater pressure to be a perfect mother.[65] Likewise, research that one of my students, Sarah Hicks, conducted for her dissertation showed that the more pregnant women used Facebook, the more dissatisfied they were with their changing body and appearance during pregnancy. Over half of mothers reported how they often compared their pregnant body to those they saw online.[66] Research has also linked too much time on Facebook to postnatal depression.[67] It's really easy to fall into a self-comparing spiral of envy and before you know it you're miserable.

Of course, half of what we see is nonsense. Anyone can be anyone on social media, including attacking others or pretending our lives are very different. In one US survey, 20% of women with depression admitted to sharing a photo or caption that didn't match their emotions. When they were feeling miserable, they shared a happy status or photo, telling everyone how great things were. I'm pretty certain this is what's behind every 'my baby slept all night, feeling blessed' post.

But don't be afraid to step back. If people's 'opinions' (attacks and judgement) on social media are making you continually tense or distressed, log off. If those people disappear once your phone is switched off, they don't have that much sway. Don't give them the power they are seeking. You don't have to justify your decisions to anyone. Least of all a profile hiding behind a cat photo on Twitter.

HOW TO KEEP INFORMED:

Be alert to the bots: check their profile or bio. Do they have real friends and followers? A photo? How often do they post? Every few minutes? Then they're either very bored at work or a bot. If in doubt, you can check them out at **botcheck.me**

Be alert to the tricks people use online. That's not to say that any large group with lots of followers should be ignored – certainly not! But be aware and keep an eye on their behaviour. How much is spin and image?

One way to check how balanced a group is, is to disagree with them politely online. Not repeatedly like the sea lions, but gently asking to discuss the topic or asking for evidence for claims. How do they react? Respectfully? Or do they shout, criticise, accuse and then block you?

5

WHO IS THE MESSENGER?

It's not just what information we see or hear, but who is giving it to us that matters. Once upon a time I'm sure we had much more respect for experts in their field – people who had spent decades researching and learning about specific topics. Although many a scientist and philosopher has met a sticky end throughout history.

However, we do seem to be at an all-time low. In an era when we think information is ours at the touch of a few buttons, and we are engaging more closely than ever with huge numbers of individuals, including those in government and positions of authority who we'd never have had the opportunity to insult directly before, our knowledge and awareness as a society seems to be going down a slippery slope. Who do we trust to give us our information?

The concept of the 'cognitive authority' – a trusted individual

You are a cognitive authority if someone trusts you to give them good, reliable information. This is all subjective. One person might put you on a cognitive pedestal, while someone else would argue with you if you said the sky was blue (though to be fair, looking out of the window in Wales in June, they might be right). Your label as a cognitive authority is also relative. You might be the only one among your friends who knows how to change a car tyre, but go to a mechanics' convention and they're hardly going to offer you a position based on your experience of five tyre changes on your own car.[1]

The problem with judgements about who we see as a cognitive authority is that they are as much to do with us as they are the authority themselves. Going back to our good old tendency for confirmation bias, we have a fairly narrow view of who we will accept as a cognitive authority in the first place. Basically they need to be telling us what we want to be true, but in a particularly convincing way... even though we desperately want to be convinced in the first place.

This does mean people can have quite a tenuous status as cognitive authorities. How many times have you seen it played out on social media, when an 'authority' with hundreds of thousands of followers dares to say something that isn't quite in line with what people want to hear? They are immediately labelled 100% bad and their authority badge is taken and destroyed. The overthrowers will then often try to convince others to villainise the authority they once worshipped.

Furthermore, individuals with very little experience or actual expertise can be worshipped as experts as they are saying what people want to hear. Some of the authors of best-selling baby and parenting books, particularly those which promote ways of caring for your baby that go against what we know to be important for attachment and bonding, have very few qualifications. They are just able to write in an appealing way, even if there is no evidence for what they say.

Consider the parenting books that tell you to put your baby into a strict routine. These books sell millions of copies and are usually right up there in the bestseller lists. However, they lack an evidence base, and the authors are generally lacking in relevant qualifications. Personal experience, yes. And often a heart-wrenching tale to explain why they wrote the book, yes. But evidence that their methods support infant wellbeing and development or even work at all? Sparse. In fact, our research shows that the methods often don't work for many parents, increase their risk of feeling like a failure and can encourage behaviours that many parents find very difficult, such as not cuddling babies so frequently or not responding when they cry.[2,3] So always stop to think about who you are allowing to be your expert.

Who do we believe on social media platforms?

Again, as we do not have full information, or time to do a detailed background search on who people are and what their experience is, we use those cognitive heuristics we discussed earlier – shortcuts. Metzger and colleagues identified six heuristics we commonly use online:[4]

- *The reputation heuristic:* we believe people who are familiar over people who are not.
- *The endorsement heuristic:* we trust people who other people appear to trust.
- *The consistency heuristic:* we trust information that appears consistent across different online and offline sources.
- *The self-confirmation heuristic:* we find people more credible if they are giving us information that fits our pre-existing beliefs.
- *The expectancy violation heuristic:* we stop trusting people if they fail to meet our expectations in any way.
- *The persuasive intent heuristic:* we dismiss information if we think it is biased.

What does this mean in a global social media, bot-dominated landscape?

1. Distrust in experts

Over the last few years, we have become increasingly sceptical about who we deem an expert and who we trust to give us our information. Trust in experts and information is generally down, worldwide, while anecdotes, news headlines and articles on social media receive more and more attention.

There's even a tool to measure the change in who we trust. The Edelman Trust Barometer tracks public trust across 28 countries on four main elements: how much the public currently trusts business, government, NGOs and the media.[5] The tool publishes trust levels per country, but also breaks down trust between different groups. One way in which it does this is to analyse trust ratings between members of the public who are considered 'informed' and those who are not. To be considered informed you must be aged 25–64, college educated, in the top 25% of income bracket for your country and report significant engagement with business news. This group represents around 13% of the population. Whether those criteria are fair or not is a different question, and of course lots of people falling outside these categories would be very well informed.

However, what is interesting is the divide. Those who are informed score more highly on trust of experts compared to those who are less informed. In the US, Canada and the Netherlands the informed group are net 'trusters', and in the UK, Australia and much of Europe the informed are net 'neutrals'. However, among the wider population, 20 out of 28 countries are net 'distrusters'. The US, UK, Australia and much of Europe, on a mass population level, are distrusters. The gap is also widening. In 2018 60% of the informed were trusters, compared to 45% of the mass public overall. In the US the gap was a difference of 21 points, 19 in the UK, and 18 in France.

This lack of trust translates into negative thinking. Those who are distrusters tend to have a sense of injustice, a lack of hope and a lack of confidence in leaders. 53% of respondents globally believe the system is failing them. Just 29% rated government officials as credible. Although this does extend across all groups: 51% of the 'well informed' also believe the system is failing.

What fuels this? Fear. Fear of corruption, immigration, eroding social values, globalisation and pace of change all predict a belief that the system is failing (exacerbated by the media, as we saw in Chapter 2). Notably, in the US 67% of Trump voters were classed as 'fearful' compared to 45% of Clinton voters. And in the UK 54% of Brexiters are fearful compared to 27% of Remainers.

The report also shows what a self-induced echo chamber we live in. Over half of respondents stated they would never change their position on social issues despite new information developing (confirmation bias anyone?). And they may never listen to that new information, as 53% state they never listen to people or organisations they disagree with. More people (59%) stated they believed information they found in a search engine compared to an editor of a news article (41%). In fact, in the rankings of 'who do you think is the most credible source of information', 'someone like myself' came top.

You can increasingly see this distrust of public health organisations, health policies and science. Often accused of having an agenda or making stuff up, these organisations are increasingly coming under attack from those who deny the worth and accuracy of large bodies of science and research. Top tip: if all the major public health organisations are agreeing broadly on promoting a health behaviour, it is likely that there is a good evidence base underpinning it. It is highly unlikely that the World Health Organization, UK Department of Health, American Academy of Pediatrics and so on are all involved in some strange racket where their policies for, let's say reducing childhood obesity or encouraging women not to smoke in pregnancy, are for murky underhand reasons. Or that they scribbled down a policy on the back of a beer mat one day in the pub. What would they stand to gain? And it is again highly unlikely that any one individual, especially one with little expertise in the area, would know better than their large staffing of many trained policy experts, science advisors and researchers. Yet still we are seeing science denialism on a grand scale across multiple areas of health and wellbeing.

2. Distrust in universities and academics

We are also changing our opinion on whether we believe advanced education and those who work within it are having a positive impact. Again these results are politically linked. For example, a survey in 2015 in the US found that 58% of Republican voters believed that universities had a negative impact on the country, with 36% believing they had a positive impact. Just two years ago that figure was reversed – 54% believed they had a positive impact, and 37% believed they had a negative impact. It's not all bad news. In the same survey, 78% of Democrats in 2017 believed universities had a positive impact.[6]

Research by Matt Motta has also shown that the less an individual trusts 'experts' or scientists (over and above 'ordinary people on the street') the more likely they are to vote for Brexit or Trump.[7] This isn't surprising, given that Trump banned the US Centers for Disease Control (CDC) from using the words 'evidenced based' and 'science based' in their budget documentation.[8] Those low in trust of experts are also less likely to believe in climate change. Interestingly, Matt found that the higher an individual's verbal intelligence, the more trusting they are of experts (whatever their own political beliefs).

Going back to Brexit again (sorry!), YouGov conducted a poll on public trust of academics and researchers giving their evidence-based statements on the likely outcomes of leave. Overall remain voters were generally trusting of a wide variety of experts. Leave voters on the other hand didn't trust anyone deemed an expert. Only 25% of leave voters trusted academics compared to 70% of remain voters.[9]

What's fuelling this distrust? Some have proposed that

the increase in tuition fees and a narrowing job market have changed the way some view universities – seeing them as selling a product, and the students as customers. Knowledge is for exams, not for the joy or benefit of learning, growth and development.[10] The situation is not helped by a lot of people not understanding what academics do. The vast majority of PhD students, for example, have had someone (usually a parent) ask them over dinner to explain again exactly what it is that they're doing.

If you've never been in a university, research or scientific environment, you are unlikely to have an insight into academic training and expertise – and you may be suspicious about how people who work there spend their money and time. We naturally do this for every position of expertise. Based on our very limited experience, we assume that we know what they do (and how they should be doing it better). How many of us have asked why our car is taking so long to be fixed at the garage? Or wondered what on earth they are teaching them at school these days? Or thought we could do a better job of being prime minister?

The rise of the internet and smart phone accessibility has contributed to this. With many people now having Google in their pocket, access to information is seen as quick and easy. Anyone can access research papers or research summaries, even if they can't actually understand them (or worse, have no idea that they can't understand them). Or check the supposed accuracy of what you've just been told. Or search for the pub quiz answers if you have no moral compass at all.

Perceptions therefore arise that experts have no real knowledge or talent, just an ability to google. But experts do more than just 'know stuff'. Years and years of expertise means that they can synthesise information, know related information, understand what is a reliable source of information, and so on – essentially the sum of their knowledge and expertise is greater than the sum of the parts of knowledge that they know.[11] While someone with no background in a subject might find one research paper online and declare it 'the truth', the expert in the subject will know how it fits in with all the hundreds, even thousands, of other papers on the topic.

For example, when such an organisation produces a health policy, they do not whip it out of thin air one day. Putting together a health policy is extremely time-consuming and usually involves numerous individuals and many, many months of work. For example, take the recent National Institute of Clinical Excellence (NICE) guidelines for the Recognition and Management of Faltering Growth in children in the UK. When such a guideline is created, a detailed search needs to be conducted of all available evidence. You search for every possible research paper, usually using many, many search terms and combinations for specific questions within the broader guideline. You then need to check and double check (usually with at least two people) whether each paper is relevant to read fully and then if it is of high enough quality to include in your review based on multiple criteria such as the type of design and any bias involved.

In the case of these guidelines, an expert committee was put together who met 13 times over 19 months. A long list of stakeholders were involved. The process of deciding what information to include was scrupulous. The number of papers they screened to decide whether they were relevant and of high enough quality to go in the review was phenomenal. Altogether 35,391 papers were identified across the searches and 576 full papers read. All this information is open and transparent and available on the NICE website for anyone to see and check the process (**www.nice.org.uk/guidance/ng75**). But oh no, Twitter-user Bob thinks the one paper he found this morning on the internet is better than this review.

Unfortunately, it appears that those who have the least experience of education and knowledge acquisition have the deepest distrust of those with the most. The higher an individual's education and experience and knowledge of science, the better their trust in scientists and other experts – and vice versa.[12] There is also a political divide. Broadly, Conservatives trust science less than Liberals. One reason proposed for this is that science often leads to changes that those with a conservative approach may not like, for example, in public health, reductions in carbon emissions, climate change… because these things are seen to limit industry and free enterprise.[13]

3. We don't trust women

There is also a very, very depressing bias against female experts, particularly younger ones. Numerous studies dating back to the 1950s show that age and gender play a role in credibility. Men and older people are seen as more credible than younger women. Indeed, one study in Switzerland looking at the perceived credibility of newsreaders found that men were seen as more credible than women. And older men were the most credible of all.[14]

One fascinating anecdote comes from transgender scientist Ben Barres. As a female undergraduate student, Barbara Barres was often told she couldn't have solved the maths problems that she did – a man must have solved them for her. After transitioning to become Ben, and continuing in the maths sciences, he overheard an audience member (who was unaware that he had been Barbara) saying that 'his work is much better than his sister's'.[15]

I have heard countless stories, and have personal experience, of people assuming that female academics are male because they are a doctor, or assuming that they must be much older than they are based on their written achievements ('I expected you to be so much older!' is never the compliment some think it is). We also know that throughout history, women have had their ideas and discoveries stolen by men – reinforcing the idea that it must be the man in the team who was in charge.

As an example, I have written a well-read paper on influences on breastfeeding duration. The work came from my PhD, and my PhD supervisors were co-authors. There are three of us: two women, one man. I am first author. My details are on the paper as the person to contact. Who gets the requests to access and discuss the paper? My male PhD supervisor, who had no experience of breastfeeding research prior to meeting me. Rather than using my email address, which is *on the paper*, enquirers take the time to search for his details instead. I let him deal with those.

Stories about men, told by men, dominate our headlines. The Global Media Monitoring Project was started in 1995 when data was collected across 71 different countries about who was presenting the news and who the stories were about. Just 17% of news or newsreaders were female. In 2000 it was repeated, and this grew to 18%... and 21% in 2005. In 2010 it was up to around a quarter – with the UK statistics reflecting this.[16]

Men also spend more time talking and explaining things in public spheres. Although we are told through the media and other outlets that women spend more time talking, they actually don't. Perhaps this is true in private spaces, but in public spaces, including online and in the media, it's men who have the majority of the words and space. They speak more, explain more and interrupt more,[17] leading to the experience that many woman have had of the 'mansplainer'.

A mansplainer is a man who feels so confident in his own ability to know and understand stuff, and so sure that his knowledge is greater than that of a woman in his presence, that he explains stuff to them. Usually their specialist subject area. The term emerged from the work of journalist Rebecca Solnit, who was so fed up of being cut off, talked over and having things explained to her by men with less knowledge than her that she wrote an essay called 'Men explain things to me.'[18]

Although there is many a joke made about mansplaining, it is actually a serious issue. Subtly, bit by bit, it reinforces the idea that men are knowledgeable and should be speaking, and women should listen to them. It slowly shuts women down, further decreasing their confidence. And most of all it encourages the general public to feel this way towards male and female experts.

Analysis of speech shows that women have been socialised to expect interruptions. When they speak they are more likely to fill natural gaps with words such as 'ummm', or use phrases such as 'like' or 'I mean' as a way of keeping talking. Conversely, men have more pauses between their ideas as they think, because they are less likely to be interrupted if they take a moment to think or pause between ideas.[19] However, these small conversation fillers that women use to defend their verbal space are then criticised as showing a lack of confidence, assurance or knowledge,[20] leaving female experts battling a vicious circle.

Emotion also plays a key role. It turns out the public don't like it when women become angry (or passionate) about their subject – but they turn a blind eye, or even find it positive when men do. Women are 'overly emotional' when they display passion or anger, and therefore unreliable.[21] Men? Well, they're just showing their expertise and passion aren't they. If women do display anger or emotion, they're also more likely to be judged as that being their regular character across all situations, while men are more likely to be excused as it being a 'one off'.[22]

What does this mean for research?

Our bias against female experts ends up affecting who is in a position to do research and which subjects therefore have a bulk of evidence behind them. Female academics are also judged as less knowledgeable and experienced compared to their male peers. One study asked psychologists (educated people, who you think would have an awareness of what they are doing) to decide whether they would a) hire someone for an academic post and b) give an academic 'tenure' (grant them permanency after doing sufficient teaching and research). The psychologists were each sent one of four CVs. Two CVs were applying for the post. Two were applying for tenure. Both post CVs were the same and both tenure CVs were the same apart from one key difference – gender. All were Dr Miller, but one of each set was a Karen and one a Brian. Depressingly, Brian was more likely to be rated as suitable for the post and ready for tenure than Karen. By both male and female raters.[23]

Ethnicity is also an issue. In a similar study, 251 biology and physics professors from eight large universities in the US were asked to read one of eight CVs for a hypothetical job candidate for a postdoctoral research position. The CVs were identical apart from the name, which was changed to denote male or female, and to suggest ethnicities that were Asian, Black, Latinx or White. Yes, you've guessed it:[24]

- The physicists saw the male candidates as more competent and appointable. They thought the Asian and White candidates were more competent and appointable than the Black and Latinx. Black women were seen as the least appointable of all.
- The biologists rated the Asian candidates more competent and appointable than Black candidates, and more hireable than Latinx candidates.

The punchline was that women were also consistently rated as more 'likeable' than men. So women are nice but not clever. Fabulous.

These attitudes are of course tied into the sexism and right-wing authoritarianism we saw in Chapter 3. Countless papers have shown that those who feel threatened by a woman acting in a position or way they view as 'male' (e.g. a leadership position, or showing her expertise) get very angry. Women who are seen to be 'deviants' from the gender norm are evaluated less favourably than men for the same behaviours.[25]

For some, seeing a woman acting competently, showing her agency or experience, or being in a leadership role, unleashes feelings of disgust, contempt, revulsion and anger.[26] These feelings are particularly strong among those who believe in hierarchy and order.[27] They can lead to individuals not supporting women in positions of power simply because they are women – regardless of their actual expertise.[28]

This can be seen in how we use words to describe the behaviours of men and women. Words like 'ambitious' or 'driven' are often used as a criticism when it comes to describing a woman but seen as desirable behaviours for men. And thinking back to childhood, how many assertive young girls are referred to as 'bossy'? How many little boys get described this way?

Women are further judged by how feminine they look. Essentially, the younger and more feminine they look, the less they are taken seriously. There is plenty of advice out there telling female experts how to dress (conservatively and mirror the male suit) and wear their hair (short preferably; if long, never down).[29] This is even more complicated for women of colour, with Black women in particular facing further racism and micro-aggressions if they wear their hair naturally. For an excellent read on this issue look up the paper by Sylvia Gray – 'To curl up or relax? That is the question.' The central message is that the expertise of women, especially women of colour, is based on their appearance.[30]

Alongside gender and ethnicity, there is also a clear bias across the field of education and academia for those who come from more privileged backgrounds in securing places and roles. We know students from more affluent backgrounds are more likely to go to university in the first place. The academic pathway is long and typically requires the very best grades as you move from degree to masters to PhD. And then getting a permanent academic role is also often a long slog. Many researchers have multiple short-term contracts, often having to move around the country before they gain a full-time role. This means that students from working class backgrounds who do attend university can feel like they don't fit in; an emotion not limited to just the students. Much has been written on the concept of academics who have come from a working-class background feeling out of place within the academy, with particular pressures again for women.[31]

But what does that mean for research? Again it can mean that only those who are privileged or who beat the odds (or both) secure a place where they can conduct research. And even if they come from communities where experience of education and research is low, their experience of being part of universities and research will invariably change their life stance and distance from the communities they came from to some extent. This means that their research topics may not be answering the needs of less privileged communities. What is really needed is a better route for more people from communities that would benefit from research to design and conduct the research themselves, with the support of those who have had research training. Do you really need a PhD and an academic post to understand, for example, the barriers in your community to vaccination? Thankfully there are now a growing number of projects to ensure this is happening – most likely with far more relevant and sensitive research findings emerging.[32]

These underlying structural issues become even more problematic when it comes to conveying evidence-based information around pregnancy, birth and babies. Women do the majority of research in these subjects (again not something I can give a reference for, but after hundreds of conferences with an audience and speaker set that is usually 95% female, that's close enough). At the last count, there were 206,870 individuals in academic posts in the UK. The gender split of those posts is fairly even, albeit weighted towards men (45% versus 55%). However, there is a clear gender imbalance across the type and level of the posts. At professorial level, just a quarter of posts are female. At senior academic level, it's a third. In terms of role, women make up 51% of teaching-only posts, despite being only 45% of the workforce.[33]

If you expand this to look at the number of women in academia who aren't White, then the situation is even more dire. Just 15% of UK academics are from Black and Minority Ethnic groups. But as you rise higher up the ranks, this drops even lower. In the UK there are just (as of February 2019) 25 Black female professors in the UK, making up just 0.1% of all current professors (and I believe there may have been some resignations since). Conversely, 68% of all professors are White men.[34]

It's not just a case of underrepresentation. If you look at who gets the funding, report after report shows men are more likely to get research grants, and certainly the bigger grants. For example, a report on funding in infectious disease research found that 72% of grants awarded went to men. Men also received 79% of the total funding, suggesting that the grants women received were disproportionately smaller.[35] Likewise, another report on funding for cancer research: 69% of the grants and 78% of the money awarded to men.[36]

One reason for this is that some data suggests that female academics apply for fewer grants. But they still have a disproportionately lower success rate. And it's not difficult to understand why they apply for fewer grants – there are fewer of them, and fewer of them in top positions (it tends to be that a professor will be the main applicant on the grant, unless it's a specific early career or development grant). And just like in the home, female academics do a disproportionate share of the 'housework' in academia. They do more teaching, particularly of undergraduates. They do more admin and committee work. They do more to care for the wellbeing of the students. They have less time to write (typically very lengthy) grant applications.[37]

What is interesting is that this pattern seems much clearer in the medical and physical sciences than it does in the social sciences. Some analyses of social science funding suggest that women get a more equal proportion of grant funding. For example, data from the Economic and Social Research council found an equal balance in the number of men and women successfully getting a grant, even though women were still submitting fewer applications (41%).[38]

Although on the surface this seems great, it is actually problematic, because social science research tends to get overlooked or not taken seriously because it is less likely to use large-scale cohorts or randomised controlled trials. It is more likely to use a qualitative approach such as interviewing smaller numbers of people, which some people deem less 'worthy', despite the fact that the social sciences offer huge input into the 'Why?' questions that are vital to understanding our society – e.g. Why do people act like this? So although women are managing to do research in the social sciences, it is less likely to be listened to or used in reviews or policy. Much more on this later.

Women are also less likely to be first author (often seen to be the lead, most influential author) on papers published in high-ranking health journals. One analysis found that just a third of papers in the top six medical journals were first authored by women. The *New England Journal of Medicine*, which is often considered the best medical journal, had a female first author for less than a quarter of articles.[39]

The upshot of all of this is that women end up doing less research and not getting taken as seriously for it. And because women predominantly do the research about pregnancy, birth and babies, this means that research in this area is underfunded and not taken so seriously – particularly the research that seeks to understand and improve women's experiences (as opposed to big prestigious randomised controlled trials that may be scientifically fancy, but often don't actually help anyone in reality). In birth and breastfeeding research, there is a sea of women with an occasional man, who is typically in a position of power rather than doing entry-level work. That's not saying the men aren't doing great work, or that we don't want them in 'women's research' (we do, as everyone is gestated, born and cared for at some point!). But it's disproportionate and not a coincidence.

The moral of the story is, if as a society we don't fund and employ women, research that really matters does not get done, meaning that we have less of an evidence base to rely on when making decisions that affect women's care. The patriarchy is alive and well in the world of scientific research.

4. We trust our friends and family

Countless studies show that when presented with competing information from experts and friends and family, we tend to believe what our friends and family tell us over the experts. One main reason for this is that we believe that they have our best interests at heart. We don't judge people only on their perceived competency, but also on their perceived character and our belief about whether they want what's best for us. We rate our family more highly than health professionals or scientists.[40]

Hendriks and colleagues developed a scale to measure how we view whether someone is to be trusted or not. The 'Muenster Epistemic Trustworthiness Inventory' measures three key elements of how we perceive people: expertise, integrity and benevolence.[41]

- Expertise: competence, intelligence, well-educated, professional, experience, qualified, helpful
- Integrity: sincere, honest, just, unselfish, fair
- Benevolence: moral, ethical, responsible, considerate

However, these elements are not equal. We are three or four times more likely to trust someone that we believe has our best interests at heart. In a study asking people who they would trust to give them information about whether the land their house was on was contaminated, people did trust scientists more than property developers. But actually they trusted neighbours, friends and family and the media more – in part because they believed they had their best interests at heart whereas the scientists did not. For some reason scientists are often viewed as being knowledgeable but not benevolent – and this lack of benevolence overrides people's trust in them.[42]

One study exploring how younger mothers could better be supported to breastfeed highlighted this. The researchers developed a counselling intervention to support younger mothers with breastfeeding. The intervention worked well to improve breastfeeding rates, but only if the mother was living away from her mother. When mothers still lived in the family home, the intervention didn't work, because the grandmothers were giving competing information which overruled the intervention.[43]

The problem is that family and friends may not have the most up-to-date information. As our knowledge increases, guidelines change. I often wonder what my own children will do differently with their (currently hypothetical and staying that way for some time please) babies, because guidelines will be different then. But I bet practically every reader who has had a baby has had a family member say to them at some point or other that 'it never did you any harm' – 'it' being whatever you are doing differently to them. It can be difficult when your grown-up child cares for their child in a different way. It can ignite all sorts of anxieties (conscious or otherwise) about whether you did it the 'right' way. Or you worry that the 'new ways of doing things' are putting too much pressure on new mothers and you want to help.

5. Who do we trust most? Ourselves

As Confucius said: *'Real knowledge is to know the extent of one's ignorance.'* Of all the possible sources of information, it turns out that we trust ourselves the most. One problem with this is that often, we don't know what we don't know. Which makes sense: if you don't know it, how do you know that you don't know it?

There are three types of knowledge:[44]

1. Known knowns – stuff you know and know you know
2. Known unknowns – stuff you know you don't know but know exists
3. Unknown unknowns – stuff you don't know you don't know (often the dangerous part)

Unfortunately, people who don't know what they don't know, are often overly confident about how much they know.

As humans we also have a tendency to make stuff up to fill in the gaps if we don't know something. To give it its more technical term, the *completion principle* is when our brain, exhausted by having to try and find out new information, pretty much makes things up instead. We make inferences about what is probably right based on our prior knowledge and thinking. Unfortunately, once it's in our brains we think it's correct, and the more we think about it the more ingrained it becomes. Then we forget we made it up. And then we use this fact to make future judgements, becoming more and more confident that we are right.[45]

To be informed you have to have two things: information and accuracy. If you have information but it's not accurate, you are not informed, you are misinformed. This is obviously contextual and not fixed. You can be informed in many areas, but still misinformed in a particular one. And lots of people are misinformed rather than uninformed when it comes to science. Misinformation (rather than a lack of information) is particularly tricky, because you believe that you have the right information and therefore anyone (like those experts) holding a competing view is wrong. A further problem of course is that once someone has misinformation, it is really difficult to persuade them to reject it and think otherwise.

When it comes to the unknown unknowns, people can be over-confident because they don't know they don't know something. Anecdotally, many people feel more knowledgeable about a subject at the start of an undergraduate degree course than they do at the end of a PhD when they've realised how complex the subject is. In everyday life, people vote a certain way because they don't know the harmful outcomes that might arise. They didn't know the impact of their voting choice on a law that affects them. Which leads, for example, to the situation in which some members of communities who received the greatest net amount of EU funding voted to leave the EU and then were angry that they would have less money.[46]

People think they have knowledge about all sorts of stuff that they don't, for example when it comes to how things work. Personally I'm particularly skilled at knowing what is wrong with my car and suggesting to the mechanic what needs fixing when it comes up with yet another of those warning lights. One day I hope he agrees with me. Overconfidence is all over the place. Many studies have shown that people usually overestimate how knowledgeable they are. In a seminal research paper back in the 1970s participants were asked a series of general knowledge questions and then after each one judged on a scale from 0 to 1 how likely it was their answer was correct. People who gave themselves a score of 1, which meant 'I am absolutely right' were actually only right 20–30% of the time. Interestingly those who gave themselves a score of 0 'I am definitely not right' were right 20–30% of the time too.[47]

We're even overly confident about what we *couldn't* know – because it's false. In another study participants were asked to rate how knowledgeable they were about a series of topics. In the list were completely made-up topics that no one could possibly be knowledgeable about because they were completely fictitious. On average participants claimed they knew something about a quarter of the made-up subjects.[48] This was confirmed in a similar study in which around 15% of participants claimed they had excellent understanding of examples of current political policies – not hampered in the slightest by these being made up.[49]

People are really overconfident about their ability to do things too. One study with medical students asked them to rate how confident they were performing different procedures. Their tutors then marked them as needing more training, competent, or having sufficient competency to teach others. Overconfidence was rife. All rated themselves as being good enough at taking blood that they could teach others, but only 10% were rated as such by their tutors. Likewise 80% thought they could teach putting a catheter in. Tutors completely disagreed.[50] This is seen all over the place. After all, how many of us believe we are better than average drivers?[51]

This may seem fairly amusing, until it isn't. Some might argue that scientific, economic or political knowledge is not needed in everyday life for many people. And there's always Google. After all, what do those experts know that I don't?[52] The serious consequences of this approach can be seen in an example like the vote on whether to remain in the European Union. After the UK Brexit vote the most commonly googled phrase in the UK was 'What is the EU'. Yes. After the vote.[53]

There are countless other examples where a lack of knowledge can really let us down and make our lives more difficult, or more expensive. Even something as simple as understanding how to work out which pasta is the cheapest in the supermarket can have knock-on effects. Our health literacy (i.e. our understanding of health and how to follow instructions) is also pretty terrible and that can have damaging effects in terms of whether we take medications correctly.[54]

Believing you have more knowledge than an expert seems particularly common when it comes to human behaviour. Once had a baby? Then you must know everything. Of course, we may be expert at understanding our own baby, but this individual expertise appears to make people question social and health science in a way they may not question a microbiologist or nanotechnologist as they don't have the same experience (or equipment) to have experienced it themselves.

It also appears directly related to well... actually not knowing. In one study into understanding of autism, 36% of participants thought they knew as much as doctors about the causes of autism, with 34% believing they knew more than scientists. However, they were then given a knowledge test about the causes of autism. Those who thought they knew more actually had the lowest scores. This overconfidence was also associated with a strong belief that non-experts such as celebrities should play a role in policy-making processes.[55]

The Dunning-Kruger effect

This brings me neatly into a fascinating yet terrifying concept that you will have no doubt seen play out across social media, and which has its own title – the Dunning-Kruger effect. This describes how it is often the case that the less competent and knowledgeable someone is, the stronger their belief that they are extremely well informed, while simultaneously believing that those who are viewed as experts in the area have much poorer abilities.[56] I'll pause for a moment while you quietly list the number of people you know who are like this.

David Dunning (whose name, along with Justin Kruger's, has been given to the effect) has explored how prevalent ignorance is in everyday life. There are countless things that you and I are ignorant about. An orthodox economist who believes that human behaviour is rational would call ignorance about subjects that have nothing to do with your everyday life entirely rational – and in fact protective. You don't need to know everything about everything and it would be counterintuitive to try, as presumably you would end up dedicating less time to knowing things that would actually help you. In fact, people who experience the type of anxiety that means they imagine every rare worst-case scenario would probably quite like some of this sort of ignorance.

However, people who exhibit a high Dunning-Kruger effect don't seem to be able to accept that they don't know everything about everything.

Dunning talks about a concept called 'Reach around knowledge' – the idea that you have knowledge (or believe you do) in one area and then just apply these thoughts to a similar sounding area. Have an opinion about a research paper on breastfeeding? Don't like it (possibly for good reason)? If you have reach around knowledge, you will simply apply this to any breastfeeding policy you then hear of, without ever reading it. You know you know it's awful. Although actually you don't know that at all. Or if you hear an expert say something you disagree with once? You then decide that whenever you see something written by that expert you will hate it – without ever reading the article, as they'll surely be wrong.

Part of this is something called *intellectual scaffolding*. You take what you think you know and build a structure for guessing about something you don't. This seems particularly true when it comes to human behaviour and ways of doing things. It is less likely for practical tasks: people won't offer to secure their own parachute before jumping out of a plane, for example. But they do like to tell people how they think they should be acting based on vaguely related personal experiences.

Then comes another issue, known as the *double burden of incompetence* – in other words, a lack of knowledge and a lack of knowledge that you lack the knowledge. If you're asked whether your results on a test are right, you need to know the correct answer to be able to confidently state that your answer is correct. And it turns out these things are strongly linked. If your knowledge is poor, your knowledge of your knowledge being poor is also more likely to be poor.

Everyone thinks they know more than they do. In one

experiment students were asked to rank their performance in relation to others from 0 (weakest) to 100 (strongest). Most ranked themselves at around 70 – well above average. Notably, those who actually did the worst in the test had the biggest reality gap, perceiving themselves as able to do far better. Many of the poorest students in the bottom 12% viewed themselves as at least above average.[57]

Even if you offer to give participants money if they are accurate in their self-ratings, to bribe them not to bluff, it makes little difference. In one study one group of participants was told that if they guessed their score on a test within 5% accuracy they would get $30 and if they were exactly right they would get $100. The other group was not promised any reward. There was no difference in accuracy between the groups – the weakest carried on overestimating the most.[58]

Those who have the least knowledge also don't realise that others have more knowledge than them. Generally, if you show a group of people evidence that others know more than them, such as higher test scores, they realise that they can't still be at the top if their score is lower. However, for those who got the lowest scores this doesn't work – they still believe somehow that they know more than most others despite the evidence in front of them. This is played out day after day on the internet. People will argue with experts who have read hundreds or thousands of research papers over many years on a topic, based on the few paper abstracts they have read that morning.

People also believe they are more accurate if they reach their answer more quickly. Speed is actually linked to accuracy. But what if the speed is false? Going back to the fact that most people on the internet speed-read a document, they may end up with false conviction that they are correct.[59] Again, people who read facts quickly on a website, or who just read the abstract of a paper rather than considering the whole thing, may be affected by this.

Judgements of knowledge and accuracy are also linked to

how much you believe you have expertise in an area. Which makes sense. If you are a history buff, you'll be more confident that you've got history questions right than if you skipped those classes. But put this in the context of parenting and you see how people can become confident in their judgements, even though really they know very little. They have given birth and raised a child, thus they are an expert. We seem to hold very strong beliefs that our own experience of something makes us an expert about other babies. One of the most common criticisms I receive from *Daily Mail* readers is 'has this professor ever been near a baby... I've raised five children and...' Furthermore, most people still overestimate their ability on subjects they have knowledge on. Did your history dissertation on Peru? Well of course you must know loads about Maori history, right? Despite never studying it...

All this links back to who people assume are experts. If someone is an expert on health, then they must be an expert on all sorts of health. I've lost track of the number of times someone has argued with me, as against respectfully debated, on Twitter about whether evidence I have presented on a topic is correct (once actually arguing with me about the content of a paper I wrote), and they then tag in another researcher to prove me wrong. Often (but not always) they tag someone with very tenuous links to the subject. Thankfully, the majority of academics are well able to say 'errr not my area of expertise', recognising that although they know a lot in their own field, they know very little about others, even if they are closely related.

Gender bias also plays a role. There is a huge body of evidence suggesting men are far more confident in their abilities than women and will judge their own performance to be far better than it is. This is particularly true when it comes to science. After all, little boys grow up being told they can be scientists and engineers – their toys and clothing say so. Women are given the subtle and not so subtle messages that they know nothing about science and this seems to carry through. In one test of knowledge of scientific concepts, women judged themselves to be far less accurate than men, despite no difference in scores. When participants were then invited to sign up for a science competition if they felt they'd done well (before receiving their scores), just 49% of women signed up compared to 71% of men.[60]

Again, this means that men are more vocal on social media about their expertise. They have had a lifetime of being told they are clever and good at science. Women are more likely to be cautious in shouting about their achievements. Unfortunately, this reinforces the misperception that men are more competent than women. And again, following this through to beliefs about research, that research conducted by men is more accurate, meaning that pregnancy, birth and baby research is particularly open to criticism.

HOW TO KEEP INFORMED:

Try to take into account a range of sources when making a decision.

Learn to spot the Dunning-Kruger effect. Beware advice from an overconfident individual who argues with experts because they once napped through a lecture on the subject 20 years ago. Enjoy spotting them among colleagues and distant acquaintances.

Read more about unconscious bias and how we fall foul of it. You can help fight it by championing female academics, especially women of colour, whenever you can.

To any female expert reading this, I urge you to have the confidence of a mediocre White man.

Oh, and you know the drill – yoga or something for the rage.

6

RESEARCH FUNDING, FINANCIAL GAINS AND CONFLICT OF INTEREST

By the time you read a science story in the news a lot has happened. Someone had to want the research to happen, secure the research funding, and most likely have some sort of connection to get the results into the news story you are reading. But how does research get funded? Who funds it? And why does it matter?

The need for research funding

High quality research can cost a lot of money. Before you even begin collecting data there are costs such as offices and heating, staff time and employing research staff. How much the actual research costs is very discipline specific. Research in the social sciences tends to cost a lot less than research in the medical sciences or engineering. Typically, the more rigorous or 'scientific' the research is, the more it costs to do it. It costs less money to construct a questionnaire and distribute it on social media than it does to conduct an intervention or a randomised controlled trial. If you need specific equipment to collect or analyse data, then it gets even more expensive.

Funding matters because without it, research will not be

completed. Why does that matter? Well first of all, knowledge and advancement should be at the heart of a forward-facing society. But mainly because without evidence, policy and practice, and investment into health and wellbeing, doesn't happen in the same way. Too often women are told 'but there's no evidence to support that' – when there is a lack of evidence rather than research that suggests whatever it is doesn't work or is dangerous (and remember a lack of evidence is not evidence that something does not work). Meanwhile money is ploughed into research that can make someone a profit.

Academics are typically under a lot of pressure to get funding for their research. If they have a permanent academic job they will often have a target set for how much research funding they have to bring in which, depending on their level, country and institution can vary hugely from not very much to hundreds of thousands of pounds each year. There have been numerous tragic cases in which academics have been sacked for not bringing in enough money, and the pressure to find funding has been implicated in suicide cases. Other experienced researchers will not have permanent contracts – they have to bring in research money to cover their own salaries. Most early career researchers have to spend a lot of time moving from research job to research job before they can get their first permanent post.

So you have hundreds of thousands of academics around the world competing for funding (and thinking back to the previous chapter, with men and their White rich men benefitting research projects more likely to get it). But where do they get it from?

Independent research funding

Many countries have independent research funding bodies that academic researchers can apply to for money. This money is (usually) not directly linked to industry (although sometimes it contributes but does not control the research).

In the UK these include UK Research and Innovation (UKRI) which brings together other specific research councils. There are also a number of other funding organisations such as the National Institute of Health Research and charitable trusts such as the Wellcome Trust.[1]

Generally this type of research funding is felt to be the most independent, as although the funding bodies have a say in who gets the money, it is mainly based on the quality of the research design and question rather than having any direction over what is studied, although as with anything politics will always be involved on some level. Sometimes the funders set priority areas or questions, but often there are open calls where you can propose all sorts of things. The downside of all of this is that the process often takes a long time (perhaps a year from application to hearing an outcome) and is extremely competitive. Estimates suggest that only around 5% of grant applications are funded and the competition is getting tougher and tougher.[2]

So researchers are left in a difficult situation. Where do they get money to fund their research? If they don't get funding then often the research can't go ahead, but that might also mean the end of their job and with it their research programme and passion. So often they turn to funding from sources such as industry.

Industry-funded research

Many researchers are funded by non-independent research funders including money directly from industry. There are a number of issues with this. It's not the case that all industry-funded research is bad – after all, industry finds the solution to many things. But it does become more complicated when you are conducting research into health.

1. Research that supports the biologically 'normal' is less likely to be funded

The problem with a reliance on industry funding is that

of course industry is unlikely to want to spend millions of pounds on research unless it benefits them in some way. Companies may have charitable donations to give, to benefit the community (or for other more cynical financial reasons), but typically they want to invest in research that improves their products or image. This is somewhat easier, although not wholly without issues, in areas such as engineering and the sciences. If you're a researcher who researches solar power, or car engines, or advanced medical devices, then your research is valuable to the company as it helps them make more money.

But who would fund research into stopping smoking? Or the benefits of walking? There's little money to be made there. And this is particularly true when it comes to birth and babies. Normal birth does not benefit industry. Nor does breastfeeding. Or baby-wearing. Yes, overall if we better understood how to enable natural options we might save money in NHS costs. But you might have noticed that the NHS doesn't have money spare to fund research.

This means that the money lies where profit can be made. Unfortunately, we know that profit and what is statistically best for health often don't go hand in hand. At the very least it means the research playing field will never be level. It means that there is much more research funding available to understand formula milk than there will ever be to understand physiological impediments to breastfeeding. It's why we have so much more money ploughed into erectile dysfunction research than we do breastfeeding 'dysfunction' – as there is a product available to solve the erectile dysfunction and therefore money to be made.

A great example is the recent drug that has been released in the US for women experiencing postnatal depression. It involves women receiving a transfusion of the drug over 48–60 hours, during which time they must stay at a medical centre. It claims in its trials to help reduce the symptoms and much more quickly than traditional antidepressant tablets.

But it costs approximately \$38,000. Suddenly there is money available as there is a profit to be made.[3]

Likewise, reducing caesarean sections is not in the interest of hospitals in the US because each procedure that happens during childbirth can be listed and added up in order to charge the woman's health insurance. Money is made from each birth, and the more complicated the birth, the more money is made. This leaves women being charged down to the very last thing. For example, one hospital (a photo of the bill was posted on social media) charges mothers to have skin-to-skin contact with their baby after birth. The argument to support the charge is that a healthcare professional has to observe the mother and baby during skin-to-skin.[4]

2. The goals of industry can be in opposition to public health

Often, industry is in direct opposition to public health. Although we do need to make sure that when formula milk or a caesarean section are needed that they are of the highest quality possible (which will be enhanced by research), when the industry that owns a product would benefit from research that finds it to be needed, then we have a problem.

Product sales and investment means that in areas where the companies are in direct opposition to public health there is often more money available, for example to pay researchers, speakers and authors. Again, this affects the messages that are promoted – and the amount of conversation. Money means that the best research can be conducted and funds made available to publish in the best journals, and then that research can be taken to the best conferences, where more people attend because places are free (and the day is well catered).

Topics like promoting lower intervention in childbirth… well where's the device for that? Breastfeeding? Where's the money to be made over and above some nursing bras and breast pumps (and some would argue that more women are expressing milk in the UK because of marketing by breast pump manufacturers). Co-sleeping? Well where's the fancy cot?

3. The funders often own the findings – and publish selectively

There is also a risk that an industry funding research will manipulate the findings, either by deciding not to release the research if it does not enhance their product's reputation, or by only releasing certain parts in certain ways. There is also less likely to be an independent body overseeing the research process (as would happen with funding from an independent research council) which could mean the research is less rigorous or even manipulated. We therefore might never get the full picture.

So industry-funded research *might* not be trustworthy. I say might. Of course research can be conducted well by an organisation that may benefit from it. But it does make it a little shady, which is why it's really important that we know who is funding research so we can judge, or at least be a little more alert, about the findings.

Of particular concern is the association between research published that was funded by industry and the direction of the finding. Research that supports the product is far more likely to be published than research that does not. The queen of exposing the relationship between industry and evidence is Professor Marion Nestle (unfortunate name share with the company: she has absolutely nothing to do with them). Back in 2015 she began keeping a log of research published by food and beverage companies into the impact or benefits of their food or related food groups. In 2015 she tracked 168 studies. Out of all those studies, 156 had findings that benefitted the sponsor. Now, did all the studies just happen to have positive outcomes? Or might it be the case that fewer negative studies were actually published?[5]

Another interesting evaluation of published studies related

to health outcomes of drinks showed that when industry funded the study, the outcome of that study was between four and eight times more likely to be favourable. To do this the researchers identified all research articles published from 1999–2003 that looked at soft drink, juice or milk consumption and health outcomes. They coded the findings into either favourable, neutral, or unfavourable for health. They then coded who funded the study – industry, no industry or mixed. They found 206 articles in all, but only 54% actually declared who funded them. Articles that were sponsored by industry were more likely to have favourable outcomes for the product.[6]

Conversely, when research is being conducted into the potential *adverse* effects of a product on health, then those funded by industry conclude that it is less of an issue than papers written independently.[7]

4. Bias can affect health guidelines

We know that selective publishing, money and influence can affect what information we see and how it is used. Increasingly, research that has industry money (and therefore a product and profit) behind it is popping up in health guidelines.

A current example of potential bias is the involvement of the formula industry in the ever-increasing specialist cows' milk protein allergy market. These specialist formulas are expensive and available only on prescription. For babies with a genuine cows' milk protein allergy they are life-saving and necessary. However, the rise in diagnoses and prescriptions for these products suggests that something is up. From 2006– 2016 the number of prescriptions for specialist formula more than quadrupled,[8] with NHS spending on the products rising from £8.1 million to over £60 million annually.[9] Although there are a number of reasons why an increase could be seen, such a rise, in such a short space of time, is out of step with epidemiological data.[9,10]

In an eye-opening piece in the *BMJ*,[11] Dr Chris van Tulleken did some digging into the many connections between the guidelines for prescribing for cows' milk protein allergy (CMPA) and the industry that produces the product. First of all he found that there were multiple guidelines available – more than for any other food allergy. Second, all of the guidelines had authors who had ties with the formula industry. In fact for two of the guidelines – the Milk Allergy in Primary Care (MAP) guidelines and the iMAP guidelines – *all* authors had connections with the formula industry. Alongside this, much of the education available about CMPA, particularly for health professionals, has ties to industry. Typically it's not the formula companies themselves promoting the products, but often organisations that look at first glance to be independent but actually receive funding from the companies.

Related to this is the funding of research by companies that ends up in guidelines, but looks a little strange. For example Coca-Cola has previously funded considerable research into... the benefits of exercise. A request for information revealed that the company had donated $1.5 million to start the 'Energy Balance Network'. It then went on to donate nearly $4 million to academic research conducted by the network, primarily for academics whose research contributed to federal guidelines on physical activity.[12]

Why would Coca-Cola fund research into the benefits of exercise? There are many reasons. One is that it could suggest that they are 'doing good' with their profits – good PR. More cynically, by focusing publicly on *exercise* and health, attention is distracted from *diet* and health. Or *sugar* and health. Or *sweeteners* and health. Suddenly we see why Coca-Cola might be interested in focusing on health guidelines that promote exercise rather than healthy diets.

There are all sorts of dodgy dealings going on in food research. You've probably noticed that in the last few years there has been an emphasis on the detrimental impact too much sugar can have on your weight and health, including illnesses that we have spent years hearing were caused by eating too much fat, such as coronary heart disease. Is sugar suddenly our worst enemy? What about fat? Do these scientists even know what they're doing?

All is not quite as it seems, however, and if you dig back through history, you'll find a rather alarming story uncovered by three academics.[13] It turns out research started to emerge in the 1950s that a diet high in sugar (sucrose) increased the risk of coronary heart disease. However, the Sugar Association (yes it's really called that) did its best to promote a link between heart disease and fat instead, as it saw an opportunity to increase its profits if everyone started eating low fat, as they'd turn to sugar instead. This is the short version – but the authors of the paper uncovered a series of communications between the Sugar Association and academics at Harvard and Illinois universities which revealed significant investment in publishing research that highlighted the links between fat and heart disease, turning everyone's attention in that direction.

In fact, a review paper was published on the causes of heart disease that deliberately downplayed the role of sugar. No disclosure was made that it was funded by the sugar industry. Records show that the industry 'encouraged' the authors to make sure the findings reflected this.

Are researchers affected by their funding?

Most researchers will argue that the source of their funding does not affect the outcome of their research. This may be true for some researchers, but there is a clear pattern between research findings and who they are funded by. A Cochrane review found that research funded by industry is more likely to report findings that support the work of the sponsor than research that is conducted independently.[14]

There are a number of explanations for this, from the Machiavellian to the subconscious. Researchers are working in a competitive climate, reliant on research funding for jobs. They may worry that if they don't publish in a way that supports the funder then they will not receive further funding or their paper won't be published as the funder will block it. They may also feel that they 'owe it' to the funder to support them.

Other academics and the public at large are aware of this. We trust scientists working in public institutions more than those in private institutions. One study asked the public in the US whether they trusted someone when it came to talking about the safety of a drug. Who they trusted depended on who funded the research into it – 59% stated that they trusted the professor if they were government funded, compared to just 41% if they were drug company funded... falling to a low of just 24% if they also had shares in the company.[15]

Should researchers who have links to industry be trusted?

A common debate, particularly in the world of researching feeding babies, is whether a researcher who has ever worked for one of the baby or formula food manufacturers is inherently biased for ever more.

Here's a common scenario: Company X makes formula milk. This isn't a bad thing in itself. After all, babies who cannot receive breastmilk for whatever reason need formula milk to grow and develop, because straight up cows' milk isn't good for them. The issue is with the way in which the company promotes its products in unscrupulous ways, or stretches the truth about added ingredients. And perhaps this company has some other nasty tricks up its sleeve in other areas of its business, such as limiting people's access to clean water.

The trouble is that this company, with its big team of marketers and billions of dollars in profits, is a big machine. It can put on big study days and seminars, fly in the best people, and generally act as though it is very knowledgeable about infant feeding. The people who attend its events can be very influential – both in industry and in healthcare or having influence over new families.

The company invites a researcher to speak at their event about how breastmilk helps protect infant health in some way. The researcher is well known for doing research into this topic. Should they go and present?

1. Some people argue that they shouldn't. They should stay away from the funder altogether and even if they go and talk about the protective properties of breastmilk they are actually promoting the products of that company by association. Some go even further and say that from now on that researcher should not be trusted as they have a bias towards the company and anything they publish might be affected by their loyalty to it.

2. Others say that a researcher should be independent. They shouldn't have a 'side' or a preference and should speak anywhere if requested, simply presenting the facts. This is quite difficult for anyone who spends a long time working in one topic area. The more you research something and understand it, depending on what the evidence says you are of course going to naturally come to some sort of professional judgement about the topic.

3. Another view is that the researcher should attend and speak (but perhaps not take any fee offered), precisely because their information should be heard by a brand-new audience. If researchers who study breastfeeding only ever talk to people who are 100% supportive of breastfeeding, they run the risk of 'preaching to the converted'. So they should go and speak as it will give them access to a whole group whose minds and knowledge might actually be changed.

4. Some believe there is no harm at all and everyone enjoys a free meal. I would suggest that these people are probably a little naïve. Industry always has a reason for doing

things, and it's never to deliberately promote something in opposition to their product.

There isn't a clear answer to this conundrum, and among public health researchers there is a range of opinion and practice.

Beware partnerships between industry and health organisations

Alongside funding research partnerships, industry makes connections with numerous organisations in order to benefit from promoting their products through this relationship. There are numerous cases of industry working alongside those who set guidelines in the very area the industry causes problems in. Some of the more eye-opening partnerships include:[16]

- Diabetes UK and Britvic (fizzy drinks)
- Academy of Nutrition and Dietetics (formerly known as the American Dietetic Association) – sponsorship over the years from Coca-Cola, Kraft foods, Nestlé, PepsiCo, McDonalds, Mars, Danone and Abbott
- British Nutrition Foundation – corporate members include Nestlé, Danone, Heinz and Ella's Kitchen
- British Dietetic Association – corporate members include Danone, Abbott and Nestlé
- Allergy UK – corporate partners include Abbott, Aptamil, Nutricia and Mead Johnson
- Eat Like A Champ (partners with Change4Life) – sponsored by Danone
- Pre-school Learning Alliance – works in partnership with Danone
- British Specialist Nutrition Association – funded by Abbott, Danone, Mead Johnson, Nestlé
- Early Life Nutrition – this is the Danone Nutricia website
- Infant and Toddler Forum – funded by Nutricia (Danone)

You can read a full report about websites and organisations

that are funded by the formula industry on the First Steps Nutrition website.[17]

Why do organisations take sponsorship and work in partnership with food and drink companies? Well, organisations benefit from the money and other opportunities these partnerships bring. For the companies it is essentially an advertising and image-boosting opportunity. Being able to partner with trusted organisations suggests that they are trustworthy, reputable and have the same ethos as the organisation. It also allows them to boost sales of their product through association. Industry representatives meet lots of people that might be useful to them – policy-makers, health professionals and potential consumers.

Many charities work with vulnerable groups in deprived areas – groups that we know are often more swayed by marketing and the food products advertised. Companies are extremely good at forming partnerships as they typically have a lot of well-paid people within their organisation working on it – departments for external affairs, PR support, company reps and a lot of money invested.

In particular, formula milk companies use partnerships because they give them an opportunity to promote their products in ways that circumnavigate advertising restrictions. The WHO Code of Marketing of Breastmilk Substitutes[18] sets out a series of rules around promotion of formula milk products. This is to protect consumers from the underhand tactics the formula milk industry have displayed over the years. The Code is not a statement against formula milk – it says that parents should not be influenced or manipulated by those who stand to make a considerable profit from their choices. Parents deserve information free from industry involvement. Education and information should be independent and in the best interests of the parents and their baby, not a company.

In short, the WHO Code states that infant formula milks aimed at babies under one year old should not be promoted.

The UK government has partially adopted this in law: in the UK milks for babies under the age of six months cannot be promoted. Industry has tried to get round this by creating 'follow-on' products aimed at babies over six months old and then heavily advertising them, as they know that lots of people can't tell the difference[19] and that brand advertising works to sell products across a range.[20] The industry often sponsors events, particularly aimed at families or healthcare providers. All the cost of this advertising – approximately $9 billion per year[21] – gets passed on to parents. For more on these issues I highly recommend that you read Gabrielle Palmer's book *The Politics of Breastfeeding – When Breasts are Bad for Business*.[22]

Many organisations are becoming more aware of the tricks that formula milk companies play. Recently both the *BMJ*[23] and the Royal College of Paediatrics and Child Health (RCPCH)[24] have formally stopped accepting formula milk advertising in their publications. More and more pressure is on companies to find people who will allow them to sponsor their events.

Unfortunately, in a climate of austerity, organisations are more and more vulnerable to needing to partner with industry. One particular example is the long-standing relationship the children's charity Barnardo's has with Danone Nutricia (which makes infant formula and other baby foods), which sponsors their 'Big Toddle' event aimed at young families. Last year Barnardo's celebrated 15 years of partnership with Danone, using the opportunity to state how much they loved helping children and families.[25]

A letter was recently sent to Barnardo's, by Malvina Walsh, chair of the Baby Feeding Law Group in Ireland, co-signed by academics and healthcare experts, to highlight how allowing an infant formula company to sponsor such family events was essentially a loophole allowing advertising and promotion of the company's products.

CEO of Barnardo's Suzanne Connolly responded, saying that the charity needed to fundraise and as part of that sought corporate sponsorships, with all funds raised by the public going directly to support its services to help vulnerable children.[26] She wrote:

> We carry out an ethical evaluation with all corporate supporters to ascertain whether a relationship is appropriate or not. Barnardo's has partnered with Danone on the Big Toddle for 16 years... This partnership, and the children and crèches who take part, have allowed us to raise €3.9m which has helped thousands of vulnerable children across the country. The partnership agreement we have in place with Danone is not an endorsement of any product under the Danone group and there is no reference to infant formula or breastfeeding in any of the materials developed for the Toddle... Danone have assured us of their compliance with the WHO guidelines.

You can see the predicament Barnardo's is in. They need funding for the event, and Danone has the funding to give them. But suggesting that Danone's products are not promoted by the partnership is naïve. Why on earth would Danone choose to sponsor events if it didn't think it would benefit the company? If they did simply want to be benevolent and support the charity they could do it anonymously.

You'll notice in Suzanne Connolly's statement a point about Danone following the WHO Code. In reality, Danone is far from compliant with the WHO code. It is a global dairy company, which made $6.9 billion from baby food products in 2016. In the UK it owns the formula milk brands Cow and Gate and Aptamil (which incidentally are almost identical, but several pounds different in price, being aimed at different types of families). The Big Toddle is not Danone's only corporate sponsorship – it sponsors many events, including study days for health professionals and the Tommy's Baby Race.[27]

There are countless examples of Danone breaking the provisions of the WHO Code, including aggressively marketing its products in 'new markets' – regions with high breastfeeding rates (and often a lot of poverty) that don't benefit from its products. In the UK the company is not supposed to target new parents but it does so, offering cuddly toys, a branded parenting club sending out emails to pregnant women that promotes a formula feeding kit, and offering nurseries money to distribute branded booklets to parents and put up posters. This is alongside idealistic messaging in its promotion of follow-on milk. For example, a shield forms part of the Aptamil logo, suggesting the milk protects babies against something, and product adverts suggest that children will develop into strong ballerinas or maths geniuses (gender specific, obviously) if they consume Aptamil.[28]

Beware expert panels

Another trick companies play is to form close alliances with academics and researchers who are invited to sit on expert panels. Again, we cannot say that a company will directly influence what is said, but we do know that the academics involved don't see any issue with accepting industry funding, and therefore may (or may not) be biased towards the industry.[29] As I am writing this the United States Department for Agriculture is putting together its first ever dietary guidelines for infants aged 0–24 months. Four of the panel of six working on the guidelines have received funding from the formula industry, including Mead Johnson, Nestlé and Abbott. Based on the discussion above, do you think the interests of those companies will end up influencing the guidelines? Again, it is not the products that are the issue, but the aggressive marketing of them by these companies that exist to make money from parents. All that marketing and advertising costs money, which is passed on to parents through the price they pay for their formula. Remove the unnecessary advertising, and formula milk could be much cheaper.[30]

The importance of funding statements and transparency

Given that there appears to be a bias in publication (and direction of findings) when a study is funded by industry, it is important for us to *know* whether it is, and whether the researchers involved have ties with industry. Again, this is not to say every researcher who receives industry funding is corrupt, or that every research study funded by industry is flawed, but given the overall pattern, it is important for us to have clear information.[31]

It is good practice – if not essential now for publication – to declare whether you received any funding for your study. This information can be hidden though, and is sometimes carefully placed at the end, as readers may not finish the whole piece. Also, by the time you get to the funding statement you've already read the piece and have it in your memory, whether you are then sceptical about it or not. Other journals place funding statements more prominently, or even encourage authors to put it in the abstract of the paper (as some people will only read the abstract).

It is also good practice for any trial that is going to be conducted to register its methods before it begins. If publication of the final results never happens, or is 'delayed' there is at least some evidence that the trial was planned.

However, there is a major issue with researchers failing to disclose conflicts of interest. A recent article published in the *New York Times* (written in collaboration with ProPublica, a non-profit journalism organisation) highlighted the extent to which some researchers twist or fail to acknowledge their links with industry.[32] It gives the example of Dr Howard A. Burris III, the president-elect of the American Society of Clinical Oncology, whose research focuses on developing new cancer treatments. Dr Burris has published over 50 journal articles over the last few years, in which he declared no conflict of interest. However, he actually received over $8 million in research funding during this time, along with nearly $114,000 from drug companies for consulting and speaking. We all want cancer treatments to be improved, and research needs money, but the failure to disclose funding raises serious questions.

Another example is Dr Robert J. Alpern, dean of the Yale School of Medicine, who published a clinical trial for an experimental treatment.[33] Dr Alpern did not disclose that he was on the board of directors of the company that produced the treatment and owned stock, therefore standing to profit personally if the trial showed the drug to be beneficial. The trial did indeed show positive results, and may be accurate, but the failure to properly disclose conflicts of interest is of concern.

According to the *New York Times*, Dr Alpern stated that he was initially told that his disclosure was sufficient and he didn't need to give further details. However, after the *New York Times* and ProPublica contacted the journal to query this, changes were made to the paper. Now, if you look it up, the disclosure is mentioned – but at the end of the paper.

D.A.B., T.H., and R.A. are consultants for Tricida Inc. (South San Francisco, CA). D.P., V.M., and E.L. are regulatory, clinical, and biostatistics contractors and consultants, respectively, for Tricida Inc. G.K., Y.S., C.L., S.M., A.L., and J.B. are employees of Tricida Inc.

Finally the article gives a further example, of research centre director Dr Carlos L. Arteaga, who did not disclose any relationship with the drug company Novartis when publishing a study about the benefits of a breast cancer drug made by Novartis.[34] He had in fact received $14,000 from Novartis. When questioned, he apparently stated it was an 'oversight' and submitted a correction. After all, don't we all forget sometimes that someone has given us $14,000?

Research into conflict of interest declarations shows a similar pattern. A study published in 2018 looked at the top 10 medical device-makers and the top 10 doctors who received funding from each of these companies. They looked at articles relevant to the funding written by 100 doctors who received compensation from device-makers in 2015, and found that only 37% of those articles disclosed the payments. And the payments weren't small. The median payment was $95,993! The results revealed another bias: 88% of the funded doctors were men.[35]

The waters are even murkier when it comes to research into public health. Trying to sell your medical device is one thing, but when you're trying to promote a product that isn't in the best interests of health, hiding your funding and connections is arguably worse. This is particularly true when it comes to the health of mothers and babies.

It is worryingly common for researchers working in infant feeding not to declare their interests relating to formula companies. For example, in a paper outlining the recommendations of an International Expert Group around follow-up formula for infants[36] (the group generally declared it a positive thing despite the World Health Organization declaring them unecessary and inappropriate), the conflict of interest statement clearly states:

> None of the authors reports a conflict of interest which would represent 'a set of circumstances that creates a risk that professional judgment or actions regarding a primary interest will be unduly influenced by a secondary interest', as defined by the US Institute of Medicine.

But there in black and white, right next to those words, is the following (the initials represent author names):

- *Z.A.B. has received support as a member of the Nestlé Nutrition Institute advisory board advising on nutrition priorities and educational activities.*
- *W.C. has received support from Danone, Mead Johnson Nutritionals, and Nestlé Nutrition.*
- *S.C. received support from Biocodex, Danone, Nestlé Nutrition, and Pfizer Nutrition.*

- *M.E.G. acknowledges support from Abbott Nutrition, Danone, Mead Johnson Nutrition, Nestlé Nutrition, and Pfizer Nutrition.*
- *G.J.F. received an author's honorarium from Nestlé Nutrition.*
- *E.A.G. received support from Nestlé Nutrition. The University of Amsterdam and the Free University, Amsterdam, and its employee*
- *J.B.v.G. have or have had scientific and educational collaborations with Abbott Nutrition, Danone, Hipp, Mead Johnson Nutrition, and Nestlé Nutrition.*
- *S.H.Q. received support from Danone. The University of Munich Medical Centre and its employee*
- *B.Ko. have or have had scientific and educational collaborations with manufacturers of FUF, primarily as part of research collaborations funded by the European Commission and the German government, from Abbott Nutrition, Dairy Goat Cooperative, Danone, Fonterra, Hipp, Mead Johnson Nutrition, Nestlé Nutrition, and Pfizer Nutrition, and receive grant support from the European Commission, the European Research Council, and the German Federal Government.*
- *B.Ku. declares no potential conflict of interest.*
- *M.M. and the Women's and Children's Health Research Institute and the University of Adelaide have received support from the National Health and Medical Research Council (NHMRC), Clover Corporation, Dairy Goat Cooperative, Danone, Fonterra, Nestlé Nutrition, and Mead Johnson Nutrition.*
- *A.W. has received financial support from Danone, Mead Johnson Nutrition, and Nestlé Nutrition.*

I considered summarising the above in a sentence, but I am shocked at the sheer number of financial associations with formula companies who produce follow-on formula, in an article declaring whether it has any benefits or not – and with a clear statement saying they have no conflicts of interest!

This is not an isolated paper. In 2018 an article was published in the *Annals of Nutrition and Metabolism*.[37] The article declared that it had 'no conflicts of interest or financial ties to disclose', but later in the article there was a statement revealing that the article was supported by funding from the Nestlé Nutrition Institute.

A group of researchers led by Marita Hennessy, including me, wrote to the editor of the *Annals of Nutrition and Metabolism* to point out that this wasn't exactly open and honest reporting, and to talk more broadly about the issue of disclosure of conflict of interest in public health. The editor rejected our letter. We instead published our letter in rapid open format in the *Irish Health Board Journal for Open Research*, reporting the issue we had with our initial letter.[38]

Generally, journal editors are taking action. They are insisting on more open conflict of interest and funding statements. However, as the *New York Times* article notes, many of those who have been identified as hiding or omitting conflict of interest statements are themselves journal editors, and have published in their own journal.[39]

Journalist Rebecca Gale recently wrote an exposure piece for Women's eNews,[40] focusing on the work of Dr Ronald Kleinman, a leading expert on children's nutritional guidelines and a physician at Harvard, who has held many influential positions, such as chairman of the Committee on Nutrition for the American Academy of Pediatrics. Dr Kleinman has numerous financial connections with the formula industry, particularly in terms of honorariums and funding received from Mead Johnson and Nestlé. Unfortunately he failed to declare these as conflicts of interest in his publications on infant feeding. This is a critical omission, because Kleinman is one of the authors of a controversial opinion piece published in *JAMA Journal of Pediatrics* in 2016 which was hugely critical of the Baby Friendly Hospital Initiative.[41]

Researchers complained to the journal and for once it responded, adding in disclosure of an honorarium from Mead (funding from Nestlé and more from Mead fell outside the disclosure period of three years that the journal had). When challenged by Women's eNews and journalist Rebecca Gale,

Kleinman said his failure to disclose was an 'inadvertent omission'.

A final cautionary tale

Occasionally, there are really dubious studies. It doesn't happen often (or at least we hope it doesn't), but sometimes scientists have been found to have completely made up their data and falsified their research. One of the most famous cases in pregnancy and baby research is that of Ranjit Chandra.[42,43]

Dr Chandra was a world-renowned nutrition scientist in Canada. He was approached by Ross Pharmaceuticals in the US, which marketed formula milks such as Similac and Isomil. It wanted to find out whether its formulas could reduce the number of babies developing allergies. The study required 288 mothers to take part with their newborns, from families where the parents already had allergies.

This was always going to be a challenge, as the data was to be collected fairly locally – in a city called St John's. Chandra hired a research nurse called Marilyn Harvey to collect the data. Even working full-time Marilyn reported that she was struggling to find enough families who wanted to take part.

While this was happening, Nestlé, which had launched a new formula called 'Good Start' that it claimed reduced the risk of babies developing an allergy, came under pressure to get some research evidence for the claims. So it approached Chandra, asking him to test their formula too. To test multiple formulas on families prone to allergies would require a large sample.

This is where it gets decidedly dodgy. By the next summer, Marilyn was still struggling to get enough participants to take part. Then she came across the published results of the study she was supposedly recruiting for, listing far more participants than she knew she had recruited – about four times as many.

Ross Pharmaceuticals saw the published study too. Not only did it claim that the Nestlé formula reduced allergies in babies, but it also drew negative comparisons with the Ross formula. This was incredible, because Ross had never provided sample formula for the trial. In a study like this researchers don't buy formula from a supermarket or warehouse – they get clinically labelled samples from a manufacturer. Tens of thousands of them.

Meanwhile, Chandra published another paper. This time it examined whether a Mead Johnson formula reduced allergies. Apparently it did. The study involved another 200 babies. Marilyn was completely unaware of them, and couldn't understand how someone else could be recruiting families far faster than she was, when it was her paid job.

Chandra's results supposedly examined three formulas. Two of which worked to reduce allergies and one which didn't. No one knew where the babies had come from… or the data. And in addition:

- Tests of the formulas showed them to be similar, raising the question of how the difference arose
- No raw data files were available
- None of the co-authors seemed to know much about the studies

In 1994 Chandra was investigated by his university and the findings suggested fraud. However, he threatened to sue and presumably, for fear of bad publicity, the university dropped the investigation. Chandra continued with his 'studies', including research claiming vitamins could vastly improve the memory of older adults that again had huge issues. The university realised this couldn't continue and asked for his data. After trying to claim he couldn't find it Chandra promptly retired.

The problem with retracting papers is that:

a. it takes time
b. you can't amend all the papers and conference presentations that cite the work

Chandra's paper in the *BMJ* on the impact of the formula on eczema has been cited 275 times according to Google

Scholar, despite the *BMJ* retracting it in 2015.[44] His other paper, published in *Annals of Allergy* has 206 citations, and hasn't been retracted.[45] These two key papers were published in 1989 and had time to become embedded in the literature.

HOW TO KEEP INFORMED:

If an article promotes a behaviour or product, always check who has funded the research. If no conflicts of interest are declared, it may be worth a quick search to check.

Research funding is necessary for researchers. They cannot avoid it. But it can influence their work. Be aware of any funding but also be open-minded – bias is not guaranteed, but do read the papers closely.

There are a lot of dubious funding partnerships. Keep your eyes open to who sponsors events and the reputation they are trying to build.

7

HOW DO YOU KNOW WHICH RESEARCH TO TRUST?

We've looked at all the tricks the press and social media can play, and why it is so easy to end up believing 'fake news' or one-sided presentations of research. Hopefully now your eyes have been opened to the challenges in this area. Hopefully you're doing yoga for the underlying rage. The next stage is to think about how you can find, understand and decide whether research is useful for you and your family and the decisions you make.

For some this section may be a refresher, for others it may be a first step in helping you develop research skills. This book won't make you an expert overnight – researchers and academics spend years building their knowledge base. And you probably don't need the in-depth knowledge that experts have in their areas of interest. But a general understanding of research and how it applies to pregnancy, birth, babies and child health is a really useful tool for anyone. With just a bit of knowledge and awareness you'll be able to:

- Look at a news headline and work out if what they are trying to tell you is useful or not.
- Understand the 'bigger picture' of the pattern of research

in different areas and know that one study doesn't change everything.

- Be aware of the different types of research and their different strengths and weaknesses, and consider how they all have something to offer in the 'bigger picture'.
- Confidently ask 'What is the evidence for that?' if you feel a procedure or option is being pushed on you.
- Feel more relaxed, because you know that no one thing we do when it comes to growing, birthing and caring for our babies is likely to definitively change their life course.

In the next few chapters we will look at research techniques and how they can help inform our decisions around birth and babies. We will challenge the idea that there is one 'best type' of research and look at how all disciplines and types of research can help us piece together a bigger picture. Importantly we'll also look at the weaknesses of current research, and at how hard it is to do accurate research when it comes to anything to do with humans.

Before we begin, here are a few things to bear in mind:

1. Research into human behaviour or health outcomes is not and never will be 'perfect'

First the bad news. There has never been, nor will there likely ever be, a perfect research study of human behaviour. That is because, unlike lab-based research where conditions can be controlled, humans… can't be. In the lab, doing experiments with test tubes and microscopes and stuff, you can make sure all factors that might influence an outcome are controlled for. But with humans, living lives and stuff? Not so much. You can try and put them into groups and encourage one group to do one thing and one group another, but it often doesn't work very well. Living human beings tend to have thoughts and preferences and other things going on. There are also ethical limits on what can be done.

Every study has its limitations but it's important to

remember that no one research paper is ever meant to be considered in isolation –it's about looking at a whole group of studies together and what they generally say, despite their different limitations, that is important. Limitations are just part of science with humans. They don't necessarily mean that the conclusions of the paper are wrong, just that, as with any paper, they should be taken with caution. Researchers are expected to identify the limitations of their work themselves. Every paper should have a section called 'limitations' or similar somewhere in the discussion. And everyone reading a paper should try to park their bias at the door, and at least try to consider it with an open mind. This means that if you want to criticise a research study, you always can. And you should. But as Trish Greenhalgh states in her book *How to Read a Paper* – '*it is much easier to pick holes in other people's work than to do a methodologically perfect piece of research oneself*'.[1]

2. Research looks at the increased likelihood of something happening – it does not say that it definitely will

There are lots of guidelines for supporting women through pregnancy and birth and caring for babies. But it's important to remember that they are based on patterns within populations – not individuals. 'Pregnant women' as a group are advised not to smoke, to try to maintain a healthy weight, not to drink alcohol, not to do drugs, to avoid certain medications... the list is endless. But it's perfectly *possible* (but obviously not recommended!) for a person to smoke, down shots every night and get stoned at the weekend... and their baby still be 'fine'. The guidelines are about likelihood, associations, the *risk* of something happening. The stoned, drunk smoker above will be at a much greater risk of something going wrong. But because of chance, risk, luck... some people will always escape negative consequences (and sadly, some people who follow all health guidelines will not).

Health is complicated and affected by multiple factors. For example, you need to be exposed to an infection in order to catch an illness. If you are never exposed to the infection you will not catch the illness, but if you *are* exposed, factors in your lifestyle can determine whether you develop it and how serious it will be. Then you need to add in further layers, such as genetics and socioeconomic status. Health is complex and multifactored – we don't all have the same risk. It's a bit like driving around not wearing a seatbelt and being absolutely fine – you will be until you crash the car. And then suddenly it matters whether you're driving a tank or a Mini.

We don't have a crystal ball, so we can't know how sick you would have been if you had acted differently. Often illnesses are not either/or – for example, if you have eczema you can have different symptoms and different levels of severity. Your experience may have meant that you still develop eczema, but you do not experience it so badly. This means you will always be able to find someone who seems to be the exception to the rule. But individual stories are not what we're interested in when it comes to guidelines – it's about bigger patterns in larger groups.

Guidelines are based on the 'healthiest' options, based on what we know about large groups of people. They tell you where to place your bets. Imagine for a moment that 10% of babies who are born by caesarean section develop a certain health issue, compared to 5% of babies born vaginally. Some headlines might dramatise this and say that babies born by caesarean are at *double the risk* of the problem. However, the majority of babies will still be fine. 90% of c-section babies would not have that the issue.

This is where the difference between public and individual health is important. In the above scenario, a baby born by caesarean still has a 90% chance of not being affected, but imagine that you are in charge of health promotion for a country where there are hundreds of thousands of babies being born every year. In the UK we have around 700,000 births a year. If a quarter of babies are born by caesarean section, and 10% of them have a health complication, that's 17,500 babies. If you can reduce the caesarean rate to 15% instead of 25%, 10,500 babies will be born with health complications – that's 7,000 fewer. It's in this sort of scenario that guidelines are issued to encourage vaginal birth.

What this means is that it's perfectly possible for someone to not follow a guideline and their baby to be fine. For example, perhaps they put their baby to sleep in a different room from day one, ignoring safe sleep guidelines. Thankfully their baby was okay. Great, we like babies being okay. But this doesn't mean that for the next baby they will definitely be okay. Public health guidelines are there to help you think about the future. The statistics show that keeping your baby in the same room as you offers your baby the best possible chance of being okay. So it's important to share those guidelines with parents thinking about making the decision as they cannot know what the future will bring. But it's not the same as suggesting that putting a baby in another room WILL cause harm or did cause harm for all babies. It's about weighing up the risks and making the best possible decision. Your lived experience and their potential future experience are not the same things.

3. Just because a study doesn't find a difference, doesn't mean there isn't one

Given that every study has limitations, just because a study doesn't find a difference in outcomes for two groups, doesn't mean there isn't one. Studies can be published without somebody spotting a weakness in their design. Study designs can mean that sometimes the wrong things are measured. This may not be immediately apparent to reviewers of papers and journal editors if they don't have specific knowledge and understanding of an area. And again, remember it should always be about a body of research papers, not the findings from any individual paper.

For example, although randomised controlled trials are often seen as the gold standard, when it comes to human behaviour they often have serious weaknesses. This is mainly because it's difficult to randomise people to act in a certain way, particularly when it's something complex that has to be repeated over time. It's much easier to tell people to take pill A rather than pill B than it is to tell them to feed their baby a specific way. People often end up feeding their baby in a completely different way from the group they were randomised to.

Also, sometimes the right outcomes aren't measured. At one point it was common for infant feeding research to only measure how babies were fed at birth and then look at long-term outcomes. Differences weren't often found, which is unsurprising given the many variations of things that could happen between the two groups over time.

Most importantly, often there is simply no research on a topic that matters to women's health. As we have seen, sometimes no one gets funding and the work isn't done. A gap in research doesn't mean there isn't something worth researching. A lack of evidence isn't the same as evidence that shows that something doesn't work or shouldn't be supported. And when we are looking at normal human bodily functions, such as pregnancy, birth and breastfeeding, the onus should be on any intervention to prove it is 'superior' (whatever that means) rather than trying to justify the biological function.

4. Developing an evidence base takes a lot of time – and is about patterns, not any one study

As noted a few times previously already (I can never stress this too much), no one study should be taken in isolation. All research has limitations, and all researchers will have collected data in slightly different ways, and on top of that people are so variable, meaning findings can vary slightly from paper to paper. What is more important is the bigger picture of what lots of different studies on a particular topic say. You need a wide overview of the area and understanding of how they all fit together. It's easy to just look up what you want to find and identify one study to support it. This is known as 'cherry picking' – choosing what you want and ignoring the rest.

This is where researchers with years of expertise in a specific area really show their worth. It is almost impossible, as an outsider to a subject area to read all the research on any one area. It would take you many years of intense study. After fifteen years researching infant feeding I, like all researchers, still haven't come close to reading *all* the papers written on the topic, despite reading thousands of the things. But what experts do have is a pretty good overview and knowledge of what is going on.

So, approach any study you do read with an open mind. Read it, digest it, explore its limitations. But never claim that one paper changes everything. It might indeed raise new questions, but is never going to be that one paper in isolation that leads to whole new policies being created or thrown in the bin. And once you've read it, ask others about it. They may well be able to place it within a wider context of other research for you.

5. Knowing why two things are associated is important

The first stage in research into a topic is to find an association between two things. We then need to know whether there is a plausible explanation – or *mechanism* – by which those things are linked. There will be more on this later, but in general correlations (e.g. a link between two things) are easy to find. However, *correlation doesn't equal causation*, as the saying goes, so your two things may not actually be linked. Just because two things are linked to one another, i.e. as one thing increases another thing increases too, doesn't mean that they have anything to do with each other.

If two things are connected, we need to understand the 'pathways' between those two things. How might they be connected and why? If drinking lots of alcohol during pregnancy is linked to lower IQ in children, *how* does this happen? Often there isn't one single explanation – lots of things will play a role. For example, in the case of alcohol and IQ there might be a direct physiological impact on brain development, but wider factors such as maternal stress, deprivation and support will likely be factors too. These can affect both the tendency to binge drink and the later environment in which the child's IQ develops.

HOW TO KEEP INFORMED:

Keep an open mind and try to leave your confirmation bias tendencies behind.

Humans are complicated creatures – lots of things will affect health outcomes including genetics, socioeconomic status and luck.

All research designs have different strengths and weaknesses. Look at the bigger picture and how they fit together.

Remember, anecdotes are not data. Research is based on large populations not individuals and just because your experience is different, it does not mean the overall principle is not true.

8

RESEARCH METHODS 101

This chapter is going to look at the basic research skills and information you need to be able to judge research for yourself. If you have studied research skills before you can probably have a little doze at this point. Otherwise, I hope it will be a helpful overview. If you'd like to dig deeper into research methods than I can here, some good books include:

- *How to Read a Paper* by Trish Greenhalgh[1]
- *Social Research Methods* by Alan Bryman[2]
- *Research Methods in Health* by Ann Bowling[3]
- *Research Methods and Statistics in Psychology* by Hugh Coolican[4]
- *Introduction to Epidemiology* by Ilona Carneiro[5]
- *Research Methods in Health* by Pranee Liamputtong[6]

What are the main types of research design?

Research studies can be broadly split into different designs, according to the type of question you want to ask, how you want to ask it and who you want to ask.

Quantitative research

This type of research tends to measure stuff using numbers. It uses 'closed' questions, tests and scales, or might take physiological measures such as heart rate, blood pressure or birth weight. Typically it has bigger numbers of participants and uses statistics. It also tends to have 'hypotheses' or ideas about what the findings might be, and tests whether these things happen.

There are four broad types of quantitative research design:

1. *Descriptive*: Data is collected at one time point without anything being manipulated (e.g. nothing is 'done' to participants). An example of this would be a questionnaire at one time point measuring how often a parent reports their baby cries. Another example would be an observation of something occurring, e.g. how many times in an eight-hour period a baby cries.

2. *Correlational design*: two (or more) things are measured, and the relationship between them examined statistically. Again, the data is collected on things that are already naturally happening; you don't ask the groups to do anything differently, or do anything to them.

3. *Causal comparative research*: this is a bit like correlational research. You measure things that are already happening, but examine differences in things that might differ between two groups. For example, you might measure stress levels in babies who are regularly carried in a sling or not.

4. *Experimental designs*: this is when you split people into groups, and ask different groups to do different things and look at the outcomes. For example, you might ask one group of women to do yoga in pregnancy, and the other not to and look at whether it shortened their labours. This is often considered the 'best' type of research, especially if you randomise who goes in each group. However, when it comes to human behaviour it can be very problematic. Some common quantitative tools include:

- *Questionnaires*, measuring quantifiable things such as how much someone smokes or drinks or their attitude towards something using a scale.
- Using *health records* to look at whether people developed an illness, or what procedures or behaviour they experienced. Examples might include looking up what procedures and outcomes happened during childbirth. Linked health record databases can link up all these different things for an individual.
- Taking *physiological measures* such as heart rate, stress levels or blood pressure or measuring how long someone took to do something.
- *Observing* how often someone does something or something happens, such as how often a baby feeds over eight hours.

Qualitative research

This type of research tends to focus more on the 'why'. It explores experiences, behaviours and emotions by asking open-ended questions rather than fitting people into boxes. Sometimes it doesn't ask anyone anything at all – it just observes. These studies tend to have fewer participants and explore their experiences in depth. Qualitative research is very much about exploring – researchers don't usually have preconceived ideas about what they will find.

There are lots of different approaches to undertaking qualitative research. These include:

1. *Ethnography*: the traditional anthropological approach in which a researcher explores a community or culture that they are interested in understanding more about. They observe behaviours that occur, traditions, relationships between individuals and things like structure and power. They might embed themselves in the community (or already be part of it). This is known as participant observation. Or they might observe from a 'distance', externally rather than part of the group, which is known as non-participant observation.

2. *Phenomenological approach*: usually this does not start with any firm idea of what it will find. It aims to describe events, lives, activities (phenomena) to understand people's experiences and the meaning they place upon things. This usually focuses on one-to-one interviews, looking at documents, or talking to groups of people to explore a certain question, with the aim of identifying themes within people's stories. The 'truth' is what people believe and say it to be, based on their experiences. For example, you might explore the question 'Why do women want to avoid induction of labour?' You might read accounts, interview women, talk to groups of health professionals and use all this information to identify the key themes in their accounts – perhaps fear, desire for nature to take its course and so on.

3. *Grounded theory*: a grounded theory approach uses similar techniques to the phenomenological approach but aims to build an understanding of the theory behind why things happen. For example, how do women make decisions around birth? Again, the researcher does not start with any clear hypothesis, but instead allows the findings to emerge from the data.

4. *Case studies*: looking at a particular context in detail, such as perhaps seeing how one single organisation treats pregnant and new mothers.

5. *Historical research*: information is pieced together from different sources to explore how individuals lived, or what practices were in place.

Some common qualitative methods involve:

- Interviews in which people are asked open-ended questions.
- Focus groups in which a group of people are asked open-ended questions, but their interactions and discussion are as much the focus as individual responses.
- Observations of what people are doing but in a more open-ended, detailed way compared to counting.

- Content analysis looking at, say, newspapers or comments on news articles, drawings children have done, or the content of message boards.

Lots of research uses a combination of methods to understand a research question. Sometimes, if little is known about a subject, qualitative research might be used to explore ideas. Quantitative research might then be used to test those ideas. Or sometimes it might happen the other way around. A quantitative questionnaire might find that women with postnatal depression are less likely to breastfeed. Then qualitative interviews might be used to explore why.

So what designs and tools do we have? And more importantly, what are their strengths and weaknesses?

1. Randomised controlled trials

Randomised controlled trials work by randomising participants into different groups and then varying the experience of those groups and seeing if any difference in specific outcomes occurs. For example, one group might take one medication and another group a different medication. Or one group might go on a certain diet and another carry on just like before. Or one group attends an antenatal class while the other is given a website to read information on. And so on.

The theory behind the randomised controlled trial is that if you genuinely randomise people to a group then, if you have enough participants, the two groups should be pretty equal in terms of everything else apart from whatever you are testing. So things like gender, age, whether they have children, income and so on should naturally end up similar in each group. This is felt to reduce any factors that might be associated with someone choosing to follow a certain behaviour in real life, that might be associated with outcome.

For example, it is often argued that if babies who are breastfed have a higher IQ than babies who are not, then this isn't anything to do with breastmilk or the experience of being breastfed, but instead to do with who breastfeeds. Mothers who are older, with a higher level of education, more money, and who have professional jobs are more likely to breastfeed. So any difference in intelligence might be down to genetic influences on intelligence or lifestyle factors that a higher education and income might bring.

Some terms you might come across in the RCT literature include:

- *Arm* – this is a fancy way of saying which group the participant is in.
- *Blinded* – this doesn't happen often in behavioural research due to it being impossible, but is more common in medication and other drug-based research. Participants take a medication without knowing whether it is active (or a placebo – a tablet with no medical properties) or what level of the drug they are taking. A trial is double-blinded if the person doing the data collection and analysis also doesn't know until the end (after the analysis is complete) which group was which. The idea is that this reduces any bias to try and interpret or measure results in a certain way. Of course, this is pretty much impossible in many areas of health research. A participant can't be blind to whether they are breastfeeding or not, or giving birth in a certain way or not. They may, however, be blind to the dose of their epidural.
- *Randomisation procedure* – People can be randomised to their groups in all sorts of ways. It might really be as simple as throwing a coin, die or drawing a card from a pack with the hope that this will lead to even numbers if you have a big enough sample. More technological versions use software that will give a random group, or even a call centre where you ring up and ask which group the individual should be placed in – reducing any bias of trying to get them in one group or another. Another way is to use block randomisation, in which, say, the first 10 people are put in

one group, the next 10 in another and so on. This approach is not without bias. If you use a block approach, it could be that 10 friends from one area, with similar backgrounds, all hear about the trial and sign up at the same time.

Another more rigorous way is to use a stratified approach. Here the researcher works out what other factors might play a role in study outcomes and tries to balance the groups based on those factors. For example, they might try to balance them on education, job, previous experience and so on. Individuals are placed into groups based on their background factors and then randomised. So you might have a high education group and half are randomly placed in one of the trial arms, and half in the other.

- *Cluster trial:* Cluster trials are popular in behavioural research when it would be difficult to randomise people within one area to different behaviours. If you are randomising people to take one dose of a medication or another then it's unlikely that they will start offering each other their medications and cause lots of crossover between the groups. But if you offered some women in one group specific antenatal classes and didn't offer them to the others, not only might one group get rather annoyed (and not take part), but also it's likely that they will have friends in the other group and might start sharing materials or things that they learned, meaning that people in the no class group also get the information.

  This is when a cluster design comes in – you might run one type of antenatal class in one city and another in another city (and hope no one has friends in that city). The challenge with this is that you need to make sure that those two cities are pretty similar in all other ways that might affect outcomes before you start.

Trials are often considered the strongest type of research evidence when it comes to health because they are seen to help reduce any other factors that might affect outcomes. However, trials do have their disadvantages, particularly when it comes to trying to measure human behaviour or outcomes that have lots of different things that could influence them. They are also not always as randomised and accurate as they might seem, often have trouble recruiting and retaining people, have big ethical issues and are very expensive and time-consuming to do right. In fact there is so much to say on the matter of trials that it deserves its own chapter (coming up next). For now I'll just direct you to the Christmas letter in the *BMJ* in 2003 entitled '*Parachute use to prevent death and major trauma related to gravitational challenge: systematic review of randomised controlled trials*'.[7]

In this article the researchers conducted a systematic review of all randomised controlled trials into wearing a parachute when you jumped out of a plane. They concluded that there were no such trials, and therefore there was no evidence that parachutes were needed when jumping out of a plane. I particularly like the conclusion in their abstract:

> As with many interventions intended to prevent ill health, the effectiveness of parachutes has not been subjected to rigorous evaluation by using randomised controlled trials. Advocates of evidence-based medicine have criticised the adoption of interventions evaluated by using only observational data. We think that everyone might benefit if the most radical protagonists of evidence-based medicine organised and participated in a double blind, randomised, placebo controlled, crossover trial of the parachute.

Of course, this is satire, albeit satire with a very important point. How many times have you heard a woman be told that there is no evidence for the way she wants to give birth, care for or feed her baby, when all she wants to do is something that is biologically 'normal'? Sometimes you don't need a trial to tell you that something is sensible or should be supported. Sometimes it would be crazy or unethical to do a randomised controlled trial, and other forms of research, expertise, or just plain common sense should be considered. Sometimes research isn't needed into the outcome, but instead perhaps into ensuring that everyone who wanted to, or needed to, jump out of a plane had the right support to do so.

2. Cohort studies

A cohort study looks at a group of individuals and follows them over time. It might measure lots of different things that happen to them and the outcomes of those things and draw conclusions. Some cohorts are of the general population to understand how frequently things occur, while others are of individuals with specific circumstances to understand what different factors affect their outcomes.

For example, one of the most well known cohort studies around birth and babies is the Avon Longitudinal study – also known as the Children of the 90s study or ALSPAC. It has followed the lives of 14,500 families in the Bristol area, tracking what happened to women in pregnancy and at birth, and then the growth, development and health of those babies. Some of those babies are now having their own babies, so the team are able to look at intergenerational effects.[8]

The ALSPAC team have published more than 2,000 papers since the 1990s on all sorts of things. They are able to look at how pregnancy, birth and early experiences affect later outcomes in a large population. The study is not randomised, so individual experiences will be driven and affected by all sorts of things, but the size of the study means it is also possible to look at how all those different things affect outcomes.

Another very useful cohort study is the Millennium Cohort Study (MCS) or 'Child of the New Century' study. It is following the lives of young people born in the UK in 2000–01. The study had 18,818 cohort members at the start.[9] Similarly, the 1958 National Child Development Study (NCDS) is following the lives of 17,415 people who were born in the UK in a single week of 1958.[10]

3. Case-control design

This design is often used to study outcomes that are fairly rare across the population. It is frequently used in areas such as Sudden Infant Death Syndrome (SIDS) or childhood leukaemia, as fortunately these things happen rarely on a population level and would therefore be rare occurrences in much smaller studies. For example, if you designed a randomised controlled trial and wanted to examine SIDS as one of your outcomes you would need an extremely large sample, as SIDS occurs at a rate of roughly 1 in 3,200 births.

A case-control study deliberately seeks out families who have experienced these things. It then looks for matching 'control cases' who did not experience the illness but are similar in other characteristics such as age and sex. It then examines the frequency of different factors that the researcher thinks might contribute to the outcome. For example, for SIDS we know that there is an increased risk if parents smoke. Therefore it might consider the rates of smoking in the SIDS cases and in the matched cases.

Case-control studies have a number of limitations, not least with recruitment issues. They are often used in situations that are very sensitive, such as when a baby has an illness or has even died. Recruiting needs to be very sensitively handled, especially when it is examining differences in modifiable factors (things that could have been different) between groups. Parents who sign up to take part may be very different to those who decline to take part, and as a whole can be very different to the control group who don't have any of these worries or feelings of guilt and so on. However, they are a useful tool for exploring risk factors for rare outcomes.

4. Cross-sectional research

This is research that is typically conducted at one time point. Participants are asked to fill in a questionnaire about their attitudes and experiences, or measurements are taken. It could include things like looking at birth records in a hospital, for example to see whether inducing labour was associated with an increased level of caesarean sections. There is no attempt to manipulate anything. The number of people in the research could range from perhaps 100 to many thousands of participants.

Sometimes cross-sectional research might have a longitudinal element in that participants are followed up at additional time points. Usually this only happens a couple of times, rather than it being a cohort design. For example researchers might ask pregnant women questions during pregnancy about the type of birth they would ideally have, and then follow up their satisfaction with their birth and their mental health when their baby is six weeks old.

A good example of cross-sectional research was the UK Infant Feeding Survey.[11] Data used to be collected on feeding practices every five years in the UK. Questionnaires were sent out to all women who gave birth in a certain time period about how they were feeding their baby, their knowledge of feeding their baby and different experiences around pregnancy, birth and the early weeks. It also collected demographic background data such as how old participants were, where they lived, and their education. This allowed for comparisons in infant feeding decisions and experiences to be compared between different groups.

The main disadvantage with cross-sectional research is that it only gives a snapshot of experiences at any one time. If you measure something when a baby is six weeks old, it doesn't tell you what happened when they were eight weeks old. It also just looks at behaviours as they occur, rather than randomising anyone into any particular behaviour. This means that outcomes could be affected by all sorts of other factors that encouraged people to choose that behaviour, although researchers can control for the effect of this (more on this later).

5. Qualitative research

As we have seen, qualitative research tends to explore the 'why' – why people make decisions – or the 'how' – how people behave – through making observations. It's all about the rich detail and exploring rather than hard, numerical outcomes. It isn't about large populations and extrapolating findings, but understanding the experiences of a smaller group of people.

Qualitative research is an incredibly useful tool. One example is the recent outbreaks of Ebola. While medical science was busy working out how to try and prevent, treat and cure the illness, social science played a big role in understanding why outbreaks were occurring.[12] It emerged, through social science researchers who had spent considerable time in the communities (and were therefore trusted), that cultural rituals around washing the bodies of the deceased were actually contributing to the spread of the disease. So social science saved lives.

Some people feel that qualitative research is biased and there's no escaping from the fact that the experiences and motivations of the researcher can affect what is asked and observed. But qualitative researchers are perfectly aware of that and roll with it. They even spend time openly reflecting on how they, as a big part of the research tool, could influence the research, and how they can try to reduce that bias.

Qualitative research includes steps to try and avoid blatant bias. This is known as 'trustworthiness' and there are several things a researcher can do to try and reduce bias:[13]

- *Credibility* – How confident are you that there is 'truth' in the findings? Techniques to enhance this include conducting research over time, tackling a question from more than one angle (e.g. asking both patients and health professionals about managing an illness), and getting another researcher to look at your findings and see if they would find similar.
- *Transferability* – Are the findings applicable in other

contexts? Lots of details about the methods used and participant background can help other researchers repeat the study in another context.

- *Dependability* – Are the findings consistent? Could they be repeated? This is enhanced by describing carefully how the data was analysed and any findings produced, such as how themes emerged from analysis of interview data.
- *Confirmability* – Are the findings shaped by the participants and not research bias? A key element of this stage is providing evidence from your data, such as supportive quotes or documents.

Is one type of research 'best'?

Some people argue that some study designs are better than others and that there is a 'hierarchy' of different types of research.[14] Research designs are typically ordered according to how rigorous and free from bias the design is considered to be. This is often visualised in a triangle shape, with the research at the top being the most 'rigorous', but smaller in quantity (because they tend to be very expensive) through to those seen as less 'rigorous' at the bottom where there are usually more studies.

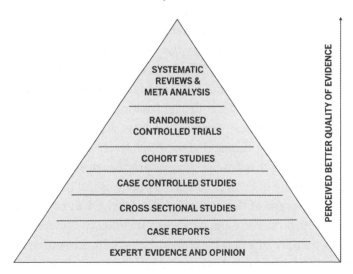

At the top of the evidence hierarchy is the systematic review or meta-analysis. Systematic reviews bring together all the different literature on one topic and consider whether, when they are taken into consideration together, there is evidence for something. Sometimes systematic reviews just include data from randomised controlled trials (more on these in a moment), and sometimes they include research from all types of design, but judge whether they are deemed strong research or not. Typically systematic reviews will judge the strength of the research according to the hierarchy of research diagram. However, more recently, qualitative systematic reviews are emerging. Systematic reviews also often try to consider how biased a piece of research might be – but that often correlates highly with the method they have chosen, with randomised controlled trials being seen as less biased.

A meta-analysis is another type of paper in which results from numerous studies are combined. It takes quantitative data from a series of studies (often randomised controlled trials but not always) and aims to mathematically compute what these data suggest when brought together. It works on the basis that every study will have limitations, but if you bring all the data together, it will help reduce them.

Looking specifically at individual study design, randomised controlled trials are seen as the most rigorous, followed by cohort studies, cross-sectional surveys and then case studies. The hierarchy of evidence was originally developed by medics wanting to know which drugs, treatments or interventions would have the best outcomes across a population. It was based on testing things that were relatively easy to compare, such as taking this dose or drug or another dose (or no drug). The hierarchy of evidence remains pretty useful in these cases.

The concept of the hierarchy of evidence has been heavily criticised, however, especially when it comes to understanding areas that are affected by human behaviour. Lots of areas of human health and behaviour are not particularly well suited to randomised controlled trials because it is very difficult to randomise people, people tend not to stick to their groups, and in some cases randomising them at all is completely unethical.

Also, the hierarchy of evidence was never meant to say that the things lower down the pyramid were not very good. The idea was that when making a healthcare decision you would start at the top of the hierarchy and see whether there was suitable evidence available, and if not move down to the next stage and so on. The layers were also meant to be considered together, as they could all add to the bigger picture, rather than ignoring research from the lower layers.

Every research design has something to offer. Trials may detect a difference, but they often cannot tell us why it is occurring, which is where qualitative research comes in. Likewise, a trial may fail to recruit well, or find that people do not adhere to the behaviour they have been asked to follow – and qualitative research helps us find out why. Ideally, a research topic would have evidence from every single step of the hierarchy and you would look at the overall picture. Indeed, a recent position paper written and signed by members of the 'Social science approaches for research and engagement in health policy & systems' (SHaPeS) and 'Thematic working group' of Health Systems Global, 'Regional Network for Equity in Health in East and Southern Africa' (EQUINET), and 'Emerging Voices for Global Health' stated:[15]

> 'I do love working on numbers... but I can only understand my findings and know how to model my data if I do have a clearer picture of the context and only after understanding the qualitative work. The latter facilitates my understanding beyond what the numbers show'. – Erlyn Rachelle Macarayan, an Emerging Voice for Global Health Philippines.

Stating that randomised controlled trials are the gold standard of research is also exclusionary. Large-scale, well-funded randomised controlled trials are predominantly (not always) led by White, male, well-paid professors in high-income countries, conducting the type of research that tends to benefit White, rich men in high-income countries. Researchers in low- and middle-income countries often lack the funding and research infrastructure to be able to conduct research that is seen as relevant by this hierarchy, but is desperately relevant and needed in their own region. Indeed, some of the best and most relevant research in different cultures and communities comes from members of those communities conducting the research through their networks – not through a large trial, but by talking to community members and understanding what is driving behaviour. This knowledge is critical to any public health policy or intervention, and more importantly still, critical to that community and culture. How dare we say that research led by a community, for a community isn't gold standard enough for our (predominantly) White, Western beliefs?

We mustn't overlook qualitative research and the social sciences

Across academia there are different areas of research, each with its own unique way of looking at the world, alongside some underlying shared assumptions. Often, health policy is based on specific data and analysis – that which is common in the medical and public health sciences – the randomised controlled trials and systematic reviews. Although systematic reviews can include more qualitative methods of analysis, many don't or consider it to be too low quality for decision-making, sticking instead to the trials and maybe some cohort studies.

This overlooks a huge body of fascinating research that can help us think about the parenting choices that are right for us. Social sciences research observes people, or events, typically without testing or manipulating anything and reports on what is naturally occurring all around us. Relationships and interactions are at the heart of what is observed, with sense-making of why things are happening and why we are reacting in such a way. Social scientists have so much to say on key topics such as politics, climate change, poverty... but their contributions are often overlooked by those who think science is all about testing things.

Let's look at some of the key social sciences disciplines to see how they can help inform our decision-making:

- *Sociology* – how communities and groups form and how people relate to each other.
- *Psychology* – focuses on how the brain works, our development through the lifespan, how individuals function alone and in groups. Psychology can tell us a lot about why we believe and think what we do and feel how we feel.
- *Social policy* – what do different groups in society need, how are they affected by different policies, and how can policies and practice better support them.
- *Human geography* – study of the world, people, communities and cultures, including how humans shape the world such as through climate change.
- *History* – what has happened to humans and communities over millennia and why.
- *Politics* – how political beliefs are formed, democracy, how people are affected by politics and what affects who is in power.
- *Linguistics* – how people communicate, what shapes language and how language is used to shape us.

On a broad topic, let's say where a woman wants to give birth, these disciplines can tell us so much:

- *Sociology* – how do the views of communities and membership of different groups affect the decisions women want to make around birth?
- *Psychology* – why do individuals want to give birth in a certain place? How does it make them feel? How do human

173

physiology and psychology interact?

- *Social policy* – who is more able to make a decision to give birth where they desire and what policies are in place to support this?
- *Human geography* – where do people give birth around the world and why?
- *History* – what was normal for humans over time? When did we start having babies in hospitals?
- *Politics* – how different political parties think about women, healthcare systems and liberal choice.
- *Linguistics* – how the language around birth, of fear and responsibility, and pressure on women not to consider their own needs shapes birth. Language such as 'all that matters is a healthy baby' and 'failure to progress'.

We're not talking about hard numbers data. But these disciplines can certainly give you context and understanding of the different influences on your decisions and why certain people might be telling you to act in certain ways.

Anthropology is particularly important

Anthropology – another key social science – is the study of people and what makes us human: how we behave and interact with each other, and how we have evolved over time to act in certain ways. Anthropology looks at both our biology (genetics, physiology) and our experiences (language, culture, traditions, religion, politics), and importantly how these two things interact and shape each other. Often anthropology looks at how humans differ (or are indeed similar) to many other animals, particularly other mammals. Sometimes anthropologists use fossil records and other archaeological tools to allow them to draw conclusions about our history, development and evolution.

Many famous anthropological studies look at our evolution and what was 'normal' for humans over different eras and generations – this is broadly known as 'biological' or 'evolutionary' anthropology. But anthropology is not all in the past. Anthropologists can study any culture around the world at any given time, and often study behaviours and rituals in the present time. This is known broadly as 'social and cultural anthropology'.

When we say that anthropologists study 'culture', some people assume that they only study 'cultures' that are in untouched, remote locations or societies that are very different from industrialised nations. Although some will, this isn't the case for all and many study current behaviours across different societies. A culture also doesn't just mean location. It can mean a workplace, or a parenting culture.

Anthropology can tell us much about what has been 'normal' for our species historically and how we have developed as human infants and caregivers. It can help explain a lot of normal infant behaviour by considering our evolution, but also by comparing us to other cultures that have less interference in their mother–infant relationships from industry, media and medical intervention.

Anthropologists don't tend to 'test' things, rather they observe. This means their research often gets overlooked when it comes to policy and our understanding of growing and caring for babies. But anthropology can help us understand what is biologically 'normal' or expected for our babies, and how this might cause difficulties in our modern, industrialised lives. This isn't to say that we will always choose to follow that, or even want to, but it does help us understand.

For example, a common concern among new parents is how often babies feed. Particularly when babies are breastfed, it is common for them to feed every two hours or more as breastmilk is very easily digested, and feeding frequently helps build up a good milk supply. We get lots of messages in Western society suggesting this is wrong – from people suggesting that 'good babies' feed less often, and parenting books saying you can put your baby in a routine. On top of this, new mothers are often encouraged to 'get their lives back' and to encourage their baby to be more separate and independent.

But if we look at data from different cultures, where keeping mum and baby together is considered the norm, babies are carried and sleep next to their mothers, and there is no 'noise' about putting your baby in a routine or getting your life back, babies naturally feed extremely frequently. Indeed, one famous anthropological study found that during the daytime, babies in one culture fed up to four times an hour, for just a few minutes at a time![17] In two other studies exploring feeding patterns in rural Bangladesh, mainly among women who were working in the fields but kept their babies close by, babies fed around once an hour.[18,19]

Obviously we can't just pick up data from one context and apply it automatically to another. But what this tells us is that when babies have free access to the breast, and there are few messages about controlling that, they feed very frequently. We can use this information to help shape our own decisions around feeding our babies, based on a combination of the reassurance of what we know is biologically normal, combined with the set-up of our lives.

To bring this chapter to a close, I am a firm believer that hierarchies of evidence don't really exist. Different methods, disciplines and data should be part of a broader jigsaw puzzle that can help inform us. And research funders and academics are increasingly recognising the importance of this through working together to answer bigger picture questions (known as interdisciplinary or multidisciplinary work). Rather than asking through a randomised controlled trial the hard outcomes of home versus hospital births, a bigger picture design would ask 'where do women want to give birth and why', bringing researchers from across disciplines to answer it.

Sticking to one discipline and research design and saying it's best is the equivalent of going to a sumptuous buffet at a posh hotel and only eating the sausage rolls.

HOW TO KEEP INFORMED:

There are numerous different research designs, each with its strengths and weaknesses. Certain designs are better at asking certain questions in certain ways.

There is no one best research method for all questions. Research topics that bring together evidence from lots of different areas and methods of research to create a jigsaw puzzle of all sorts of different knowledge will be the best.

Social science research, particularly qualitative research, is often overlooked. This has implications for what research gets done and what gets funded and noticed, and supports a system where only the most privileged researchers get to answer questions that further their privilege.

Some people will continue to tell you that there is a hierarchy of evidence and only the things at the top matter. Ask them when they will be jumping out of a plane without a parachute.

9

LIES, DAMNED LIES, AND STATISTICS

If the author H.G. Wells was still alive today, I think he would be rather disappointed. Back in 1903 he wrote in his book *Mankind in the Making* that he hoped that '*statistical thinking will one day be as necessary for efficient citizenship as the ability to read and write*' – or at least he wrote slightly more complex words to that effect. That quote is actually a paraphrase of the extract by Samuel Wilks (a mathematician) some 50-odd years later to describe the work, but the meaning is the same.[1]

Instead we've ended up in a place where experts aren't necessary and statistics are misused all over the place. To quote another expert, '*There are three kinds of lies: lies, damned lies, and statistics*' – Disraeli. But understanding statistics is a really important part of understanding research.

Now before you recoil in horror, perhaps with memories of skipping maths class, I'm not going to spend pages and pages deep in statistical theories and workings out. But I am going to give you an overview of some of the terms and tests you might come across and how they can be misused. If you want more detail, I recommend the following books:

- *How to Lie with Statistics* by Darrell Huff[2]
- *A Field Guide to Lies and Statistics* by Daniel Levitin[3]
- *The Art of Statistics: Learning from Data* by David Spiegelhalter[4]
- *Statistics for Dummies* by Deborah Rumsey[5]
- *Naked Statistics: Stripping the Dread from the Data* by Charles Wheelan[6]

Note: thinking back to our earlier point on who is leading research and writing the books, there certainly appears to be a tendency for men to be dominating the statistics literature.

Some basic terms

Lots of research will report differences between two or more groups by describing the average or most common finding within each group, for example how much babies who were born by caesarean section weighed versus how much babies born vaginally weighed. There are different ways of expressing the average, most common or middle figure depending on the data you are looking at.

- *The mean:* the average score in a set. If 10 women all take a test examining their symptoms of postnatal depression and have a score out of a potential 20, you can find the mean score by adding everyone's score up and dividing it by the number of people (in this case 10). The issue with the mean is that it brings everyone to the average point. You get the same mean if, out of your 10 people, most people score around 10 out of 20, or if half score nothing and half score full marks. Virtually no one in that second set of scores scored the mean score.

One casualty of the tendency to report means is when considering something like breastfeeding duration. You'll often get a finding that the average duration of breastfeeding is six weeks or something. In reality, this will be skewed by a tendency for many women to encounter difficulties in the early days and weeks and stop then, while others, once breastfeeding is well established, breastfeed for much longer. It doesn't give a full picture.

- *Standard deviation:* this is a measure of how much a data set varies, so it can help tell you if everyone scored around half marks, or in fact there was a much wider range. A smaller standard deviation means there is less spread in the data, and a larger standard deviation means a bigger spread. It is based on the square root of the variance of a sample, but there are tests that work that out for you!
- *Median:* this is the figure 'in the middle'. So if you have five people who score 1, 2, 3, 4 and 5 then your median is 3. Again if they are not so evenly distributed then all it tells you is what's in the middle.
- *Mode:* the mode is the one that happens most often. So if you have 10 women breastfeed and one does it for one month, two do it for two months, and one does it for three months, your mode is two. This is a lot more useful when it comes to stuff around babies, but you don't see it very often.

A word of warning – means and medians are used to illustrate the central or average point in a sample. However people's interpretation of the midpoint in a sample as the normal point or something everyone should aim for is rather problematic. One of the best examples of this is baby weights. How often have you heard someone suggest that all babies should be around the 50th percentile on their growth charts? It's a big cause of concern for many parents, when in reality only 1% of babies are expected to be on the 50th percentile.

When babies are weighed and measured they are plotted on centile charts. These charts are based on the weights of many thousands of babies across the whole weight spectrum. They take into account a wide range of *expected and healthy* weights, with some concerns at the very top and bottom that a baby might sometimes be at risk for under or overweight, but this would take into account other factors too such as how long they are and how tall their parents are. Some people are just bigger than others. If we say all babies should be on the 50th centile, it's like saying something is wrong with a woman if she isn't exactly 5ft 4in tall and 170 pounds (the average stats for a woman in the UK). It's clearly nonsense.

Based on weighing and measuring thousands of babies, the charts rank expected weights from the lowest weights (1st percentile) up to the heaviest babies (the 99th percentile). Over a large population, roughly 1% of babies will be on each of these percentiles. Although the 50th percentile is the mean point, there should be no more babies there than at the 30th or 70th percentile. A baby on the 40th percentile is heavier than 40% of all babies. A baby on the 85th percentile is heavier than 85% of babies. And the 50th percentile baby is just heavier than 50% but lighter than 49%.

Testing whether something is 'significantly different'

On a basic level there are two main groups of statistical tests: those that tell you whether there is a difference between two (or more) groups, and those that look at whether two things are related to each other (if one goes up does the other go up or down). Each of these tests will look to see whether the difference between groups or the strength of relationship between two things is big enough to be 'significant'.

Significance testing considers the strength of the data and gives a percentage calculation of how likely it is that those things (a difference between groups, or a relationship between them) have happened due to chance. There is a general consensus that researchers are happy with a risk of this happening 5% or less of the time. So they set their significance level (known as a p value) at 0.05 (or 5%). Some will set it at a lower level – sometimes 0.01 (or 1%). You will be able to see this written in any statistical test outcome as p= followed by a number. So p=0.034 would be considered a significant difference or relationship, but p=0.161 would not be. Sometimes researchers will write p=<0.05, which means p= less than 0.05, or p=>0.05, which means p= greater than 0.05%.

P value really does matter, and it is bad practice to suggest that data 'is almost significant' or 'approaches significance'. Although 0.05 is pretty arbitrary, it's a cut-off, and even if the value comes back at 0.04 it should mean you have less faith that there is a strong relationship. As the number gets closer to 0.05, the chances of it being a 'false positive' increase – if your significance is just under 0.05, there is around a 30% chance your finding happened by chance. However, this doesn't stop some researchers from declaring that they have found differences or associations in their study (small print – even though not significant). For example, one study looking at the impact of acupuncture on colic highlighted values between 0.05 and 0.1 as 'approaching significance', as if this was important. In reality, growing numbers of researchers are calling for the significance level to be brought *down* – to 0.01 or even 0.005. The lower the significance level, the more confident you can be that the findings reflect a real difference and not chance.

It is also important to consider 'real-life' significance as well as mathematical significance. Significance is asking whether there is a big enough difference or association between groups, and how likely it is that this is a fluke based on the pattern of scores. But things can be mathematically significant, especially in big samples, when in reality that significance might not seem important at all. In one study that compared timing of introduction of solids to babies, looking at early and late introduction, the researchers declared that early introduction had a significant impact on sleep. SIGNIFICANT! Parents' ears pricked up across the land. What, giving my baby solid foods early could make a significant impact on their sleep? Let's break out the baby rice! 'Significant', in this case, turned out to mean an average of seven extra minutes of sleep per night.[7] Maybe pop the champagne back in the cupboard.

In another example, headlines screamed that eating a junk food diet delayed how long it took women to get pregnant. In reality, those who didn't eat much fruit took 0.2–0.6 months longer to get pregnant than those who did, while those who didn't eat their greens took 0.4–0.9 months longer.[8] So days then. Differences measured in days are not of real-life significance when it comes to getting pregnant. And junk food does not act as a contraceptive!

Independent and dependent variables

You might spot these phrases when statistics are discussed. Simply, a dependent variable is whatever is *being measured* – it is the data, or outcome. So if you are measuring how much babies weigh, how many women breastfeed, how many women have forceps deliveries – these are all dependent variables.

The *independent variable* is the potential *reason for variation* in the dependent outcomes – so groups you are measuring a difference in dependent outcome between. This could be experimental groups, or natural groups. For example, if you were measuring the duration of breastfeeding associated with three different birth types – caesarean section, assisted vaginal delivery and unassisted vaginal delivery – then the birth type is your independent variable. And the breastfeeding duration is the dependent variable. If you assigned pregnant women to two types of antenatal class and looked at how anxious they were about giving birth after taking the class, then the class type is the independent variable and the anxiety levels are the dependent variable.

Types of statistical analysis

There are a few different tests in each of those groups. Which test is used also depends on the type of data that you have. Broadly, there are three types of data:

Nominal data

This is when you don't really have numbers at all, but you have measured things and in order to explore them statistically you have to give them a number. So if you were measuring birth modes you might assign a caesarean section to be 1, an unassisted vaginal birth to be 2, and forceps or ventouse to be 3. These numbers just act as labels and mean nothing else. A forceps delivery isn't 3 times a caesarean section for example. And although you could find the modal birth type you couldn't work out a mean. A 1.3 birth would be nonsensical.

If you only had this type of data you would only be able to look at associations between things. And this would affect the type of test you could do.

Chi square

The first of these is called a *chi square* test. Imagine you have type of milk given at birth (breast milk, formula milk – coded in your data set as '1' and '2') and then ethnicity (let's say Black, South Asian, Chinese and White – coded in your data set as '1', '2', '3' and '4'). If you wanted to look at whether ethnicity was associated with milk type, you would do a test of association. Chi square is a common one. It looks at whether any one ethnic group is associated with any one birth outcome more than others by producing a crosstabs box such as this one, using data from the UK Infant Feeding Survey:[9]

	Breast	Formula
White	78%	22%
Black	96%	4%
South Asian	95%	5%
Chinese	97%	3%

The chi square test essentially looks at whether each method of feeding is associated with any ethnic group. As you can see there is a significant association: women from White groups are less likely to breastfeed at birth in the UK.

Odds ratios

Another test you could do would be to look at *odds ratios*, which look at the association between an event/exposure and an outcome. These are often used in health research. Imagine you have two groups of pregnant women and you assigned one group to eat fish oils during pregnancy and the second to be the control group (no fish oils). You then measured how bad their back pain was. The odds ratio allows you to look at how much more likely the intervention group was to experience pain compared to the control group. It measures the outcome for one group in relation to the outcome for another group. This allows you to say, for example, that 'Compared to women who didn't take fish oils, women who took fish oils had a 70% lower chance of severe back pain'.

To calculate the odds ratio, you put the intervention result as the numerator (the top number) and the control result as the denominator (the bottom number).

	Severe back pain	No severe back pain
Fish oils	3	27
No fish oils	10	20

To calculate the odds ratio you would calculate:

$$\text{Odds ratio} = \frac{\text{Fish oils pain/All who took fish oils}}{\text{No fish oils pain/All who didn't take fish oils}}$$

If both groups had equal 'odds' of having severe back pain, the odds ratio would be one. Anything *above one* means that the intervention is scoring higher than the control, and anything *below one* means that the control is scoring higher than the intervention. In the example above, the odds ratio is 0.3: those in the intervention group have a 70% lower chance of experiencing significant back pain.

When you compute odds ratios you don't measure statistical significance, but rather how confident you are that the odds you have calculated are 'precise'. This is known as calculating the '95% confidence interval'. It gives you two values through which you can be sure, if you repeated the research, that you would find an odds ratio lying between these two variables 95% of the time. Sometimes this measure can be taken as a measure of significance. If the confidence interval does not overlap the 1 (e.g. the equal outcome) then this is taken to be significant.

Ordinal data

This is when the data that you have has some kind of order, or rank – but the distance between each data point is not necessarily an even gap. For example, imagine new mothers were asked to rate their experience on the postnatal ward and given the following options:

- ☐ Loved it, it was like a luxury holiday
- ☐ It was alright I suppose
- ☐ I didn't like it
- ☐ Hell on earth

You can see that the options have some kind of order to them, where the top option is the most positive and the bottom option the most negative. However, we can't tell just how different 'Hell on earth' and 'I didn't like it' are.

Another type of ordinal data would be positions in a race: first comes before second and second before third, but the times in between would not be equal. Imagine a set-up where five pregnant women have their labour induced in five different ways. The recording of who gave birth 'first', 'second' and so on would be ordinal data (and a rather dubious experiment ethically).

Frequency or interval data

This data occurs when the difference between each data point is standardised and meaningful. Birth weight is a good example of frequency data: 2.5kg is half of 5kg. If you measure how frequently something happens, or how much of something is given, that is also frequency data. For example, the amount of donor human milk used to supplement a premature baby. Or estimated blood loss after a haemorrhage. Scores on tests such as the scales used to measure postnatal depression or maternal self-efficacy are usually frequency data too.

Both ordinal and frequency data allow you to do statistical tests, but which version of the test you use depends on the type of data you have.

Tests between groups
Both ordinal and frequency data can be used to test whether there is a difference between two or more groups in an outcome. Depending on the test used this might use a mean score (for frequency data) or the ranked position in the data (for ordinal data). For example, you might compare estimated blood loss between women who have an injection to deliver the placenta after birth and those who don't. Or the mean score on the Edinburgh Postnatal Depression scale (a test used to measure depression in postnatal women) among depressed women who had been prescribed counselling, medication, or a combination of both. Thinking back to the example of how women would rate their postnatal ward experience, you might compare responses from women who were based on a large ward or in a private room.

Depending on the type of data you have, you would use a different test. Some examples of tests you might see in research include:

- *T tests:* these are used to compare mean scores of two groups when frequency data is used. They might be two different groups, or one group with two measurements over time.
- *Analysis of variance (ANOVA):* these compare the mean score of more than two groups. Again they could be separate groups, or the same group over time. If you compare more

than one outcome measure then you could put them into the test at the same time and have a MANOVA – a multiple analysis of variance.

- *Mann Whitney U test/Wilcoxon rank sum test:* this looks at differences between two groups when the data used is not ordinal data. It compares the median score between groups.
- *Kruskal Wallis test:* like the Mann Whitney U test but for three or more groups. Again uses the median score.

Associations between two scales or scores
The other type of test you might want to do when you have ordinal or frequency data is to look at the relationship between two or more scales or scores – known as a correlation. For example, if you have a measure of breastfeeding duration in days and a postnatal depression score, you might want to look at whether if one goes up, the other goes up or down too. If a correlation is positive, as one variable increases, the other does too. If a correlation is negative, as one variable increases the other decreases. However, just because two things are correlated doesn't mean there is necessarily any relationship between the two. It might be completely random.

Tests you might do include:

- *Pearson's r correlation:* a correlation for frequency data looking at how scores on each scale are associated with each other.
- *Spearman's rho:* a correlation for ordinal data, looking at how rankings on each measure are associated with each other.

How are statistics misused?

Let me count the ways:

- They can be misused accidentally, because those conducting them don't quite know what they're doing.
- They can be misinterpreted accidentally, because those interpreting them don't quite know what they're doing.
- Or they can be misused and abused through a combination

of a desire to attract readers and just enough ignorance about how they work not to feel guilty about that.

Here are some tests you can use if you suspect that someone is trying to pull the statistical wool over your eyes:

1. Are they trying to give you only one side of the story?

This one is very common. A reporter only gives one side of the story, without putting in the context of the other side. Knowing only one side of the story means nothing. If 5 out of 1,000 babies who had a certain vaccination still developed the illness they were vaccinated against, that tells us very little. We need to know how many who *didn't have* the vaccination developed it. But that's the part that is often left out, resulting in a scary-sounding headline like 'Babies become ill after being vaccinated', when in fact the data may actually show that far fewer babies become ill after being vaccinated than if they don't receive the vaccine.

As I write this, a story is circulating that claims breastmilk is full of toxins. The headline in the *Telegraph* is 'Cocktail of chemicals found in UK mothers' breastmilk due to home furnishings'. Pretty terrifying, right? Should we all stop breastfeeding immediately to save our babies from the chemicals? Definitely not. The headline was taken out of context, in this case a report by a parliamentary select committee on the environmental health impact of chemicals, especially one which makes furniture flame retardant.[11]

In the report we find that these chemicals have been found in the bodily fluids of adults and children, including blood, urine, umbilical cord blood and I assume something to do with male fertility, as male infertility has been linked to higher levels of these chemicals. The main point is that these chemicals are already in all of us: babies are affected in pregnancy and just by living in our houses, regardless of how they are fed. So the real issue is why these chemicals are getting into our bodies in the first place – not whether they happen to be in breastmilk or not.

Sometimes, research doesn't even properly use a control group for comparison. More on this later, but a control group is a group you compare outcomes to, if you have manipulated another group to do something. It is your reference point. Let's say you give a colic treatment or sleep intervention to one group, but not the other (your control group) and then measure not only whether things improve before and after the treatment in your intervention group, but also whether any improvement over time happens in the control group. In this way you can see whether it is the intervention that is making the difference, or something else.

Another example is that everyone has natural rises and falls in their levels of cortisol (a stress hormone) during the day. Just because it has risen, doesn't necessarily mean you are stressed. It rises after we wake up and falls after we fall asleep. However, the natural resting level it sits at has been observed to fall throughout the first year and into childhood.[12] So if you measured changes in cortisol level over time, you'd see an improvement in stress levels regardless of any intervention. Similar things happen with how much babies cry, how much they wake up and how highly women score on tests for postnatal depression. They all get slightly better naturally over time (in the majority of cases, but not all) so if you want to assess an intervention, you definitely need a control group to compare against, otherwise you might be attributing natural changes to something you have done, rather than nature taking its course. But if you want to mislead, just use the data from this one group: Look! Our intervention led to stress levels falling!

2. Are they trying to dazzle you with rankings?

We naturally assume in a ranking that 1 is highest, followed by 2, followed by 3… and so on. But while this might be technically true, ranking things doesn't tell us anything about whether the gap between the ranks is significant. If someone wins a race, how much better are they than the person who came second? If I rank all my favourite types of cake in order (for reference I'm going for coffee cake, followed by carrot cake, then chocolate brownie) that doesn't tell you anything about how much more I like coffee cake than carrot cake. In reality there's barely any difference at all. But people fall for a good ranking.

In his book *How to Lie with Statistics* Darrell Huff illustrates perfectly how rankings can be used to deliberately confuse people.[2] He refers to a *Reader's Digest* article that included a survey of the levels of chemicals in different types of cigarettes. The findings showed that there was basically no significant difference in the levels of chemicals between the different brands. However, it placed the results in a table, in order of content. The one at the top technically had the highest levels of poisonous substances in it and the one at the bottom the least. But the actual differences were negligible – they were all as bad as each other.

However, in a list, something needs to be bottom, and the company who manufactured the cigarette brand at the bottom – Old Gold – leapt on this and started marketing its brand as the least toxic, carefully omitting actual numbers and just saying that it was placed at the bottom of the toxicity rankings. Advertising Standards caught up eventually and told the company to stop it, but of course by this point the adverts had been published and people remembered them.

3. Do their graphs look a bit suspicious?

People like visuals. But they rarely look at the minor details. The two graphs below show exactly the same data, but the reference points along the x (vertical) axis are different. Imagine a study in which the researchers (perhaps funded by a baby food company) want to test whether giving a baby 'perfect porridge' before bed helps them to sleep or not. They really want to show that it does.

The researchers know that if they ask mothers 'How long did your baby sleep last night?' they run the risk of everyone rounding up or down to similar amounts, so 'eight hours' could actually mean closer to seven or closer to nine. So they decide to ask how many *minutes* the baby slept (yes, researchers have actually asked sleep-deprived parents to report their baby's sleep in minutes). They will then get more variation in their data: eight hours is 480 minutes, and 450 minutes (7.5 hours) sounds a lot less than that. I'm surprised they haven't had a go at asking parents to estimate their baby's sleep in seconds.

What's really 'clever' (aka deceitful) is that they can then manipulate the data on a graph. As we've seen, though every minute counts when it comes to how much your baby sleeps, small variations don't make much difference in everyday life. Imagine that the researchers didn't have much luck and everyone reported that their baby slept for pretty much the same length of time whether they'd had porridge or not. The average sleep duration for babies who hadn't had porridge was 475 minutes, compared to 480 minutes for those who'd had the porridge. A five-minute difference. Doesn't sound too impressive, does it?

But you can make it look much more noteworthy on a graph. In the graph below, the data is exactly the same, but on the left the x axis is set to cover a 10-minute sleep range, whereas on the right it is set to cover a much wider potential sleep time from 0–10 hours. I know which one I'd be using in my news article if I ever become an unscrupulous journo.

By the way, there isn't any evidence that giving your baby porridge before bed will help them sleep. Why would it? Babies wake for all sorts of reasons, just like adults, and it doesn't mean that it's because of hunger.

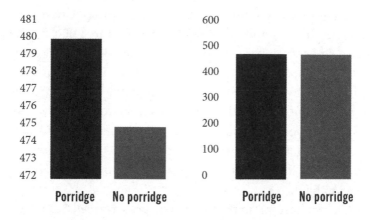

| Porridge | No porridge | | Porridge | No porridge |

4. Are they trying to scare you by telling you 'your risk triples'?

This is my favourite bad way to use statistics. I say *favourite* with heavy sarcasm. I see it virtually every day. Technically there is nothing wrong with it from a statistical perspective, but there is a HUGE amount wrong with it when it comes to public communication.

Nearly every day a newspaper will run a headline that states that something to do with our health increases the risk of some illness or other. You know the type, 'Drinking three nights a week triples your rate of cancer', or something like that. These headlines are both accurate and deliberately misleading at the same time.

The risk that these headlines are quoting is called the *relative risk*: compared to people who don't drink, how much more likely are people who drink every day to develop a certain cancer? Fair enough. But what is usually ignored is something called *absolute risk*: the actual percentage chance of something happening. Yes, drinking every day may well triple your risk of a certain cancer, but if the risk of developing that cancer was only 0.2% in the first place, then you've only got a 0.6% chance of it now (or a 99.4% chance of not).

Relative risks have less meaning for individuals, but more meaning when governments are looking at population-level risks: in this example the rate of cancer is 2 in 1,000 for the non-drinkers compared to 6 in 1,000 for the everyday drinkers. Over a population of 70 million individuals, encouraging drink-free days may lead to a reduction in the number of cases of cancer, but most individuals will still be fine. Relative risk doesn't tell you much about your *individual risk*. If we know, for example, that 1 in 100 people will get a certain type of cancer, then there is on average a 1% risk of any individual developing it.

A recent headline in the *Sun* newspaper screamed that babies born by IVF were eight times more likely to have 'dangerously high blood pressure' as adults.[13] In fact the study was based on ICSI as well as IVF, and there were only 54 adults in the study who had been born by ICSI/IVF, matched with 54 of their friends.[14] The actual results showed that the mean blood pressure in the ICSI/IVF group was 120/71 mmHg, compared to 116/69 mmHg in the control group. And while eight people in the ICSI/IVF group had high blood pressure (above 130/80 mmHg), just one in the control group did. So that's where the 'eight times' came from. But the sample size was very small, and so were the real differences. After all, 44 of those in the ICSI/IVF group didn't have high blood pressure – 81% of them. But that doesn't make such a good headline, does it.

5. Are they pretending that because two things are linked, one must affect the other?

Just because two things correlate doesn't mean that there is necessarily any relationship between them. Lots of things completely unrelated to each other correlate. The website **www. tylervigen.com/spurious-correlations** has some great examples, including significant correlations between the number of people who drowned by falling into a pool and the number of films Nicolas Cage starred in per year. And per capita cheese consumption and the number of people who died becoming tangled in their bedsheets. And the exceedingly worrying per capita consumption of margarine... and the divorce rate in Maine. So if you see a significant correlation being reported, always ask yourself *why*. And maybe avoid eating too much cheese in bed. Just in case.

Back in 1965 Sir Austin Bradford Hill came up with nine steps that he believed indicated *causality* rather than just *correlation*. These became known as the Bradford Hill criteria.[15]

1. *Strength of the association:* if the association between two things is particularly strong, then it's more likely to be causal.
2. *Consistency:* if the same thing keeps being shown across studies, then it's more likely to be causal (remember – findings across numerous papers are more important than just one).
3. *Specificity:* does something have a specific influence on another where the mechanism can be defined and explained?
4. *Temporality:* do things happen in the right order for causation to be implied?
5. *Biological gradient:* does more of something have more of an effect?
6. *Plausibility:* does it actually make sense that it could be causal? Do we have a mechanism to explain it?
7. *Coherence:* very similar to plausibility – does it make sense? Is it easy to accept?
8. *Experiment:* can you test it? By changing the exposure?
9. *Analogy:* is something similar known to have an effect?

HOW TO KEEP INFORMED:

Mathematical significance is not always real-life significance. Check what the actual mean scores are, or what the increase/decrease is.

Correlation is not causation. Always question and think about the mechanisms.

Check graphs carefully, especially if they appear in advertising material.

Ignore statistics that tell you that you have ten times the risk of something – always find out what your initial risk was and what ten times that actually refers to.

10

HOW TO UNDERSTAND
A RESEARCH PAPER

Once researchers have conducted their research, they publish it in scientific journals, of which there are many of varying quality. Research should be written up in a set expected format. Journal editors will then send the paper out to be reviewed by other researchers, and, if positive comments return, publish the paper. The research is then ready to be read and interpreted by others in the field and the general public.

However, there may be flaws in this process, from the initial research work through to where the paper is published, which can skew how the research is eventually interpreted. Understanding what to look for in a paper (and what might be missing) and being able to make a judgement about the quality and reliability of the journal it is published in, are important skills.

Unfortunately for the general public, a lot of research is behind paywalls. Although some papers are open access (free to read), others you have to pay for, unless you are part of an academic institution with a subscription to the journal. Some papers are open access because the researcher (or more likely their institution or research funder) has paid a fee for this to happen so more people can read it. This fee can often be thousands of pounds, so you can see why not many researchers can afford it – and why research published by industry that supports industry is more likely to be open access (and therefore more likely to be read and shared).

Somehow, these paywalls and prices have become acceptable in the strange crazy world of research publication. Researchers do not get paid for publishing their research papers. If you pay to access the paper, all the money goes to the publisher. However, researchers are expected to publish frequently as part of their academic contracts. As they and their students need to read the papers, their institutions then pay the publishers for everyone at the institution to be able to read it for free. Yes, the institution pays a publisher for its staff to be able to read work that the staff wrote in the first place.

The good news in all this craziness is that the author of the paper, although not allowed to share the full paper publicly on their website or social media, can respond to a personal request to send it to an individual. So if you want to read a paper, email the researcher – their email should be on the paper (and remember, email that author, not their male co-author!).

Also, there is another loophole. All journals allow researchers to freely share the copy of their paper that they submitted to the journal (the unedited version). Some even allow them to share the version after the reviewers have commented. Lots of academics now make these copies freely available, so as long as you're happy not reading the fancy edited version, you can still access the results. If you can't find details on Google, try contacting the author. Most are happy to help.

Reading and understanding a research paper

Pretty much all research papers, whatever the discipline, follow the same structure. They are made up of specific sections, each with specific details in, although sometimes the sections are called different things in different journals. Here's an overview:

Title

This is brief, usually up to 20 words. This means the title often implies that the paper might be far more generalisable than it is, by not including sample size, location, participants or other details.

Abstract

This is the summary at the start of the paper. These are usually around 200–300 words and should cover a brief introduction to the topic, the research question, the methods and an overview of the findings and conclusions. As you can imagine, given the short length, it is easy to emphasise or highlight specific parts of a paper and to ignore others. The abstract is there to give an overview and should not really be used instead of reading the full paper. The problem is that many people do only read the abstract, and sometimes researchers even end up citing papers based on the abstract, magnifying the problem. If one researcher writes a paper misinterpreting another paper based on its abstract, there is a real possibility that a second researcher will simply use that citation too, and so on until the paper is being used to cite something very far removed from what it actually said.

Highlights

Some papers will have highlights, which are brief bullet points about what is already known on the subject and what this paper adds. These are tricky to write as they often have strict word limits, so they may not be able to convey the details revealed in the full paper.

Introduction/background/literature

This should set the scene for the rest of the paper, presenting what is already known on the question. It should discuss the limitations of existing research and point out the research gap that the paper addresses. It should give enough details about the existing research in an area that you can judge whether the research is relevant, such as mentioning sample, location and methods (for example, 'One study with 300 pregnant women in Germany used a questionnaire to…').

Unfortunately, 'cherry picking' of the literature is possible and some researchers mention only those studies that support their argument, or that they feel are incomplete and need furthering or contending, ignoring the ones that are inconvenient.

Methods

This section should give you details of what the researchers actually did, in enough detail that you can judge the quality of work and so that other researchers could repeat the work using the same measures if they wished.

You should find details of participants, with both the criteria for someone being able to take part (known as *inclusion criteria*) and the criteria that would stop them from taking part (the *exclusion criteria*). Inclusion criteria might be things like demographic details such as sex, age, location and health details, such as being pregnant or a new mother, or having a certain health issue or experience. Exclusion criteria are important too as they describe who wasn't included, such as babies born before 37 weeks, low birth weight babies, or those classed as failure to thrive.

Details of what the researchers did should be included. What type of study was it? Did it use questionnaires? Interviews? Was it an RCT? What did they actually measure? If they were measuring infant feeding, when did they measure it? At birth? At six months? Did they measure the degree of exclusive breastfeeding, formula use and how babies were fed, by bottle or breast? If they used measures of mental health, what tools did they use?

There should also be details of how the study actually happened. So how were participants recruited? How were they randomised? This can tell you a lot about whether the sample might be biased or not. If researchers just went to antenatal clinics to collect data, an obvious limitation is that they might miss women who have specialist appointments at a different time, or who can't or won't attend antenatal care.

Also look out for a statement about whether the researchers got ethics permission to do the study, and who they got it from. All research involving humans should seek permission from an ethics committee and agree that it will abide by certain ethical standards (for more details see Chapter 13). If this is missing, what does that say? Is there a reason? I once reviewed a paper that didn't include a section on ethics and when I read the methods it was clear why. They wanted to do some research on body image and wellbeing among young women (university students) and found it hard to recruit because they wanted to weigh the participants and most people prefer not to be weighed in front of others. To get around this the researchers decided to conduct the study before students took an exam, making it compulsory to take part. So they force-weighed women in front of all their peers in the exam hall.

Results (may also be called findings)

This should give you details of precisely who took part, with numbers and hopefully their background details such as age, education and so on. This should also be the part where the main findings are presented – which will look different depending on the type of paper and what the findings are. In a quantitative paper there should be numbers and tables or graphs showing you what the data looks like, alongside the statistical tests performed. If it is qualitative you would also expect evidence of what was found, such as participant quotes.

Discussion

Watch out for this bit. Here researchers should summarise their key findings again, often in plainer English than previously, and consider how their findings fit in with previous research that has been published. Again it can be difficult to spot whether they are being selective unless you know the whole field. Sometimes authors will deliberately omit discussion of studies that they don't agree with or that their work contrasts with.

The discussion should always include a section on the limitations of the study, which is really important. This should be where the researchers highlight issues with their sample or methods, but they don't always do so.

How do I judge a paper's quality?

Different research designs need different judgements about whether they are of sufficient quality that you can rely on the conclusions. There is a series of checklists you can use to decide whether a paper is high quality according to its design, known as CASP framework lists. CASP stands for the Critical Appraisals Skills Programme and is designed to help you judge how reliable/trustworthy and relevant research is. You can find the checklists for all kinds of papers from systematic reviews to qualitative work here: **casp-uk.net/casp-tools-checklists.**

For example, for a qualitative paper it will ask you to think about things like:

- Was there a clear statement of the aims of the research?
- Is a qualitative methodology appropriate?
- Was the research design appropriate to address the aims of the research?
- Was the recruitment strategy appropriate to the aims of the research?
- Was the data collected in a way that addressed the research issue?

- Has the relationship between researcher and participants been adequately considered?
- Have ethical issues been taken into consideration?
- Was the data analysis sufficiently rigorous?
- Is there a clear statement of findings?
- How valuable is the research?

Taken together these questions will help you consider the overall importance of a research paper, helping you decide whether it is relevant for you and your family.

How do papers get published?

The general procedure for a paper being published goes like this:

1. Researcher submits a paper to a journal. If they are anything like me, no matter how closely they follow the rules of the paper, it is then sent back for them to format it correctly. Paper gets amended and resubmitted.

2. Editor decides whether it looks like it will be suitable for the journal or not and either passes it through to review stage, or rejects it. Some journals get so many papers submitted that only 10% might ever end up being reviewed. Others might review almost all of them.

3. The paper gets sent to 'peer reviewers'. These are other researchers in the field who have agreed to read papers and comment on them. For some very prestigious journals these may be absolute experts in their field with lots of publications themselves. Other journals might ask anyone with an interest in the area, including PhD students or those with few publications. The job of the reviewers is to read through and make comments on the paper and judge whether it should be accepted for publication or not. Most journals will send the paper out to at least two reviewers.

   This system is fallible. Some reviewers are a lot kinder and more constructive than others. Unfortunately, not all are helpful, or indeed correct in their reviews and, depending on the journal, may not even have particular expertise. Some researchers also hold biases or grudges against others. Some might be bitter and not like other people having success. Some might not have true expertise in the area and thus not spot mistakes. Others are just rushed off their feet. That's before you add in the politics of what they do and don't want to publish. Or how much they think people will want to read your paper.

There are a lot of jokes circulating about reviewers' comments. One goes 'A reviewer walks into a bar and complains it's a terrible library' meaning that some reviewers are renowned for criticising papers for not measuring something well... when the paper was never anything to do with that. Others insist you include their work in the paper, no matter how tenuously linked. There are also numerous jokes (and indeed even a dedicated Facebook group) about how critical 'reviewer two' always seems to be. Somehow you can have reviewer one love the paper and suggest small changes, while reviewer two pretty much says you should never darken the door of research ever again.

Some journals have introduced 'open review', in which the reviewers' comments are published alongside the paper with their names attached. This can work both ways. Some reviewers are probably kinder and more careful in their reviewing style. Others may be too worried to be properly critical (no matter how positively worded) because they don't want Professor Big Name to hate them forever. Indeed some may be positive because they want Professor Big Name to love them forever. All in all, review is not necessarily the straightforward process it might be. Just because a paper has been peer-reviewed doesn't mean it is perfect.

Some journals have introduced an option for the researcher to suggest reviewers for the paper. They should choose people with expertise who they think will have the time to review their work. In reality they probably choose their friends or people they know (who may of course still conduct a fair review). Sometimes you have an option to list 'non-preferred reviewers' too, meaning you can ask the journal not to consult the academic you just got into a fight with on Twitter and whose work you are criticising heavily, just in case they wouldn't be objective and fair.

4. The reviewers send their comments back to the editor who decides whether to a) accept the paper, b) ask for changes to the paper based on the comments, or c) reject it from being published in that journal. If b), the researchers are asked to make the changes. They aren't required to make them, but they need to justify why not. The paper is then either published or rejected.

How do I find journal articles?

Many will pop up in a Google search. If you know which journal you are looking for you can go to the journal homepage. Alternatively, there are a number of databases that you can use to search for topics or specific journal articles. Some trusted ones include:

- Google Scholar scholar.google.co.uk
- PubMed (National Institutes of Health) www.ncbi.nlm.nih. gov/pubmed
- Web of Science wok.mimas.ac.uk
- PsycINFO www.apa.org/pubs/databases/psycinfo
- Medline www.medline.com
- EMBASE www.elsevier.com/en-gb/solutions/embase-biomedical- research
- Cochrane database www.cochranelibrary.com

To find journal articles on a specific topic you can enter your search terms into the box. These days searches are so good that you can pretty much just put your question in. Many let you set the date range. You can also use set words known as Boolean operators in most search engines to limit or broaden your search. These are:

- AND – to search for things that have two characteristics, e.g. Pregnancy AND Flu
- OR – to search broadly for one or more topics, e.g. Pregnancy OR Childbirth
- NOT – to exclude things, e.g. breastmilk NOT breastfeeding

Does it matter where a paper is published?

There are many hundreds (thousands?) of reputable academic journals in which papers are published. These tend to be fairly subject specific, although there are some broad methodological journals. Formally and informally some journals are considered better than others. One measure that can be used is a journal's 'impact factor'. This is based on the average number of citations papers in it get – or in other words, how often its journal papers are referenced in other journal papers. The argument is that the more a paper is cited, the more important it is.

The most cited journals in health are the *New England Journal of Medicine*, *The Lancet* and the *Journal of the American Medical Association* because they publish topics that appeal to a broad readership and are therefore more likely to be cited. Conversely most journals that focus on birth and babies have a lower impact factor as they have a smaller readership and are therefore cited less often.

This is unfortunate, because there can be academic snobbery about impact factors, with pressure out on academics to publish in high impact factor journals. Impact factors can even be used in promotion or offering a job. Academics can be judged on what is known as their 'H index'. If you have published one paper, with one citation, you have an H index of one. If you have 10 papers with 10 citations you have an H index of 10, but if you have 10 papers and only six have been cited six times you only have an H index of six (still with me?). If you publish in a field which gets lots of citations, and in big teams where you publish lots of papers, your H index will be higher.

Impact factors and citations are far from a perfect measure, as bad papers can also be cited (as examples of being bad!) and review articles might be cited more than basic research as everyone cites them. It also means that fields where there are lots of researchers get far more citations than fields where there are fewer researchers. This again puts baby and birth research down the list of perceived 'importance'. High impact journals are also more likely to publish certain types of research, such as randomised controlled trials, over other types, which as we have seen can mean that social science research is sidelined. A paper published in a lower impact journal is not necessarily a less good paper.

Other indicators of whether a journal is a good one are their rankings. Each journal will usually report on its webpage where it sits within certain discipline rankings. For example, let's look at the popular journal *Maternal and Child Nutrition* (onlinelibrary.wiley.com/journal/17408709).

It has a current impact factor of 3.3 and ranks 33 out of 86 nutrition and dietetic journals and 14 out of 124 paediatric journals. That's good. Most of the decent journals (but not all) belong to big publishing houses. Ones to look out for are Springer, Wiley, Sage and Elsevier. Mary Ann Liebert is another one.

Predatory and fake journals

Some journals, however, are not so reputable. Based on researchers' need and desire to publish, numerous 'fake' or predatory journals have popped up. These publish literally thousands of papers each year, including some from well-known researchers. The list of these predatory journals grows daily – and although academics try to keep track of them it's an almost impossible task. Many of them have made it onto a blacklist found here: scholarlyoa.com/list-of-standalone-journals

If you're not paying close attention, their attempts to appear like a genuine journal can catch you out. One study found that over 5,000 scientists in Germany alone had published papers in these journals. The research estimated that over 400,000 scientists worldwide had been involved with them.[1]

It's easy to see why. Many have very convincing names, often something like the *International Journal of...*, as they know there is pressure on academics to publish in international journals. Without an understanding of the field these can be difficult to spot. For example, the *International Journal of Nursing Studies* is a well-ranked genuine nursing journal. Yet the *International Journal of Nursing* is a predatory journal. If you didn't know the field you might think that was the other way around.

Another paper published in 2015 that sought to calculate the number of papers being published by these journals found that in 2010 an estimated 53,000 journal articles were published, rising to 420,000 in 2014, across 8,000 journals. Around three-quarters of authors publishing in these journals were based in Asia and Africa.[2] A paper published in 2016 examining the issue in nursing (which would cover research into pregnancy, birth and baby care) found 140 different predatory nursing journals from 75 different publishers. Some of the main topics these journals covered were obstetrics, gynaecology and women's health, including breastfeeding, paediatrics and community and public health.[3]

Predatory journals spam academics (and PhD students) with 'invites' to publish (an actual invited publication from a proper journal is seen as prestigious). They may have fake journal editorial boards and lie about where they are based. They may put misleading or false information on their web pages about how well read their journal is. Advances in technology have enabled this to happen: anyone could set up a supposed journal by the end of the day and publish pages on their website. Some have even posed as real journals, creating fake websites and collecting the money the researchers pay to have the piece published.

The main catch is that apart from the fact that publishing in a predatory journal won't be recognised in academia as a genuine, established publication (quite the opposite, it has a detrimental effect on reputation), the fake journals also charge a hefty fee of thousands of pounds. Sometimes they approach established researchers to write a piece for their journal for free, hoping to benefit from that researcher's reputation.

These journals spam researchers many times a day. Most emails start with 'Hey' or 'Salutations' or something equally odd. Usually the invite is nothing to do with your field whatsoever: I am regularly invited to publish on engineering or dentistry, or ageing. It is infuriating when less experienced colleagues get excited about being invited to write for a journal only to find that they have been duped. There is also an issue with genuine invites then being overlooked. I once ignored a prestigious medical journal for some time before I realised it wasn't fake. That was an awkward conversation.

Predatory and fake journals are not peer-reviewed, and are unlikely to be read by knowledgeable readers. Many promise an exceedingly fast publication time (which can sound very appealing), with papers published within days of being submitted. Some will publish absolutely anything. There have been cases of academics managing to publish absolute nonsense in these journals, which would be funny if it didn't expose how corrupt these publications are. Back in 2009 researchers used a software programme to generate a grammatically correct but nonsensical paper and it was accepted for publication (as long as they paid the $800 fee).[4]

In another case, a researcher submitted a paper about the anti-cancer properties of a chemical that they had supposedly extracted from a specific lichen to the *Journal of Natural Pharmaceuticals*. It was nonsense and full of methodological weaknesses and other craziness. It was also submitted from the Wassee Institute of Medicine (which doesn't exist) by the eminent researcher Oocorragoo Cobange (who also doesn't exist). It was accepted after very minor changes, such as to referencing style. Real-life researcher John Bohannon has submitted this paper to 304 open access journals. More than half accepted it straight away.[5]

There's also a delightful study entitled *'Get me off your fucking mailing list'* which has that phrase repeated over ten pages, with a flow diagram and scattergram included (it's a thing of beauty). It was accepted by the *International Journal of Advanced Computer Technology* (sounds legit, doesn't it?). They wanted $150 to publish it.[6]

Of course, if your research is dodgy, you want it to be published quickly, and you don't want anyone to review it, so these journals are very appealing. The study of predatory nursing journals examined mean time to publication. For those that advertised this in days the mean time was 3.45 days and for weeks it was 3.17 weeks.[3] Anyone who has ever had a paper properly reviewed knows that publication takes many months. There is no way that credible peer review can be done and decisions made within three days.

Because the authors are charged, the papers in predatory journals are open access and everyone and anyone can read them. That study in Germany found that the journals are incredibly popular among pharmaceutical companies.[1] Almost half of companies listed on Germany's blue chip stock market index have had papers published in these journals, or participated in conferences organised by them. They are also incredibly popular with climate change sceptics.

This is obviously a problem, because those who are finding and reading articles do not realise that they are spam journals and trust what has been written in them, using them in arguments online and in other places as 'evidence'. It really has got to the stage where it seems you can publish anything you like and trick some people into believing it is actual science.

HOW TO KEEP INFORMED:

Check which journal research is published in. Is it a well-known, indexed journal from a major publishing house? Or might it be a fake journal? Check how many previous issues it has had. Genuine new journals sometimes appear, but many of the brand-new ones have suddenly popped up out of nowhere. The journal website can tell you a lot. Does it look professional? Who is on the editorial board? Are they real academics? If in doubt google the journal name – you may well find warnings or complaints!

You can look at a checklist of how to tell a journal may be predatory here: **thinkchecksubmit.org**

Read a paper carefully. It should give you full details of how the data was collected and what the findings were. Think about what might be missing. Look at the limitations – they can be telling, especially if there aren't any!

If you can't access a paper, drop the author an email. Their contact details will be on the paper.

11

WHAT ABOUT OTHER TYPES OF WRITING?

Back in 2011 an article in the *BMJ* caused significant debate about the best time to introduce solid foods.[1] I had a four-month-old baby at the time and first heard about it when an acquaintance waved a copy of the *Daily Mail* at me (yes, we still bought newspapers back then) and victoriously proclaimed, 'See, I told you so... and I'll be telling my health visitor so too.' She went on to tell me that the age for weaning was being changed back to four months because the experts had found that waiting until six months was harmful, and there was a big study into it all over the news.

Fortunately I didn't have to buy a copy of the *Daily Mail* to find out what on earth was going on. Which was that four academics had written a position piece, published in the *BMJ*, entitled 'Six months of exclusive breast feeding: how good is the evidence?'[2]

The actual article was nowhere near as strong as the newspaper headlines suggested. It was not a new study at all, nor was it presenting specific findings from a study. Instead it was a position piece debating whether six months of exclusive breastfeeding should be promoted. The authors put forward a number of positive and negative arguments for six months' exclusive breastfeeding, and concluded that a review of the evidence was needed. Three of the authors, including the lead author, had been involved in consultancy work or received research funding from companies manufacturing infant formula and baby foods (which would stand to benefit hugely if the guidelines were changed to four months).

This is another great example of what can happen when the press seizes on something to report, often manipulating the actual research. As I write this, a similar position piece has emerged but with a different conclusion – that we should stick to promotion of six months' exclusive breastfeeding based on the evidence.[3] This was also the conclusion of a recent review of the evidence by the UK Scientific Advisory Committee on Nutrition.[4] But the newspapers didn't choose to run with that as a headline.

Another example of a position piece that caused waves was one published in the *Journal of the American Medical Association* in 2016 entitled 'Unintended Consequences of Current Breastfeeding Initiatives'.[5] The paper proposed that the UNICEF Baby Friendly Ten Steps to Successful Breastfeeding might be having unintended negative consequences for infant health and even mortality. The headline was alarming, and the article was widely shared on social media, despite it being behind a paywall. Few people were able to access anything more than the abstract (which of course did not give the full picture). They just liked the title, decided it said what they wanted, and shared it.

Again, *reading the actual paper*, it was based on the views of three medical doctors. It was not a formal or new evaluation of the Baby Friendly Initiative. This is not to say the doctors' views were wrong, or that these individuals were not qualified to publish the paper, but the paper did not directly relate to a specific research study.

The Ten Steps is a UNICEF Baby Friendly Initiative policy

based on evidence supporting normal bonding processes between mother and baby in the early hours and days.[6] It encourages hospitals to take steps that are known to promote successful breastfeeding, such as skin-to-skin, keeping mother and baby together and not using pacifiers. Evidence from around the world shows that it helps improve breastfeeding rates, particularly if all of the steps are taken, including links with support in the community.[7]

Three of the Ten Steps are specifically critiqued in the *JAMA* article, namely skin-to-skin contact, keeping mother and baby together after birth and not using pacifiers. The authors proposed that these behaviours were inherently risky and should not be so widely promoted.

However, each of these steps has an evidence base that explains why it promotes successful breastfeeding, and impacts on wider infant health and wellbeing. For example, babies who have skin-to-skin have better temperatures, steadier heart rates and breathing and better oxygen levels. They are more likely to breastfeed as they are naturally close to the breast.[8] Babies who are kept close to their mothers are more likely to be breastfed, probably because they are fed more regularly and responsively. Separating mother and baby increases the risk of difficulties with breastfeeding.[9] The evidence is a little more mixed for pacifiers, with some studies suggesting a negative impact upon breastfeeding[10] because it reduces nutritive sucking, and others suggesting that as long as mothers are motivated to breastfeed there may be no impact.[11]

However, despite this evidence the authors of the paper stated:

> It is important to be certain that the basis for the recommendations has been documented in reproducible scientific studies and that the benefits of the practices recommended outweigh the risks. Unfortunately, there is now emerging evidence that full compliance with the 10 steps of the initiative may inadvertently be promoting potentially hazardous practices and/or having counterproductive outcomes.

One of the arguments that the authors put forward was that skin-to-skin promotion as per the Ten Steps increases the risk of 'sudden unexpected postnatal collapse' (SUPC), which refers to babies who collapse unexpectedly (not because of illness or prematurity) in the first few days of life. Let's unpack that a little.

• Firstly, thankfully, SUPC is rare. Estimates from two studies in Germany, cited in the paper the authors refer to, suggest a risk of around 3 in 100,000 babies.[12] This is obviously traumatic for those who have a baby who collapses, but in terms of individual risk, the likelihood of not collapsing is 99.97%. Babies do not commonly collapse.

• The paper also shows that only one-third of these cases happen in the first two hours of life (the key time for skin-to-skin is around an hour after birth). The likelihood of not collapsing is therefore 99.99% in skin-to-skin care post-birth.

• The other two cases described happened on the second day of life. The babies just happened to be having skin-to-skin with their mothers at the time.[12] The authors of a paper on those specific cases said there was no causal explanation that they could think of.

• Oh and it's skin-to-skin: *mothers holding their babies*. Like they have been doing since the dawn of time.

The second issue the doctors raised was that keeping mother and baby together through rooming-in might increase the risk of babies falling out of bed. In the US (where the study authors were based), hospital nurseries still exist in some places and there is a lot of debate over the move to encourage mother and baby to stay together. From speaking to older colleagues and mothers, I know this debate also happened in the UK when practices were changed. However, it is now accepted practice. Fears in the US are mainly around mothers being exhausted after birth and babies being accidentally dropped.

The authors of the *JAMA* paper refer to a US research paper which estimated the risk of babies falling out of bed in hospital at around 1.6–4.1 in every 10,000 births – again a very low individual risk.[13] This is obviously traumatic if it happens to your baby, but should we be stopping more than 99% of babies who do not fall out of bed from staying with their mother as nature intended? Falls are not an issue due to mother and baby being together, but due to a lack of postnatal care that could prevent mothers from being so exhausted their baby falls. Indeed, the authors of the falls study did not conclude that mothers and babies should be separated, but that there should be interventions put in place including: *'Monitoring mothers more closely, improving equipment safety, and spreading information about newborn falls within the state and throughout the hospital system'.*

I searched for similar statistics in the UK about babies falling but did not find them (although apparently 20,000 adults in the UK attend A&E after falling out of bed each year). However, one key study in the UK that looked at baby sleeping position in hospitals, comparing babies being in bed, sidecar cribs and standalone cots found that no baby experienced an 'adverse event'. Importantly, there were also no differences in mother or infant sleep,[14] which challenges the notion that separating mother and baby will promote rest.

If you look at any behaviour closely enough you will find a risk. Risk is part of our everyday lives. Getting in the car, walking down the street or even walking down the stairs. Indeed, over 30,000 adults die from falls every year in the US. You can look at statistics and argue risk for home births, while someone else can show risks from giving birth in a hospital. It's all about balancing individual risk against potential individual benefits and for the vast majority of babies, skin-to-skin, not using pacifiers and keeping mother and baby together will have the best outcomes.

The authors of the *JAMA* paper highlight rare risks. I argue that reducing these risks should not be down to the Ten Steps, but long before. We need to do three things: enable normal birthing practices where possible, provide far more postnatal care and support new mothers better in general. Many new mothers might feel too exhausted and unsupported to care for their babies according to the Ten Steps, but that is not an issue with the Ten Steps, it is an issue with our society.

Birthing practices can make caring for a newborn more difficult, and in the US the risk of intervention during birth is high, increasing the chances of mothers feeling exhausted, medicated and unable to care for their baby immediately after the birth. The overall rate of caesarean section is 32.2% in the US[15] compared to 25% in the UK.[16] The epidural rate in the US is 61%,[15] while the UK has a rate half that.[17]

Caesarean sections and epidurals increase the risk of the mother being immobilised for longer postnatally. These interventions (albeit life-saving for some) can also affect normal hormone patterns after birth, increasing stress hormones and reducing oxytocin levels.[18] This can make it more difficult for a mother to have her baby close to her. However, we should not consider mother and baby being close together as the issue that needs solving, rather the high level of birth interventions creating this situation in the first place. Promoting normal birth where possible would allow more mothers to feel able to care for their baby immediately after birth.

Further, you would have to be living under a rock to be unaware of staffing crises in hospitals. Midwives and doctors are rushed off their feet and have little time to sit and care for new mothers. Each of the articles used by the *JAMA* authors to critique the Ten Steps raises the issue of poor postnatal care as a key focal point. Again, skin-to-skin and keeping mother and baby together are not the problem – a lack of support and care for new mothers during the postnatal period is. We need to invest in postnatal care if we genuinely want to improve the health and wellbeing of our mothers and babies.

Finally, if our new mothers are too exhausted to spend time having skin-to-skin, getting breastfeeding off to the best start and keeping their babies close, the answer is not to separate them, but to support them to care for and bond with their babies. As a society we need to start to 'mother our mothers' better so that they can care for their babies without these statistically rare perceived risks.

Industry-funded position pieces

Opinion-style position papers are sometimes influenced by industry. The *JAMA* paper we have just looked at was co-authored by Dr Ronald Kleinman, who we discussed in the chapter on conflicts of interest, and who has been funded by the formula industry. I am not saying that this article was funded by industry, or that his opinion was definitively swayed by his links with the companies, and indeed the article states none of the authors have any conflicts of interest (although we know of Kleinman's industry links from other sources).

However, I personally know that industry will seek to publish research to its benefit through academics because a few years ago I was approached to do so. I had an innocuous sounding email from someone wanting me to write a journal article, but they would only give me more details over the phone. It turned out they specifically wanted me to write an opinion piece saying that my research showed that there was too much pressure on women to breastfeed. Aside from the minor issue that my research didn't show that, they offered:

1. To write the paper for me and then I could simply submit it to a journal of my choice with my name on it.
2. They would pay me – from a budget which different formula companies had contributed to.
3. They would also pay open access costs so everyone could read it for free (how kind).

In shock I said no – and wished I'd said a lot more in hindsight.

I'm still keeping an eye out for that paper with someone's name on it. I haven't spotted it yet. It's a murky world.

Books

Pretty much anyone can publish a book. Even if you can't find a reputable publishing house to publish it for you, with options such as Amazon self-publishing, and a raft of other publishers – many of them predatory – anyone can publish anything. I often get spam emails telling me that they can make my publishing dreams come true, and I won't even have to pay them anything (side note – I also wouldn't get paid no matter how many sell). Others even charge authors to publish with them.

This isn't to say all self-published books are nonsense. Some authors choose to self-publish to publish quickly and not involve a publisher and their interests. An excellent example of a brilliant self-published book is *You've got it in you* by Emma Pickett – a lovely guide to supporting breastfeeding. It is one of the most accurate breastfeeding books out there. There are a number of ways you can think about whether a self-published book will be useful. Who wrote it and what are their qualifications or experience? And also look at the reviews. Are they good *and* giving useful information about the content of the book, suggesting they are genuine? Word of mouth is also useful. Good books will be supported by other experts in the field.

Academics tend to publish their more academic books with the big academic publishing houses such as Sage, Policy Press and Routledge, which have a rigorous publication process. Potential authors have to submit a proposal which will be reviewed by a panel. The finished book is then often peer-reviewed by experts in the field – just like a paper – before publication. Other non-academic publishers are less likely to have peer review in the same way, but often send out drafts of books to experts for their opinion. Others will not do this, essentially relying on the authors to be accurate and evidence-based in what they say.

You can tell a lot about a book by looking at the publisher. Of course, every big publisher will have its dodgy books, and every tiny publishing house will have its big sellers. Generally you can trust the big names – the academic publishers and names such as Penguin, but it's always good to keep a critical eye as their reviewers may not be subject experts. There are a number of trusted publishers when it comes to books about babies. Of course I'm going to suggest books by my own publisher, Pinter & Martin (I read numerous books of theirs before publishing my own with them, I promise). Praeclarus Press in the US, headed up by Dr Kathy Kendall-Tackett is another reliable choice.

Conversely, there are the publishers who are quite happy to publish work that is not evidence-based because they know it will be controversial, and they know it will sell. In fact, if you are able to ignore all evidence, you can make a lot of money appealing to audiences by writing what they want to hear.

One way to consider whether a parenting book is evidence-based is to look at the list of references, resources and further reading that it provides. One word of caution here: not every book aimed at parents is going to have lots of references in it, simply because when you're frazzled and sleep-deprived you may not want to wade through tonnes of academic reference works. This is when looking at the credentials of an author can help – are they an expert in their field?

However, when they promote very clear ideas about caring for a baby, especially if this deviates from being responsive to their normal needs, you should expect there to be justified explanations for this. If a book is saying it is okay to let a baby cry, that it's okay to let them sleep in another room, or that how you feed them has no impact – you should expect evidence to back this up. After all, remember that the burden of proof is on them to prove that deviating from the biological norm is beneficial, or at least not harmful.

For example, let's look at books that advise parents and practitioners on infant sleep. One of the most respected books in this field is *Holistic Sleep Coaching* by Lyndsey Hookway, who provides the evidence for normal infant sleep and nighttime needs, and what works in gently supporting sleep in older babies. The book has over 600 references, the majority of them peer-reviewed articles.[19] Another highly respected book, *Nighttime Breastfeeding: An American Cultural Dilemma,* by Dr Cecilia Tomori, has many hundreds of peer-reviewed references.[20] Conversely, many of the more controversial 'cry it out' or strict routine-based parenting books have very few peer-reviewed references... or none. Something to hide?

Another way to consider the reliability of a book is to consider the credentials of the author writing it. This isn't to say that you have to be a professor or health professional with 40 years' experience before you can write a book, or that qualifications or professional positions are everything – they certainly are not. But considering the background qualifications and experience of the author is still worthwhile. Just because someone has a PhD in one field, doesn't make them a fountain of knowledge in anything they choose to write about.

If I decided tomorrow to write a book about astrophysics and aliens (hey, that's a catchy book title!) I would be taken more seriously because a) I have a PhD and b) because I've published work before. We could pop 'Professor Brown, global selling author' on the front and unsuspecting people would buy it. Maybe they'd read my other books and were genuinely interested in my thoughts on astrophysics and aliens. But most likely not.

But this happens all the time in academia. People from one discipline use their existing skills to write about subject areas they have no context-specific understanding of, and therefore do not recognise (or deliberately misconstrue) the subtleties of research that can be vitally important. There are a lot of context-specific details that need taking into account when you research a specific area of behaviour. Just because you are an expert in one field, doesn't mean you are automatically an expert in another or across many subjects.

Another thing to consider is whether there is balance within the book. For example, any book on breastfeeding worth reading will highlight risk factors for not being able to breastfeed and be able to signpost the reader, if not give information within the book, to what to do if you are struggling to breastfeed, and perhaps how to safely make up a bottle. Any decent book on childbirth will recognise that there are different ways that women want and need to give birth, and include information on those. Any balanced book providing evidence for a certain way of doing things, such as responding promptly to a baby's cries, will recognise that there are certain gaps in the literature and consider the reasons why parents may want to leave their baby to cry.

Beware what an individual might be trying to sell you. Is it just their book or something else? Of course, people need to earn money. People deserve to be paid for their products and time. But it is worth keeping one eye open when people are telling you to act in a certain way, or that their product is vitally needed.

One perfect example was a spate of headlines in 2011 that told readers to 'Ignore official weaning guidelines'. An expert stated that:

> In a developed country like the UK where we know about sterilising milk bottles and preparing food in a hygienic way, there's no real risk of weaning before six months... You can talk to your health visitor, but anybody who knows anything about baby nutrition will say you can introduce solids from 17 weeks.[22]

The 'expert' was not a scientist or researcher who had developed a wealth of high-quality evidence to challenge World

Health Organization recommendations, but Annabel Karmel, writer of baby food books and seller of products that focus on giving your baby puréed foods. Annabel is not a dietician or health professional by background, and developed her recipes cooking for her own children when she was worried about her baby being a fussy eater.

That's all well and good – and her books have helped many a parent come up with new meals for their babies and young children. But straying into weaning guideline territory without professional training and when you are promoting something that would increase your sales, in spite of the evidence, is decidedly dodgy.

Annabel went one step further. With her range of recipe books and products that were based around making and storing purées behind her, she took part in a debate with parenting author Liz Fraser on ITV's *Daybreak* programme. She was vehemently against baby-led weaning, stating that it was dangerous and babies would be at risk of not getting enough nutrients. In particular she said of baby-led weaning (you can watch it in the clip):[23]

> *My children would store the food up in their mouth for up to 20 minutes after they've eaten and the danger is that sometimes you'd go out of the room and they'd still have food in their mouth... They could bite it off but then they don't know what to do with it... sucking is a natural reflex and learning to swallow it something that has to happen gradually. But the danger is really that babies at six months are just not efficient at feeding themselves and from six months babies need much more than milk, particularly iron, so baby isn't going to get the nutrients they need if it's just solely baby led weaning.*

Anyone interested in the topic of introducing babies to solid foods may have raised an eyebrow five years later when Annabel published her *Baby-Led Weaning Recipe Book: 120 Recipes to Let your Baby Take the Lead*. On the Amazon page it states:

Championing a flexible approach to feeding, this book makes for the ideal stand-alone guide for those wanting to explore baby-led weaning (BLW) exclusively... self-feeding offers a prime opportunity for babies to discover their natural abilities to explore a wide variety of tastes and textures, encouraging independence and good eating habits.

Maybe Annabel had a change of heart after reading all the evidence carefully. Or maybe her book aimed to cash in on the popularity of baby-led weaning. Who knows?

Blogs and websites

The blogosphere is a huge realm, with blogs ranging from the very informative to the completely insane. Many of the same rules we've discussed above apply. Check the credentials of the author, and consider why they are writing. Do they back up their writing with evidence? At the end of this book I have compiled a short list of trusted bloggers and websites, but there are a few examples of excellent blogging and website-based resources here:

1. Dr Sara Wickham **www.sarawickham.com**
Sara is a midwife and researcher who collates evidence-based information on pregnancy and birth, particularly around the real risks for different options, as well as writing on a range of current topics in midwifery.

2. KellyMom **kellymom.com**
The KellyMom website is a huge resource of evidence-based articles on infant feeding, written by Kelly Bonyata, IBCLC and other invited authors. All the pieces are well referenced and serve as excellent tools for answering all sorts of infant feeding questions.

3. Evolutionary Parenting **evolutionaryparenting.com**
The site is run by Dr Tracy Cassels, who has a wealth of knowledge across early parenting. Her focus is on attachment

parenting, heavily supported by evidence in the area and she has a wide range of articles on different aspects of infant care.

4. Baby Sleep Information Source (BASIS) **www.basisonline.org.uk**
Led by Professor Helen Ball at Durham University, the BASIS team conducts research into normal infant sleep and shares the findings, alongside other research in the area, as a resource for parents and health professionals.

5. Lactation, Infant Feeding and Translation (LIFT) **www.swansea.ac.uk/humanandhealthsciences/research-at-the-college-of-human-and-health/research-centres-and-groups-at-human-and-health/lactation-infant-feeding-translational-research**
This is my own research centre's website. The LIFT website is new, but will act as a resource for all the infant feeding research that comes out of our university, specifically sharing articles, infographics and animations communicating the science in a way that is easy to follow at 3am when you are desperate for information but can only open one eye. Aimed at both parents and professionals, it aims to answer questions such as 'How much should my baby feed?' or 'Is baby-led weaning beneficial?' by bringing together the research and evidence in the area.

6. Conversation UK **theconversation.com/uk**
Increasing numbers of researchers are also turning to writing for the public through blogs. This is a developing skill for some, as writing scientific articles is a very different skill. Many academics have developed personal blogs, but one excellent resource to sign up to is the Conversation UK. This news-based website is made up of articles written by researchers at different universities about their specialist subjects. All articles are edited and checked for content.

Encouraging more academics to write for the public is vitally important, as some do have a habit of either not sharing their research, or sharing it in a way that makes no sense whatsoever to anyone who doesn't live and breathe the subject. This was echoed in recent research that showed that mothers really wanted to be able to access scientific evidence, but what they came across was too complex or detailed for their specific question (especially at 3am). In a great quote from the study one mother described how she ended up with *'journal level detail'* when she wanted *'mom level detail, but [ideally] you want "mom level detail" from an expert.'* This goes to show the real importance of academics writing at a non-technical level so everyone can benefit from their knowledge and research.[24]

However, we still have a long way to go. Most researchers trained at a time when not many people were reading journal articles outside of academia, education or policy. When writing them, they were writing for other researchers, not those directly affected by their work. The internet changed all of this – now you can search for papers easily online, many are open access and the readership has changed dramatically.

Writing style and language has often not caught up. 'Significance' means something very different in scientific language than it does in real life. Academics are taught to 'big up' their findings to get space in the journals. And with further pressure on them to now 'engage' and share their findings with the public, this means that the messaging is not always particularly useful. They are often not writing with a parent in mind, or may not realise the myriad of pressures parents experience. It's all very well to do your trial that suggests that mothers should breastfeed, but sharing that in the press without considering all the reasons why so many mothers struggle to breastfeed is unfair.

Likewise, sharing your findings that are really interesting on a scientific level but you don't fully understand the reasoning behind why it is occurring can be unhelpful. Universities may put pressure on academics to release early stage findings and in fact the public can put pressure on universities to show what they are doing with their funding. But this leads to headlines such as ones in the press as I am editing this book around paracetamol during pregnancy damaging babies. For example, the *Daily Mail* have just run a story with the headline 'Pregnant women who take paracetamol risk giving birth to a child with behavioural problems study claims'. The article went on to claim taking paracetamol in pregnancy could 'damage the development of children in the womb, with studies linking it with asthma, infertility and autism'.

How is that headline helpful? In an article about the paper, the lead author concludes *'It is sensible to suggest that pregnant women should reduce their intake of drugs, including over-the-counter drugs, whenever possible, since no drug can be proven to be entirely safe for the unborn child'.*[25] Maybe true but paracetamol are not a lifestyle choice. They are not sweets or drugs pregnant women take for fun. They are presumably used when women are in pain and needing relief. Where is the woman in all of this? Where are the articles and research looking at how we can ensure both outcomes: mothers who are not in pain and babies who are healthy?

Importantly it noted in the article that many scientists argue that it is not the paracetamol but rather illness, e.g. infections, temperatures and inflammation, for which the paracetamol was taken that could have an impact. Which are things that paracetamol can help to reduce. Moreover, there were a number of weaknesses in the study including few women in the study taking paracetamol regularly and the fact that the researchers looked at the link between paracetamol use and 135 different cognitive and behavioural outcomes.[26] Remember from the statistics chapter, doing so many tests for one measure means that it is likely you will find some significant findings by chance.

Returning again to the ongoing issue that journal articles were never meant to be read in isolation. They were meant to be read by those reading across the topic, who could piece together the bigger picture of evidence. Instead we have journalists picking up one paper and shouting it from the rooftops as if it were the only evidence. Again, check out the NHS Choices 'Behind the Headlines' page to see literally hundreds of news headlines unpicked **www.nhs.uk/news**. But the papers love research that will grab attention. And academics are increasingly being pressured to release their research findings to the press, in press releases of a few hundred words where all the background, bigger picture, limitations and nuances of the research gets lost.

HOW TO KEEP INFORMED:

If a sensational story is being circulated in the media always check the actual research article to see whether it is new research or simply an opinion piece.

Do not dismiss other types of writing because they are not published in journals – they can be useful summaries, bringing together all the evidence in an easier to read way. Beware those pushing opinions without backing their findings up with the research evidence. The onus is on authors to provide proof, especially if they are arguing that interventions against the norm are important.

Check the credentials of any author. What is their background? Their motivation? What are they trying to sell?

Follow some trusted blogs. Exploring what a range of experts have to say on a subject can be illuminating and reassuring.

12

RANDOMISED
CONTROLLED TRIALS

Irritating person on Twitter: '*Well actually I think you'll find that randomised controlled trials are the best type of evidence there is – the gold standard in fact – and if you don't have data from this type of study to support you, you have no reliable evidence at all*'.

We've already looked briefly at randomised controlled trials in the section on research methods, but this is something that keeps coming up. Does data from a trial really 'beat' any other type of evidence? Short answer: No.

Randomised controlled trials certainly have their place. But they were never meant to be the only type of research you should consider, especially outside of clinical medicine. Often they don't find significant differences because they are really difficult to do well when it comes to human behaviour. And I'll go as far as saying that sometimes they do a lot of harm, because their conclusions are interpreted as something not being important. So when you read that a trial says something is 'not significant', always think about what it has really measured.

When can trials be useful?

It all depends on what the question is. If whatever you are asking your participants to do requires little effort on their part, then trials can work really well. Imagine for a moment you are a scientist wanting to know whether a lower dose or a higher dose of a medication brings down blood pressure best in pregnant women. (For now let's ignore the fact that ethics mean you can't usually do trials with medicine and pregnant women). You give half the women in your study with high blood pressure one tablet and half another. All they have to do is take it.

Now, to be fair, there is a problem with people remembering to take medication in general, but this should apply to participants in both medication groups and those in any control arm. And these are pregnant women wanting to bring their blood pressure down, so they are likely to want to try to remember to take the pills.

This type of trial works well because it is so simple. It doesn't involve people having to do complex things that are additionally affected by lots of other factors outside of their control.

Other simple trials that have been published have also worked well because they are fairly simple. For example, one recent study examining whether a probiotic solution could help babies with colic over and above a placebo managed to retain 76% of participants in the study who adhered to the protocol (their instructions). The study was relatively simple – give a few drops of solution on a spoon once a day. Parents volunteered for the study and were motivated to keep up with the treatment because they wanted to find a solution for their baby's colic.[1]

There are reasons why participants might not give their baby the solution – perhaps their baby didn't like it, or maybe those in the placebo group didn't see a benefit so stopped, or maybe they just forgot. But there are no complex psychological or social factors getting in the way of you giving your baby the drops if you really want to.

Trials are also great if they don't require the participant to do anything other than consent. For example, in a recent trial giving routine antibiotics to women who had a forceps or ventouse delivery, women simply had to consent and then they were either given a one-off dose of antibiotics or a placebo (saline solution). Women didn't have to do anything. Nothing in their external environment prevented them from following through. It was a straightforward, one-off medical procedure, not a long-term behavioural intervention. The outcome wasn't subjective – it was a factual infection rate.[2]

Incidentally, the antibiotics pretty much halved the rate at which infections developed. However, as only 19% in the placebo group went on to develop an infection, you have to worry, in this climate of antibiotic resistance, what routine use of antibiotics might do. Also, some women can react negatively to antibiotics, so it's not a straightforward win-win situation. But in terms of a trial having a useful outcome and being well conducted it's a great example of how useful trials can be.

So if the trial you are reading about has a straightforward method, then the study is more likely to have gone to plan. Higher numbers of participants are more likely to have stayed in the study and the results are therefore less biased by who drops out or too small because so many people couldn't follow the instructions. This doesn't mean there aren't other limitations to the research – and you should check things like what they actually had to do, the sample size, and the funding. But it means the methodology is suitable – it stands a chance of working.

The picture isn't quite so clear when it comes to research that tests more complex human behaviour, and particularly when it comes to anything to do with birth and babies. So here are some top questions to ask yourself when considering trial data:

1. Did it measure something simple?

Take the previous example of antibiotics (or a placebo) being given to women after an instrumental delivery and looking at whether they develop an infection or not. This is a fairly simple question. Infections in wounds after birth are caused by pathogens such as bacteria. Antibiotics fight bacteria. Infections are not caused by multiple complex factors. Someone might get sicker due to multiple complex factors, but infections are caused by pathogens. So if you are testing whether something works to prevent them taking hold in the first place, then giving an antibiotic is a simple (and turns out effective) way of doing this.

But lots of other things aren't that simple. Take obesity for example. Literally hundreds of different factors can increase the risk of someone being overweight, and they are often interlinked. Although basically weight is a consequence of how much energy you eat versus how much you need, many things affect both what you eat and what your needs are. Genetics. Illnesses. Bacteria in your digestive system. How much Vitamin D you get. Stress. Sleep. The list could take up half this book. Here is my favourite diagram about obesity.[4]

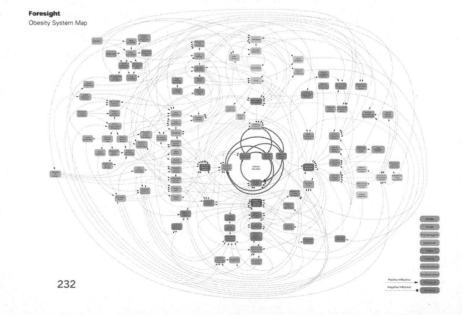

Foresight
Obesity System Map

See all those boxes? They are things that influence obesity. The lines between them are how they are connected. You can also see an interactive version on YouTube.[5]

If all these things affect obesity, and you do a trial that looks at changing one of them, what will it tell you? Can any one thing make that much difference when so many things are involved?

Of course, the logic of a randomised controlled trial is that if you have a large enough sample and make sure you measure enough things, your groups may end up similar in terms of all the other factors. But often this is not the case. The real issue is still that even if you do change one thing, it's only likely to have a small effect. It won't miraculously make all the other things go away.

Here's a probably incomplete list of things that have been associated with infant weight in one study or another: maternal weight in pregnancy, maternal diet in pregnancy, maternal smoking in pregnancy, growth restriction in pregnancy, gestational diabetes, genetics, birth weight, speed of growth, birth type, microbiome, early milk feeding, later milk feeding, timing of solids, protein density of the diet, maternal body image, maternal feeding style, poverty, maternal age, maternal education, how active babies are, maternal mental health… basically the list goes on and on.[6-8] It seems that almost everything is linked to infant weight, and they're probably all linked to each other. And now my head hurts.

A randomised controlled trial to look at whether how you fed your baby affected their weight (e.g. baby-led weaning versus spoon-feeding) would have to ensure that all these factors were equal in the two groups, which is a big ask. And imbalances between the groups could affect the outcome of the trial. Furthermore, the researchers would have to look at and measure all the factors – which would be so time-consuming, expensive and downright irritating that it's never happened. There are so many gaps in our knowledge. For example, I recently asked Twitter (as it always has the answer somewhere) whether anyone knew of a trial looking at infant feeding and weight outcomes that had measured genetic susceptibility to over-eating and overweight. One small study was offered, but it wasn't actually a trial, just a study looking at those two things.

In scenarios like obesity and infant weight, what's probably more important is the overall pattern. More researchers are starting to ask questions like 'How do multiple factors affect obesity?' They are using data from cohort studies to look at the risk of a baby being overweight if they have two risk factors or ten risk factors. How do different risk factors add up? If a baby is a normal birth weight, is born vaginally, has skin-to-skin contact, is breastfed, is introduced to solids at six months, is allowed to eat at their own pace, is offered healthy foods, their parents have plenty of money, their parents are healthy... (and so on and so on), what is the outcome? This kind of work cannot be done through trials.

2. How many people stuck to what they were told to do?

Just because you recruit people into a trial doesn't mean they will do what you ask them to do. One of the key parts of considering whether the results of a trial are meaningful is to look at something called the 'adherence rate'. Did people stick to what they were asked to do?

Even in medical research where you're just asking people to take a pill, some forget. Or they experience real or imagined side-effects. Or get bored. Or even want to sabotage your research. If they are being asked to do something far more complicated, every day, maybe multiple times a day... will they stick to it?

Unfortunately, 'not doing what you're told' is common in trials, especially when the behaviour isn't straightforward or could be affected by lots of different things. For example, in the recent EAT study (Enquiring About Tolerance), which often makes the news headlines, mothers were randomised to introduce solids (particularly allergenic foods) to their baby at either three months or six months. The researchers believed that early introduction of foods babies are more likely to develop allergies to would help reduce food allergies in susceptible babies. But when the study was published, the adherence rates were really low, particularly in the group who were randomised to start solids at three months old. Just 43% of mothers followed the guidelines for that group. One of the biggest reasons for non-adherence was 'maternal distress' (presumably due to trying to persuade a baby that can't even sit up to eat solid foods). That's *a lot* of non-adherence.

Another example is in a trial of baby-led weaning versus spoon-feeding in New Zealand, comparing weight and eating behaviour.[12] The researchers had hypothesised, based on other research, that baby-led weaning would lead to a lower risk of overweight and greater ability of babies to regulate their appetite compared to spoon-feeding. But the findings showed no impact of weaning approach on weight,[13] despite observational research comparing different approaches showing a difference.[14,15]

Again, adherence was a potential issue. Just like many other behavioural trials, the baby-led and spoon-feeding groups weren't completely distinct from each other. It wasn't as if in the baby-led group all babies just fed themselves and in the spoon group all babies were spoon-fed. In fact, at seven months, 52% of food eaten was 'fed by adult and child' in the control group compared to 44% in the baby-led group. So in fact around half the babies in each group were fed in a similar way. The difference came for the other half – 27% of meals were fed by an adult in the control group compared to 2% in the other group, and 9% of meals were self-fed by the baby in the control group compared to 40% in the other group.

There is no way around this. In both cases it is possible

that the results would be different if everyone had actually stuck to their group. But unless you took the babies away at three months, kept them locked in cages for the next year and rigidly fed them according to their designated arm... you could never ensure a fair test. Ethics review boards would have an issue with that approach. And even if it went ahead, the set-up would be so different to real life that your results wouldn't be generalisable. Researchers can never win.

All this shows why qualitative research is important. It can tell you *why* people didn't stick to the protocols. Okay, so you could do a tick box questionnaire – but to really understand people's motivations and experiences you need to go deeper. What were they struggling with? Or could they just not be bothered? We could learn a lot from that.

So, you've looked at the adherence rate and checked how low or high it is. The next question to ask is '*Whose data was analysed?*' In a trial you can do two different types of analysis:

- An *intention to treat analysis*: this is where you analyse the outcome for everyone in each group anyway, regardless of whether they took part or not. The problem here is obviously if people aren't sticking to what they were meant to be doing, what are you actually examining the outcome of?
- A *per protocol analysis*: this is where you analyse the data only for those people who stuck to what they were meant to do. Which of course means you are measuring your two different things. But unfortunately your groups are no longer randomised. The people who stay in their group and adhere are likely to be very different from those who didn't. You might as well have spent your time doing a big cohort study instead.

In the EAT study researchers ran both types of analysis. First they ran their intention to treat analysis as planned, and found no difference. Which is not surprising given the adherence rate. Then they went on to compare outcomes for those who stuck to their arm, finding some differences. But given the huge non-adherence rate, those who adhered in the three-month group are likely to be very different to those who didn't, so any difference might be down to other factors that perhaps enabled or motivated them to stick to what they were doing. Eliminating the effect of these was the point of doing the randomised controlled trial in the first place.[11]

The final part of this question is to ask how much adherence you need. Unfortunately, one study looking at adherence rates in medical trials found that once the non-adherence rate reached 20%, the results were significantly more likely to show no difference between the groups. Unsurprising, as they might be pretty similar.[10] One way around this is to recruit more people until your adherence rates are better. But this can be difficult – it costs more, takes more time and means the study findings can be seriously delayed. Roughly speaking, if 20% of your participants are not sticking to their instructions, you'll need 60% more participants to get the same power. And 40% of non-adherers? You'd need 180%. You can see why this gets problematic – and very time-consuming. And expensive.[9]

3. Is it possible to randomise the behaviour the researchers want to investigate?

Research into breastfeeding is often criticised for not being based on randomised controlled trials. One reason for this is ethics. It is recognised that infant feeding can have a significant impact on infant and maternal health and wellbeing, so randomising is not allowed (more on this in the next chapter). However, let's imagine researchers could randomise 500 women to either breastfeed their baby or not. Women are given instructions and a year later the researchers pop back and measure whether there are any differences in health outcomes between the two groups. They find some difference for some illnesses, but not for others, and declare that breastfeeding makes no difference to babies' health.

This sounds simple, doesn't it? But it's not. How many of those women, particularly in the breastfeeding arm, do you think exclusively breastfed their babies for six months followed by continued breastfeeding until the researchers came back at 12 months? Probably not many of them at all. And not because they couldn't be bothered, or forgot, or wanted to sabotage the study. But because there are so many physiological, social and cultural barriers to breastfeeding that even among the most determined mothers, many will stop before they are ready. In the last Infant Feeding Survey in the UK our exclusive breastfeeding rates at six months were just 1%. And that wasn't through choice. 80% of women who stop breastfeeding in the first six weeks are unhappy and not ready to do so.[16] So even if you could randomise how mothers fed their baby, very few people in that exclusive breastfeeding arm would be able to stick to it, thanks to the specifics of our UK culture.

One way in which researchers have attempted to tackle this is by randomising support to help mothers breastfeed for longer rather than breastfeeding itself. The hope is that this will naturally mean they have one group of mothers who breastfeed much longer than the other group. Allocation to the breastfeeding support is random, so it still counts as a randomised design.

One such well-known trial is the PROBIT trial (Promotion of Breastfeeding Intervention Trial), which aimed to compare the outcome of different durations of breastfeeding.[17] To do this researchers used a cluster approach, in which women in certain cities were given a more intense package of breastfeeding support compared to the usual support in another area – in the hope that breastfeeding duration would increase in the intense support group and they could then compare outcomes.

All women in the study intended to breastfeed. And those in the intense support group were more likely to do so and for longer. However, in real terms the difference was not huge.

At three months 73% of babies in the intense support group were receiving any breastmilk compared to 60% in the control group (and 19.7% versus 11.4% by 12 months). Which meant that at three months the majority of babies were breastfed, but at 12 months the vast majority of babies were not breastfed. The intervention also increased exclusive breastfeeding until six months, but again the differences were not huge – 7.9% in the intense support group compared to 0.6% in the control group. A significant difference in *exclusive* breastfeeding was seen at three months – 43.3% versus 6.4%. But we know from other studies that although exclusive breastfeeding provides the best protection against infectious illnesses, partial breastfeeding still helps as the baby is still receiving important antibodies and other immune factors.[18]

So this was a group of women who wanted to breastfeed and were given greater health professional support at birth and postnatally. Yet the majority still did not exclusively breastfeed, or indeed do so partially until 12 months, even in a country with higher breastfeeding rates than the UK. The vast majority of babies in the study had formula, or were exclusively formula-fed by 12 months. Why? Because even if women want to breastfeed, and get professional support, there are still lots of factors that get in the way of them being able to do so. It is not as simple as a medical trial telling them to take one medication or another – it is a complex behaviour, with many influences, that then has to be maintained every couple of hours or so for months on end.

Despite the quite minor differences in breastfeeding between the two groups, differences in rates of gastrointestinal infections were seen. Babies in the intense support group, which had the higher rates of any and exclusive breastfeeding, had lower occurrences of gastrointestinal infections (9.1% versus 13.2%) and atopic eczema (3.3% versus 6.3%). Or, in terms of those babies that developed those illnesses, roughly 60% of gastroenteritis cases were in the lower breastfeeding group and 65% of the eczema cases.[19] It is logical to hypothethise that if the groups had been more distinct, greater differences would have been seen.

However, this trial really raises the question of whether a randomised controlled trial will ever be the best study design for behaviours such as breastfeeding. It might show some differences, but given the overlap between the two groups they would probably be much bigger if you were actually comparing two distinct groups. Researchers might be better off spending their time elsewhere, looking at large cohort data, for example. This is why you won't find many trials looking at health outcomes in babies breast or formula-fed. Importantly, this doesn't mean that there is a lack of evidence about breastfeeding (despite what people on Twitter might say). It just means that relevant randomised controlled trials are few and far between, for good reasons.

4. Check how many people withdrew from the study

Alongside looking at how many people adhered to their study arm, another important piece of information to look at is how many people didn't want to take part in the first place, particularly if they withdrew between being randomised to their group and starting the study. Why is this important? If the numbers are large, it tells you that certain people may not have wanted to take part in the study (meaning the study is less representative of the general population) or people only agreed to take part if they were randomised to the arm they wanted to be in (meaning the randomisation part of the trial is much less random than it appears).

If the trial is looking at behaviours that people feel very strongly about (like pretty much everything to do with babies) it is likely that the group of people who decide to take part are fairly ambivalent about that topic – and therefore might be different to the general population in lots of ways. For example, if you approach mothers and say you'd like them to sign up to a study that compares different ways of giving your baby solid foods, such as baby-led weaning or spoon-feeding, you'll find that those who have already decided on a preferred way are unlikely to take part as they don't want to be randomised. Or, you might have some who agree to be randomised but only agree to stay in the trial if by chance they are given their preferred option. If someone who would prefer to spoon-feed is placed in the baby-led weaning arm, they might drop out before the trial begins.

So look at how many people were invited to take part. Often you can find this in the methods section of the paper – there is likely to be a flow diagram of the number of potential participants at the start through to how many were still in the study at the end. Looking again at the EAT study,[11] of 3,716 mothers who contacted the team for more information and who were eligible to take part in the study (so already a select group who were interested in taking part in such research and actually remembered to contact the team):

- 2,397 chose not to take part (64.5% of those initially interested).
- 1,303 were actually enrolled and were randomised – 651 to standard introduction and 652 to early introduction.
- After randomisation 43 withdrew from the standard group and 69 from the early group. So 6.6% of the standard compared to 10.6% of the early.
- In terms of adherence data, 81 in the early group had *missing data* compared to just 31 in the standard group (13.9% versus 5.1%).

By the time the analysis was completed, the early group had just 486 participants compared to 564 in the standard group. And that was before adherence was checked. Although some dropped out for unrelated reasons, such as family issues, emigrating and wider family health issues, the number who dropped out because they were unhappy with participating or who simply disappeared without giving a reason was much higher in the early group (n=49) compared to the standard group (n=27).

Similarly, in a study looking at how to support breastfed babies who had lost 7.5% or more of birth weight, researchers proposed randomising babies to either have formula milk top-ups or to carry on exclusively breastfeeding. Out of 543 babies who met the inclusion criteria, 379 mothers declined to participate (70%). Of those who declined, 63% didn't want to risk being randomised to using formula milk.[20]

These low rates of mothers actually agreeing to take part in the research in the first place are important because they mean that even if the trial goes ahead and finds a significant difference, how useful is it going to be in supporting mothers in real life? If 63% of mothers approached didn't want to take part in the trial because they may have had to give their baby formula milk, this suggests that a better solution needs to be found, or there will be a lot of women in real life either refusing care offered, or giving formula when they are not happy to do so.

In both cases those who were entered into the research had different views on infant feeding, and potentially different backgrounds and concerns, than those who didn't want to take part. This self-selection limits the scope of any findings.

5. Check the actual numbers of participants who had a 'good' outcome

It is all too easy to get distracted by overly simplistic public health messages or deliberately misleading newspaper headlines that try to tell you that just because a study is 'significant' then the results will apply to everybody. Nope. Trials look at outcomes between two groups and if one group has higher numbers than the other, that is deemed significant. But it certainly doesn't mean that all those in the higher group had the good outcome.

For example, take the ARRIVE trial. This trial randomised women to either be induced at 39 weeks of pregnancy or be 'allowed' (ha!) to stay pregnant for longer. The main outcome was significant complications or infant death (thankfully very low and not different between the two groups), but one of the paper's significant findings, which was then widely shared, was that women who were induced at 39 weeks were less likely to have a caesarean section.[21]

Interesting? Well, kind of. When you look at the actual study 18.6% of those in the early induction group had a c-section compared to 22.2% in the 'biding their time' group. So even with early induction, 18.6% of women still had a c-section (there are lots of different indicators that could lead to a c-section). You could say that statistically speaking 3.6% of women in the waiting group had a c-section because they weren't induced (actually, you can't really generalise like this because there are other issues with the study that we will look at in a bit). But induction didn't suddenly magic away the need for c-sections in all women.

This sort of study is useful for policymakers. If you are in charge of making sure there is professional care available for the 700,000 babies born each year, and you know that c-sections cost more money, you might like to do something to reduce that (if you think you have that power and the right to play with women's lives, obviously). If you see women as statistics, you'd be thinking: 'Right, for every 100 women, if we induced them all at 39 weeks we'd save 3.6 sections per 100 women which is... um... 25,000 fewer sections per year! Let's do it.'

Or not. Because there are many other ways to reduce c-section rates, including continuity of care, one-to-one support in labour and listening to women. And birth isn't all about getting the baby out. Women and their experiences actually matter too. And of course this was just one study, which would never be enough evidence to base health guidelines on. *Stern look*.

So when a headline tells you that a trial has reduced a health risk or increased a positive outcome, always ask, how much by?

6. Remember that trials often only measure the 'big outcomes'

You know, the ones deemed important by those White, middle-class male scientists. Trials are expensive. A decent-sized trial can cost more than many people's homes to conduct. After all you are paying for salaries, recruitment costs, participant costs and so on. Therefore trials are often conducted to measure 'big things' that could be shown to save or make money in the long term. It always comes back to money. Which means that when Twitter sea lion comes clapping and barking you have nothing to throw at them, not because a trial has shown the opposite, but because a trial of that question has never been conducted.

But sometimes, hidden in the paper, you might find more of the type of outcome that might be important to you. This struck me recently as I was reading a paper about a study in the US which randomised women who were having a straightforward pregnancy to either have the support of a doula or not during their labour. Having a doula present significantly reduced emergency caesarean sections and epidurals. For caesareans, 13.4% of women with a doula had a caesarean section compared to 25.0% of those without a doula (incidentally a bigger difference than in the ARRIVE trial). And for epidurals, 64.7% of those with a doula had an epidural compared to 76.0% of those without.[22]

Lovely stuff. Especially if you're that person looking at outcomes for the population as a whole. But this study also took some measures of how having a doula made women *feel*. The final line in the abstract reads '*On questionnaires the day after delivery, 100 percent of couples with doula support rated their experience with the doula positively.*'

Now that to me is a successful piece of research.

7. Sometimes trials just can't be done

'*Parachute use to prevent death and major trauma when jumping from aircraft: randomised controlled trial*'. In this small trial, researchers found parachute use did not prevent death or serious injury when jumping from an aircraft. They asked participants to jump from a plane wearing either a parachute or an empty backpack and found no difference in outcomes. Wait... what?!

I should point out at this point that the aircraft was not a jumbo jet, but a small aircraft and it was at an altitude of... zero. It was on the ground. In their conclusions the researchers declare that caution should be applied when extrapolating the findings to high altitude.[3]

Of course this is satire, but it illustrates a valid limitation of trials. Some things can never be randomised, or shouldn't need to be because we have evidence from other sources about their efficacy, including plain (plane?) common sense. Of course, parachutes have never been tested in a randomised controlled trial (at high altitude). We couldn't randomise people to jump with or without one. Sometimes understanding the mechanisms is enough – you don't need a trial to prove it.

Sometimes you can't do a trial because of ethics and general human decency. No ethics committee will let you randomise women to breastfeed or formula feed, or to have a caesarean section or vaginal birth. These things have important outcomes for women and families and it would be unethical to tell them what to do.

Likewise you would get a very strange look from a research grant panel if you proposed putting one group of women on a starvation diet so they became underweight and over-feeding another group so they were obese... then encouraging them to get pregnant... then following up what happened to them (all the time still starving them or feeding them up). And what about age? Could you approach a group of women at age 16 and ask some to get pregnant immediately, with others waiting until their mid-twenties and still others until they are 35 or 40 so you could measure the outcomes for their babies?

In conclusion, randomised controlled trials are an important part of the bigger picture, but they are not the only part worth looking at. Caution should be applied and questions asked. Look at the details and make up your own mind.

HOW TO KEEP INFORMED:

Remember that randomised controlled trials may be the gold standard in medical research, but they do not necessarily work well for behavioural research.

A lack of trial data doesn't mean there is no evidence for something. Likewise, one trial does not win over a whole bank of cohort studies just because it is a trial. It's about the bigger picture.

Always check the adherence rate, the crossover in behaviour between groups and what type of statistical analysis was performed. Remember that low adherence rates can mean false conclusions.

If a behaviour cannot be randomised for ethical reasons, as with breastfeeding, isn't that enough reason to believe that it is important? Instead we should invest research money into understanding how we can better support mothers.

If we want to do research in order to understand a desired behaviour that has low take-up in a community, why do we think we can randomise people to that behaviour when there are major barriers preventing them from following that behaviour in the first place?

Randomised controlled trials tend to be conducted by those in big institutions with lots of money and are dominated by certain demographics. They often do not answer the questions mothers and families want answers to.

13

MORE ABOUT
ETHICS

Another day, another Twitter sea lion: *'But where is the evidence from randomised controlled trials that leaving a baby to cry for hours harms them?'*

The answer to this, as we saw in the previous chapter, is that there isn't any evidence like that because of research ethics. You can't go around leaving babies to cry, telling women to give birth a certain way or telling women to feed their babies a certain way. Thankfully. So there will never be data from randomised controlled trials on these issues.

Why are ethics important?

Researchers are bound to do no harm to their participants through the data they collect. This means that when we already have a body of evidence for a topic (or a bit of common sense), you cannot randomise people to an arm that might harm them. Nor can you cause distress through your research questioning. This means that some areas of study will never be randomised, and some areas of study need years of data collection, training and sensitivity to conduct.

A brief historical overview of research and ethics is important to remind us just how much this matters. Researchers did not always need ethical permission. Individual countries had some guidance, but this was often not upheld. Although not all took advantage of this, many undertook research which ranged from inappropriate to barbaric. This came to a head after World War II when the atrocities of the experiments that scientists had conducted came to light during the Nuremberg trials.

From December 1946 to August 1947 Nazi researchers and medics were put on trial as part of a series of trials for war crimes. This was known as the Doctors' Trial. Twenty-three scientists were held accountable for the experiments they had conducted during the war. It transpired that scientists had killed, disfigured and disabled many, many victims in concentration camps – in ways that would now be termed medical torture.

Experiments on twins, and on people with disabilities and those from Jewish communities were particularly common. Research on children was also common. In research led by Josef Mengele, almost 3,000 twins were thought to have died. Often experimentation was done on one twin, and comparison made with the other twin – as a control. If the twin being tortured (a more fitting phrase than 'experimented on') died, the other twin was often killed at the same time to compare the state of each.

The 'rationale' for these experiments was to aid the German military, for example by understanding the effect of extreme cold temperatures on the body, or exertion, or medications. The doctors and scientists justified this by saying it was the same as Allied troops bombing them and causing casualties – in other words, the subjects were collateral damage. I won't go further into the specific details here – they are too distressing and also freely available to read online. However, the trials found 16 of the 23 guilty, with seven receiving death sentences and the rest imprisoned, several for life.[1]

The result of this trial was the Nuremberg code – a set of 10 ethical principles for researchers and scientists to adhere to when conducting research with humans.[2] At a later date the Declaration of Helsinki was developed by the World Medical Association based on these principles.[3] The declaration is a series of guidelines that any researcher conducting a study with human participants should follow. It is not legally binding as such, but adherence to it is a generally accepted standard. The declaration is long, but the basic principles are:

1. The wellbeing of any participant always takes precedence over the need for research. If it cannot be conducted in a way that does not harm the individual it should not be done, or should be stopped if harm emerges.
2. Respect for the individual and their dignity must be at the heart of the research. This is one reason why the research community now uses the word 'participants' rather than the word 'subjects', which implied the individuals were being subjected to the research.
3. The participant should never be put under any pressure to take part. They can withdraw at any point. They must receive sufficient information about what the research involves to allow them to make an informed decision about whether to take part.
4. Individuals who may not be able to give informed consent, such as children or those with physical or mental disabilities, should have someone who cares for them to give consent (although they should also be asked, where possible).
5. Research should bring a benefit to others (even if just a small specific group) and therefore those conducting it should have a good understanding of the issue and how to collect data that will be useful. The researcher should have an informed belief that a benefit will arise.
6. Any data from the research should be as anonymous and confidential as possible. Every effort should be made to report on aggregated findings across a sample if possible.

If a participant might potentially be identifiable (e.g. they have a specific rare medical condition) this risk should be explained to them.

Do we need such strict ethics codes?

Yes. Even outside of war, a number of researchers have had dubious ideas about what is acceptable in the pursuit of greater understanding of human behaviour. And not just medical scientists developing medical treatments. A brief trawl through the history of psychological research brings up some eye-opening examples. In particular, there was a whole raft of psychological experiments, often conducted with the consent of parents, carried out on children in the middle of the 20th century. At the time they were seen as acceptable (although I'm sure not everyone felt that way). But they are very good examples of why strict ethics codes are needed.

Little Albert

Little Albert was a nine-month-old boy whose mother was paid $1 for her son's participation in Watson and Rayner's research study at Johns Hopkins university in the US in 1920. They wanted to know how we learned to become fearful of things. Having watched Pavlov's experiments conditioning his dogs to learn to associate a light or noise with food, they wanted to know whether fear could be transferred to different situations.

They let Little Albert play with a tame, fluffy white rat – which he quite happily accepted. Then, when he was calmly playing with it, they crept up behind him and made a loud, sudden noise that made Albert cry. They kept doing this – giving him the rat, then making the noise. As predicted, after a few tries, Albert became very fearful of the rat even without the noise. He went on to become fearful of things that reminded him of the rat, such as big white beards.

Long term we do not know what happened to Albert. Attempts to trace him found he had died aged six of acquired hydrocephalus. There were also suggestions that Albert already had some kind of neurological impairment before the study started, but despite any of that, terrifying children in the name of science is not something you can now get away with.[4] Thank goodness.

The Bobo doll experiment

This is another 'classic' taught in psychology. Short version of a longer story: children were invited to watch a video of an adult beating up a large human dummy. The adult spent at least 10 minutes hitting and shouting at the dummy. The researchers then let the children loose on the dummy to see what would happen. Children, regardless of whether they had shown previous aggressive tendencies, started to hit and shout at the dummy in the same way. Teaching kids to be violent – yay![5]

The Monster study

Dr Wendell Johnson wanted to disprove a theory that stuttering was genetic. He wanted to prove it could be caused (and cured) by interactions. He took 22 young orphans (this isn't off to a great start, is it?) and split them into two groups. One group had 'normal speech' – they didn't stutter. This group got lots of praise and positive encouragement about their speech. In the second group, half were stutterers and half 'normal', but they were all told they were stutterers. They were 'treated' by continual criticism, and told they must stop stuttering.

By the end of the treatment, five out of six of the 'normal' children in the stutterer group had started stuttering. Just one child in the normal group had worse speech issues after the study. Unfortunately, despite the attempts to reverse the experiment, it didn't work and the children who had become stutterers remained so. The researchers also didn't debrief the children, who found out about the whole thing 60 years later when the story was uncovered and reported. The findings were never published in a paper out of fear they would be compared to the experiments in the concentration camps (did that not tell the authors their experiment might not be so great?!). Six of the participants have since been awarded damages by the University of Iowa, where the study was carried out.[6]

The triplet study

This study followed the lives of three triplets separated at birth. I am not going to give details here as the film has just been released on DVD and is on Amazon Prime in the UK and I'm not going to spoil the plot. Let's just say, that all the data is held by Yale University until 2065. And you can read details on the linked reference if you wish.[7]

These are just a few examples of the work which went on before ethics committees were a thing. People used to argue that the 'science discovered' provided more benefit to society than the harm that was done, which we thankfully now realise is not the case. I feel I need to apologise on behalf of my psychologist ancestors.

Based on this history, researchers are now required to seek ethical permission to conduct their studies (if they are collecting data from human beings). The vast majority of research you see published will have received permission from an ethics committee to go ahead. Research funders typically require projects to have ethical permission, and good-quality journals often ask authors to provide a statement on their ethical permission and how they ensured their study was ethical. This information should be found in the methodology section of a paper. Some journals ask for this to be under a separate heading, while others might include it in the participants section. If you spot a journal article without a statement, it's perfectly reasonable to ask the editors why.

This process of obtaining ethics permission involves completing an ethics form that asks specific questions about the research and how it plans to adhere to ethical factors such as those described in the Declaration of Helsinki. The basic underlying principle is that the research will do no harm to the participant. It will also include questions such as:

1. *How will you recruit participants?* – Correct answer: no one will be pressurised to take part.
2. *How will you ensure participants are able to give informed consent?* – Sufficient information about everything the study involves will be given to the participant before they take part. If the research involves anything the participant may find distressing or time-consuming, they should be given time to reflect on this and not have to take part immediately.
3. *How will you make sure participants' identity is not revealed?* – Obvious stuff like not including names and addresses in your dataset.
4. *How will you ensure participants' data is kept safe?* – No leaving data on trains…

Who gives ethics permission?

Universities have their own research ethics committees. This might be done in different ways at different universities, but often there are several committees specific to broad subject areas, so they have some understanding of the research in a field.

Depending on the type of research done, further ethical permission may be needed. For example, if research is conducted with participants in the NHS, permission will need to be sought from the ethics committee for each hospital board. If the research is going to be completed across health boards, permission often has to be sought individually from each health board – which as you can imagine can be very time-consuming (but important).

Sometimes, if the researcher works in the hospital and the research is directly related to their job, the research board will decide it is 'service evaluation' rather than research, and permission is not needed from the hospital board. Permission should still be sought from a research ethics committee though, so if the researcher is linked to a university they will usually seek permission from there instead.

Sometimes research will fall through the gaps. It may be funded by a private company who do not ask for ethics approval, it may be published in a journal which doesn't pay attention to this, or it may be published as a report for a company (circumnavigating the need for peer review).

What are the consequences of needing ethical approval for research?

Obviously, researchers cannot conduct experiments that could potentially harm people. The consequence of this is that we will never know the scientific answer to many questions about medications in pregnancy and breastfeeding, birth interventions, or health outcomes. For example it wouldn't be ethical to:

- Test a medication on a pregnant woman
- Randomise women to breast or formula feed
- Give a pregnant or breastfeeding woman a drug and see what happens
- Conduct a trial into different sleeping locations (e.g bed, sofa, cot) to see how many babies die of SIDS
- Test whether a method of introducing solid foods leads to more babies choking or not

This means that research in these areas will always be criticised for not being 'robust enough'. As we have seen, there is no ethical way around this. We can only look at what happens among those who choose to adopt a behaviour, do so accidentally, or have a tragedy happen to them. This means that it is likely that we do not know the full picture, or get a slightly skewed picture, as these situations will be measured in terms of who took part in the research, rather than who they happened to.

Does this mean that all research ends up being biased?

At this point a Twitter sea lion will probably tell you that only randomised controlled trials remove bias. Of course, after reading the previous chapter you'll be able to neatly put them straight on how not all RCTs are as unbiased as the researchers would like to think. But there are also a number of things you can look for in a paper which will tell you whether the researchers took any particular steps to try and reduce bias in their sample. These details are usually found in the data analysis section in the methods section of a paper.

1. Did they try to naturally increase a behaviour in one group?

As discussed in the previous chapter, in the PROBIT study that wanted to look at the impact of breastfeeding on health, enhanced breastfeeding support was offered in one region to try and raise breastfeeding rates in one group over the other. This does have the limitation that support won't work for all women – there are many other factors which will determine who actually goes on to breastfeed. Which then reduces how random those who go on to breastfeed actually are.

2. Did they 'control for covariates' (sometimes known as confounders)?

Another way to reduce the bias in your sample is to identify the other factors you think might lead to any outcome and take them into account in your statistical analysis. For example, going back to that common suggestion that mothers who breastfeed are more likely to have a higher level of education, and it is the education that leads to any improved health outcome, not the breastfeeding, most good studies will now take maternal education (and age, and often income or job) into account in their analysis.[9] Researchers might measure all sorts of different factors that they think could affect their main outcome (the covariates or confounders) and 'control' or 'adjust' for them by mathematically taking into consideration their effect on the main outcome and considering whether the other factor you are looking at still has an influence.

For example, if you were reading a paper about whether timing of introducing solid foods affected babies' weight, you would want to know if the researchers had controlled for other factors that might affect both when a parent introduces solids to their baby and a baby's weight. These might include parent age and education, baby birth weight, maternal own weight, whether they were breastfed and so on. Good research will control for things like this. If it doesn't you might be more cautious with the findings.

So to sum up, sometimes we just have to accept the fact that ethical considerations mean some research questions will never be examined in RCT format... *and move on*. Other research designs, especially as part of a bigger picture, can tell us lots about the potential outcomes of different behaviours.

HOW TO KEEP INFORMED:

The first rule of research is to do no harm. Therefore many research questions cannot be answered using the methods that some might like us to use. Some behaviours will never be randomised. We have to work around that.

There are ways of reducing bias by including the influence of other factors in the analysis. They are not perfect, but no research ever is.

If a behaviour cannot ethically be randomised because randomisation may be harmful, then why on earth do we need research to prove the benefit of that behaviour?

14

CHANNEL YOUR INNER FIVE-YEAR-OLD AND ALWAYS ASK 'WHY?'

'Eating lots of fish in pregnancy is linked to obesity risk for kids' – Reuters 15/02/16[1]

Hang on, what now? Isn't fish meant to be good for you? (See countless other headlines berating pregnant women for not eating enough fish). Don't panic. Let's look at the actual research and data behind the story.

This headline came from a study that looked at fish consumption in 26,000 women in 10 different countries and concluded that if women ate more than three portions of fish a day then their child had a 14% increased chance of being overweight by age four.[2]

The problem with the study, and the headline, is that even the researchers didn't have a reason for *why* this was the case. They hypothesised that pollutants in fish somehow interfered with development and metabolism. But when they looked at whether child weight was linked specifically to oily fish consumption (pollutants accumulate more in oily fish), there was no more risk than for white fish. Also, they didn't compare obesity rates between countries, even though women in the study reported huge variation in how much fish they ate. Women in Belgium only liked to eat fish on average once a fortnight, but those in Spain were eating it nearly every day. And they didn't look at the rest of the diet. Or how the fish was cooked. And whether it was in batter with chips. Nor did they consider factors such as maternal education and health awareness (women in the UK and many other countries are advised to eat no more than three portions of fish a week because of the accumulation of toxins). And so on, and so on…

All in all your five-year-old self would be mightily unsatisfied. But that doesn't stop the media circus. However, you can look for the logical explanation yourself.

Understanding how something works – having a plausible mechanism for how it has an effect – is really important. If you're reading a paper from a big, expensive trial and they're trumpeting a significant difference, then great, but why did that difference occur? How did it work? Which bit worked and which bit wasn't necessary? Is that logical based on what they actually measured? And would it work for a different group of people living in a different place?

This last one is really important. Too many studies are done in one place, let's say Sweden, and then the findings are used to make changes in a completely different area. Just because something works in Sweden doesn't mean it will work in Hull. Or if it was conducted with women who have lots of money and support, it doesn't mean it will work for everyone. Too much research is conducted with one group of people (often those who have many layers of privilege) and the results used to form knowledge about everyone (who likely do not). This is why it's important to know the full details of the study.

This is another reason why qualitative research is really important alongside any study that tests the impact of something. It helps you understand how it helps, or doesn't help – or how able participants were to follow instructions and actually adhere to the behaviour suggested.

So what should you be looking for in a study to understand

how it is logical, how it might apply to you and which parts are important?

1. Look at whether there is a plausible causal mechanism

A headline or article tells you that a behaviour in pregnancy or birth promotes healthier outcomes. How do you know if this is true or just a coincidence? One way is to look at the *causal mechanism* the researchers are – hopefully – proposing. Causal mechanisms are also really handy when it comes to research questions that can't ethically be part of a randomised controlled trial. Here are a couple of examples:

Breastfeeding helps reduce the likelihood that a baby will get an infection
There are hundreds, probably thousands, of papers linking reduced ear, respiratory and gastro infections in babies to breastfeeding.[3] Some people say that this is nothing to do with breastfeeding at all, and is just down to who decides to breastfeed. The logic runs that mothers with higher education and more money are more likely to breastfeed, and their babies are also less likely to get sick.

However, what we know about the content of human milk and how it helps fight infections counters this argument. Human milk scientists have found a number of properties in human milk that they know can help fight infection. These include:[4-6]

- *Immunoglobin A*: binds itself to bacteria
- *Leucocytes*: white blood cells that help fight infection
- *Epidermal growth factor*: helps cells repair themselves after any attack from infection
- *Human Milk Oligosaccharides (HMOs)*: stop bacteria from reaching cells
- *Lysozyme*: destroys bacteria
- *Peptides*: encourage mucin production in the digestive system, which then stops pathogens (harmful substances)

being able to attach themselves to the surface of the intestines.

This helps explain why research in cohort studies often finds a link between breastfeeding and different health outcomes, and makes it less likely that those who believe it's all down to who breastfeeds are right. There is a biological, logical explanation for how human milk protects babies.

Skin-to-skin helps improve health outcomes for babies
Although there have now been multiple trials showing the benefit of skin-to-skin, and a Cochrane review bringing all these studies together,[7] some medical professionals are still sceptical. Although long-term studies have shown that especially for premature babies it can reduce hospital stay,[8] and promote cognitive development and lower stress reactivity in childhood,[9] some still do not see the benefit and view it as a delay in 'finishing' the job of childbirth.[10]

Therefore, understanding the mechanisms by which skin-to-skin contact protects and supports babies is helpful in conveying its importance. It's not just a 'nice thing'. Skin-to-skin contact after birth helps:[7, 11-15]

- Stabilise babies' heart rate
- Regulate their breathing
- Increase blood glucose levels
- Increase breastfeeding initiation (and continuation)
- Reduce crying
- Reduce infant pain during procedures
- Promote oxytocin release in mother and baby
- Reduce maternal stress

If we understand the biological mechanisms by which something works, our belief in the accuracy of the findings increases. And knowing these biological mechanisms helps in helping others understand the importance.

2. Ask what the specific risk factors are and why

'Revealed: nearly three babies are accidentally dying every WEEK while sleeping in their parents' bed with 141 fatalities in the past year alone' – Daily Mail 29/01/18

Headlines like the one above can sound pretty scary (although 141 babies a year is 0.02% of all babies born, a thankfully low number, although obviously beyond devastating if it is your baby). Even though the data in the headline is accurate, it is far, far too generalised and one-sided. Another reason to go digging into the mechanisms is to not only understand *why* two things are linked, but to understand more about the *very specific factors* involved.

The concept that sharing a bed is inherently dangerous is misguided. And again different disciplines and scientific approaches can help us understand why. Firstly, the concept that sharing a bed with your baby automatically puts them at some kind of high risk is nonsense. Anthropology will tell you that around the world, sharing a sleep surface with your baby is actually the norm. SIDS deaths are low in regions that naturally co-sleep. Why? Because sleep surfaces are simple, without huge fluffy pillows, duvets or even waterbeds for babies. Beds are low to the floor, or even are the floor. It is not the bed-sharing that is risky, but the contexts that bed-sharing occurs in.[16] Yet all too often research looking at the tragic cases of SIDS doesn't take into account factors such as whether safe sleep precautions were taken.

It is not just the sleep surface that is the issue, but also parental behaviours. Co-sleeping is not one simple behaviour in one location. However, in a number of overly simplistic studies (and certainly in the headlines) all co-sleeping deaths are lumped together regardless of where they occur. However, sleeping with a baby on a chair or sofa is far more dangerous than co-sleeping in a bed.[17] This is because whoever is caring for the baby can fall asleep, suffocating them, or the baby can fall and get caught in the sofa and suffocate. Ironically, the headlines shouting 'never bedshare with your baby' probably *increase* the risk of sleeping on a chair or sofa with a baby. Parents worry that they shouldn't bring their baby into bed, so they sit on the sofa with them, exhausted, and then fall asleep.

This is where the value of qualitative research comes in. A trial doesn't tell you why parents make the decisions that they do. But qualitative research can tell us so much about why parents co-sleep, how they do it, and the wider cultural and social influences on their decision.[18] Likewise, a recent report told us how many parents were hiding the fact that they were co-sleeping from their health professionals, as they were worried they would be judged. So rather than having an opportunity to discuss safe sleeping practices, they were trying to pretend it didn't happen.[19] Thankfully, guidelines now state that health professionals should discuss safe co-sleeping with mothers who wish to co-sleep.[20]

Research has gone further in exploring which babies might be at greater risk if co-sleeping. Research into the mechanisms of what appears to increase the risk of SIDS has shown that the safety of bed-sharing is affected by maternal alcohol and drug use, parental smoking and maternal morbid obesity. For example, in one study it was found that for babies aged up to three months the risk of SIDS was:

- 18 times greater if the adult sleeping with the baby had consumed 2 or more units of alcohol
- 4 times greater if the adult sleeping with the baby smoked

A recent case-control study has shown that when unsafe sleep location, alcohol consumption and smoking were taken into consideration, sleeping in a bed with a baby in the absence of these factors *was no longer an increased risk of SIDS*.[17] Also, sometimes, babies sadly just die. Not every baby who dies in bed will have died because they are in bed. In fact the majority of babies who die of SIDS actually do so in a cot, but you don't see headlines calling for cots to be banned.

Moreover, breastfeeding was found to be protective of babies who were co-sleeping, compared to babies who were breastfeeding but slept alone. But not every study thinks to include (or has the data on) feeding, meaning the risk for breastfeeding mothers is probably lower. Again, bioscience research into how breastfeeding and breastmilk protects babies can help explain this. One explanation is that because breastmilk contains immune factors, babies who are breastfed may be less likely to develop infections. Research has shown that an underlying infection can increase the risk of SIDS. Also, it then actually increases the risk of unsafe co-sleeping as parents who do not plan to co-sleep (and therefore may not understand how to do it safely) might bring their unwell baby into a bed that is not safely set up to bed-share. Again, qualitative research can tell us all of this[18] – potentially saving lives.

Blanket bans on co-sleeping are therefore unnecessary and may do more harm than good. Some research shows that mums who co-sleep get more sleep themselves and are more likely to carry on breastfeeding. Also, when a baby sleeps next to their mother their heart rate, breathing and temperature is all likely to be more stable.[16] These things have advantages to babies too.

3. Before you make changes, dig out details of the specifics of the findings

It's too easy to read a study headline, or even the abstract or results section of a paper, and miss the details of what actually happened in any trial and intervention. This means that the findings can be extrapolated beyond what they really found.

One good example of this is the trial that looked at either supplementing breastfed babies who had lost over 7.5% of their birth weight with formula milk for a few days, or letting exclusive breastfeeding continue. In a pilot study and full trial the researchers reported that formula supplementation had no impact on whether mothers continued to breastfeed or not (measured at one week and one month).[21] These findings are really interesting as previous research has shown that supplementing with formula can increase the risk of breastfeeding difficulties and low milk supply, leading to breastfeeding stopping.[22]

However, the results of the study were taken completely out of context in the press, with numerous articles being written that claimed that giving your baby formula top-ups in the early days didn't affect your chances of breastfeeding. And that isn't quite true. There were a number of important details in the study that could mean the findings are only relevant in certain circumstances:

1. Mothers were counselled about giving formula milk supplements. They understood the specifics of the study, had the opportunity to ask questions and were generally listened to. This is in distinct contrast to many women's experiences on busy postnatal wards.
2. Women in the supplement group gave their baby *just 10ml* of formula after each feed – not large amounts. This meant that their baby was getting a small boost of milk, but likely not so much that they drank less from the breast, with the risk that milk supply would be reduced. In comparison, those ready-made bottles of first-stage infant formula milk come in *70ml portions*. This is a big difference and if you started topping up with this much milk after each breastfeed, then your risk of ending up with low milk is likely to be much higher.
3. A specific hydrolysed formula was used, which is different in smell and appearance to many first-stage formula milks, perhaps creating a separation between formula as a medical intervention versus a long-term decision.
4. A syringe was used for the feeds. This is a really important detail. There is some suggestion that using a bottle for feeds can lead to some babies then preferring to get their

milk from a bottle because the milk flows easily. Using a syringe allows tiny drops of milk to be given, slowly, with no association with a bottle. It suggests a brief intervention, not a switch to bottle-feeding.

5. These women were older than average (mean age 31 compared to 28 in the general population of new mothers) and had a lower c-section rate than average for the US (26% versus a national rate of 32%).[23] Older mothers and those who have a vaginal birth are more likely to continue breastfeeding.[24]

6. Participants were very motivated to breastfeed. Over a third had prior experience of breastfeeding and mothers planned to breastfeed on average for around 8–9 months or more. At one month 88% were still breastfeeding, many exclusively, which is a far higher percentage than those who even start breastfeeding in the US.[25] This is really important as maternal motivation may be key – mothers who really want to breastfeed will do what they can to keep going, even if their baby has been supplemented. However, others who are less motivated may struggle, finding it more difficult.

The data itself is interesting in terms of best practice on how to support mothers who want to breastfeed but are not producing enough milk. Although ideally there would be the option for mothers to choose to use banked donor milk, the study shows that when supplementation is needed and very carefully managed it may not have an impact on breastmilk supply. The devil really is in the detail though – and a blanket message that you can just supplement with no impact on milk supply has the potential to cause harm. Many articles were published that declared that you could give your breastfeeding baby formula and it would be fine. We don't know that – it's not what the study showed.

Another example of how the details really matter is the difference between recent headlines and findings in a study that looked at progesterone treatment for women at risk of miscarriage. The *Daily Mail* published an article about the 'risk being slashed' and 'thousands of lives could be saved'. But in the main planned analyses of the study, there was no difference in live birth rates for women who had early bleeding and took the progesterone and those who didn't.

What the papers picked up on was a small sub-analysis (one of 10), which looked at women who had already had three miscarriages (suggesting a genetic or physiological issue). Here, progesterone treatment did reduce the risk: 71% of those who took the treatment went on to have a baby compared to 57% who didn't. But this group of women made up less than 10% of the study participants, and the researchers hadn't planned for this to be a main analysis, so the findings were not as strong as they could have been in a larger planned analysis. The newspapers ran with the 'big' story, talking about a study of thousands of women... misrepresenting the findings completely.[26]

4. Consider whether the mechanisms might be transferable to different situations

If you understand how something works, you can apply that logic to different situations – perhaps your own. For example, the body of evidence in general suggests that breastfed babies are less likely to be overweight compared to babies who are formula fed.[27] Remember, not all babies, other things matter, and generally it's a small difference. But it is one influence that is important.

That information in itself isn't very helpful if you aren't able to breastfeed. However, the research that has been conducted over the years into *why* this difference exists is extremely useful. One reason identified was that infant formula, as it was made from cows' milk, had a higher level of protein than breastmilk.[28] Humans and cows have different growth patterns and therefore cows' milk evolved to prioritise body size, while human milk prioritises brain development.

Protein is associated with faster weight gain, so one theory was that babies who were receiving cows' milk formula were getting lots more protein, hence the greater weight gain. Around 15–20 years ago scientists started trying to manipulate the amount of protein that was in formula milk, lowering it so that it was closer to the level in breastmilk. They then did a trial to understand whether giving babies this lower protein formula milk resulted in a weight gain similar to breastfed babies.[29]

The short version is that it did. Babies who were given the lower-protein formula milk were less likely to become overweight compared to those who had the standard formula milk, and this followed through to school age.[30] Although of course, as with every study, this was a lowered risk, not a definitive one; some babies in the low protein group still became overweight, but they were less likely to. More research was done to test this, and many companies are now offering lower protein formula milk. This is great news for babies who need to receive formula.

While we're on the subject, another explanation for why babies who are bottle-fed might be at increased risk of being overweight is the *way* in which they are fed. Research shows that overall, when bottle-feeding, there is a tendency to try to convince the baby to finish the bottle, and mothers who bottle-feed are more likely to start worrying and tracking their baby's milk consumption. Some parents specifically choose to bottle-feed because they want to try to persuade their baby to take in more milk. However, we know that generally, a responsive feeding style, in which babies are allowed to set the pace of their meals, promotes healthier eating behaviour and weight gain.[31]

So although more research is needed, if you are bottle-feeding for whatever reason, doing so responsively can help make sure your baby doesn't get more milk than they need. Just little things like being alert to when they seem to have had enough, not trying to persuade them to take in bigger feeds, and not worrying too much about them finishing a set amount in their bottle. Again, knowing the specific mechanisms by which something happens stops us from taking a broad brush approach and announcing that all bottle-fed babies are overweight. And as we discussed earlier, other stuff matters when it comes to weight. Genetics and poverty are big predictors and less easy to change. But some small things are modifiable.

Related to this concept, although there is not a large amount of research, it seems that a baby-led weaning approach (in which babies feed themselves rather than being spoon-fed) might be associated with lower levels of fussy eating in older babies, and possibly a lower risk of overweight (although the evidence is quite mixed).[32] However, not all families want to follow a baby-led approach, or there might be developmental reasons why their baby can't. Fortunately, we know that baby-led weaning is associated with lots of other things that can promote healthier weight and eating behaviour, such as:[33]

- A longer breastfeeding duration
- Introducing solid foods closer to six months
- Lower anxiety around how much baby is eating
- Joining in family meal times
- Letting your baby set the pace of the meal
- A slower pace of meal
- Having the opportunity to touch, handle and play with finger foods

All these have been shown to help reduce the likelihood of fussy eating or overweight, and it is not clear how much of any outcome of baby-led weaning is due to the actual feeding practice or these associated elements. Certainly, a baby-led weaning approach encourages these things to happen, but they are certainly transferable to a spoon-feeding approach. The Department of Health in the UK recommends babies have finger foods from the start of introducing solids, so even if a predominantly spoon-fed approach is used, a baby can still sit at the table as part of meal times, eating some of what the family is eating, and playing and experimenting with how different foods feel and taste. You can still ensure that babies are spoon-fed slowly and responsively rather than it being a simple case of them finishing a meal. And so on.

A final example is thinking about the adaptations that can be made at a planned caesarean section. We know that for some, there is an increased risk of feeling dissatisfied with their birth experience, including feeling very anxious during the caesarean birth.[34] How much of this risk could we mitigate if we understood the mechanisms by which dissatisfaction is caused?

Research is exploring the impact of a 'gentle planned caesarean section', at which a series of steps are put in place to mitigate any negative impact of the experience. These could include meeting the obstetrician (or team) beforehand, and having a chance to look at the room. During the procedure small changes such as putting any pulse-monitoring devices on a woman's foot rather than her hands, running any electrocardiogram leads away from her body rather than across it, and putting an IV in her non-dominant arm so she can more easily have skin-to-skin with her baby when they are born may make a difference.

During the actual birth, the baby's head is brought out first, and they are allowed to 'rest' in this position (and naturally cry) before the rest of them is born. Cleaning the incision of blood, lowering the screen to let the mother watch (and offering the opportunity to her partner), and allowing the pressure of being in the uterus to help the baby clear their lungs can also be done. The baby is then brought to the mother's chest to allow skin-to-skin. And her partner can still cut the cord if they wish. Perhaps this approach is not for everyone – but for those who would prefer these steps to happen, we can learn a lot from understanding what can increase risk in a caesarean section and transferring this knowledge to how we can then reduce it.[35]

5. Double-check that the headlines – and the researchers – are focusing on the *most* plausible mechanisms

Sometimes researchers design studies that involve an intervention that has lots of different parts to it. Sometimes they will be most focused on one part (accidentally or deliberately), and when they find their intervention works, they concentrate on that, giving all sorts of plausible (and less so) explanations for why it works.

One good example is a well-publicised study that looked at the outcomes of controlled crying. The researchers randomised different areas of Victoria in Australia to be intervention sites or control sites. Women living in those areas were recruited into the trial if they reported that their baby had a sleep problem at 7–8 months old (note – this was a self-defined sleep problem). Researchers measured maternal mental health and infant sleep issues before and after the intervention.[36]

Those in the intervention group were offered guidance on two forms of sleep training – controlled crying (leaving their baby to cry for increasing amounts of time) or 'camping out' (sitting with their baby until they fell asleep). The control group was not offered any intervention.

The findings showed that at 10 and 12 months the intervention group number reported fewer sleep difficulties than the control group, with lower incidences of postnatal depression at 10 months (but just a lower score at 12 months). So the sleep training worked?

Possibly. But we can't tell. The issue with this study is that the package of support offered to the intervention group didn't just include guidance on controlled crying/camping out. It also included:

- Information about normal sleep patterns in babies age 6–12 months
- Learning about sleep associations
- A nurse to talk to about their baby's sleep issues

- Opportunity to make a sleep plan with the nurse
- Filling out a sleep diary
- Advice on how to look after their own wellbeing

When asked which elements of the intervention mothers found helpful, 78% found the controlled crying information useful and 17% the camping out info. But what was most interesting was that 93% rated 'having someone to talk to' as helpful. Other things mothers found useful were:

- Learning about sleep associations (79%)
- Normal infant sleep info (70%)
- Having sleep cycles explained (60%)
- Filling out a sleep diary (59%)

Mothers in the intervention group were also far more likely to proactively seek support from others with their baby. So a better conclusion for this study would be – mothers of frequently waking infants benefit from having further specialist health professional support, predominantly from having someone to talk to. That is not the same thing as controlled crying supporting maternal wellbeing and infant sleep!

A better design would have been to offer all mothers the basic package of normal infant sleep information and someone to talk to, and have those in the intervention group practise the controlled crying. Then we would have been able to pick out any difference. Would the intervention have worked if women were just counselled and cared for? Did the intervention work because women felt happier, calmer and had more realistic expectations of infant sleep? I'd bet my life savings on it.*

6. If a headline seems too good (or insane) to be true, check that any mechanism is actually plausible

'Like it or loathe it, but Marmite could help prevent millions of miscarriages and birth defects around the world' Daily

---

* As a millennial in today's housing market I don't actually have any life savings, but I do very much believe this is the reason why the trial 'worked'.

Telegraph, 10/08/17

This was a small case-study based design, with just four families included who had children with birth defects, three of whom also happened to have had repeated miscarriages. The researchers were looking for genetic clues, mainly for the birth defects, and reported that these four families were examples where the children had a genetic mutation that prevented the production of an enzyme responsible for cell signalling.[37]

So... how is that linked to Marmite, exactly? Working backwards...

a. Vitamin B_3 is needed in the production of this enzyme
b. In mice who had the same mutation and had previously had miscarriages (where you find these specific mice I am not sure), vitamin B_3 supplements reduced their miscarriages
c. Marmite has a lot of vitamin B_3 in it

So if you're in the 'loathe it' camp and are looking to get pregnant, you'll be relieved to know that there's no need to start mainlining the Marmite.

HOW TO KEEP INFORMED:

Always ask why: why have the findings emerged? What is the mechanism or theory of change? Or is it caused by another factor?

Understanding how things work can tell us a lot that we might not necessarily be able to show in a trial (due to ethics or low adherence rates).

Asking why helps us transfer knowledge from one context to another, for example by understanding that responsive feeding is important across all stages and methods of feeding.

Asking why lets us hone our interventions to make sure we are not recommending practices unnecessarily.

15

WHO TOOK PART?

True story: a friend of mine at university once collected data for a mini research project (thankfully not published) looking at public perceptions of football. It was during a World Cup year, so, clearly inspired by the building passion, she thought she'd ask how much people liked football and whether their gender mattered. She of course spent most of the term procrastinating, so handily collected the data one afternoon among fellow students... at the regular uni football matches. Strangely enough, most people liked football. And 'even the women' (gender stereotypes aplenty there!) liked it too. Who'd have thought?

Now we can hope that this example is just an amusing anecdote, but unfortunately many research samples don't look anything like the population the researchers want to generalise the findings to. So knowing who took part in a research study is really important, as it can tell us whether enough people were included for the results to actually mean anything, and who if anyone they might apply to.

In research we can never ask everyone in the world to take part. What we have to do is measure or explore things in a smaller group of people (which could range from around eight to 800,000 or more) and hope that they have enough similarities with the wider population that we can extrapolate or generalise the findings from our sample to the wider group. In some cases this might be the general population, but in others it might be smaller (for example pregnant women), or even more specific (pregnant women with pre-eclampsia).[1]

What should you look for in a sample?

Hopefully, the researchers will have collected lots of background data on their participants and offered it to you in a table in their paper so you can judge whether you think it can be applied to a wider group. Every research paper should have a section on who took part, including things like how many participants overall, their sex, age, education, location and any other defining characteristics. Often papers will state what the 'inclusion criteria' are (what characteristics participants must have to take part) and also the 'exclusion criteria' (what characteristics would stop them taking part). So what should you look for specifically?

1. Look at who took part – how closely do they represent the general population?
Unfortunately, every research study has some degree of bias in who decides to take part, unless perhaps they have used clinical records. Even then, not every woman will have full data, and some of those may be women who haven't attended health appointments. These women are those most likely to be living in deprived or stressful circumstances, immediately adding a layer of bias into who has taken part in every study.[2] Ideally, you want to see that the sample has a wide spread. Some things you might want to look for are:

- *Maternal age:* often women who are older are more likely to take part, but this means that the sample could have a different physiological and psychological profile compared to younger women. Why? Maybe the topic appeals more, or they feel more able to share their experiences. Has the study in some way put younger women off? Sometimes, however, you will find that women will be much younger than average, which can also suggest there is a reason why older women are declining to take part.

- *Maternal education:* as with maternal age, often women with higher levels of education decide to take part. This means that the findings may only be applicable to those with a higher level of education. If researchers have looked at health or developmental outcomes, the women's higher education level might be skewing things. If the researchers designed an intervention, such as perhaps an antenatal class, and found it worked but the women in the sample were very well educated, you have no idea whether those with different educational qualifications will find it relevant or useful.[3]

- *Ethnicity/race:* so much research is conducted without a diverse range of participants, particularly in the UK. Often data on ethnicity isn't even collected and, when it is, is often skewed towards White participants. Research in the US usually has more diverse participant backgrounds, but often seems to collect data only to make comparisons between ethnic groups about 'problem behaviours' such as obesity or smoking, rather than working with a diverse range of participants to ensure findings are relevant to all. Often participation is low because the research topic does not appeal, or people do not feel included or valued, or indeed feel judged by participation. This is exacerbated by very low levels of diverse representation across researchers, and a long history of White men turning up to collect data from 'different cultures' (communities of colour), rather than researchers coming from within the communities. This is a huge topic in itself and I suggest you read something much more detailed such as *White Logic, White Methods: Racism and Methodology*, edited by Tukufu Zuberi and Eduardo Bonilla-Silva.[4]

All of this means that our research understanding is skewed towards White participants (and outside of perinatal research towards men[5]), which in turn contributes to statistics such as those that show Black women in the UK are five times more likely to die during childbirth.[6]

2. Where and when was the study conducted?

Where was the data collected? This is really important, particularly in research that is calculating the risks of something happening during pregnancy, birth or with your baby. You need to read something that has data collected in whatever country is relevant to you. For example, rates of birth interventions are far higher in the US, so if you give birth in the US you will want to put your risk in that context.[7] Meanwhile, if you are wondering what your chances of breastfeeding are in Scandinavia, support for breastfeeding is much higher there, meaning breastfeeding rates will generally be better.[8] Likewise, it's important to think about the date of when people took part. This is not to say that older studies are not relevant, but given healthcare practice and behaviours change over time, the findings might no longer be so applicable.

One good example of the importance of location is a review paper that collected data on how many breastfed babies become dangerously dehydrated in the days after birth. There have been many scary headlines in the press recently about babies who have died because they didn't get enough breastmilk. Often there is a complex story, and tragically families haven't received the support and information they needed. But increasingly I see statistics from specific studies in the US used to tell women more generally that the risk of their baby becoming dehydrated is much higher than it is.

When babies don't get enough milk in the early days after birth, the risk is that their sodium levels will rise to a dangerous level. Medics generally consider a level of ≥ 150 mmol/L to be dangerous and needing treatment. When this happens due to a low intake of breastmilk it is called breastfeeding hypernatraemia.[9] One sign that babies aren't getting enough milk after birth is that they lose a lot of weight. It is normal for babies to lose some weight after birth, but if this goes over 10% then it is a potential sign that they may be becoming dehydrated (and that their sodium levels are rising).

Firstly, it's important to recognise that if a baby loses over 10% of birth weight it *might* be an issue – it isn't always. It is a warning sign to check what's going on. Some babies will lose more weight after birth if their mother had an IV drip during labour, it was particularly hot on the ward or they emptied their bladder just before weighing.

So what is your individual risk of your baby having breastfeeding hypernatraemia? It turns out that it differs according to where you live. I summarise the research on the topic below:

1. Study in Italy of 686 healthy breastfed babies:[10] 7.7% lost more than 10% of birth weight, but only 2.8% of those babies had a sodium level ≥150 mmol/L.
2. In a retrospective study in the UK,[11] the risk of a sodium level level ≥160 mmol/L was 71 per 100,000 breastfed infants (1 in 1,400).
3. In a Dutch national study looking at records for all babies readmitted during the first year of life:[12] roughly 58 in 100,000 babies were readmitted for dehydration, with the number who were at serious risk of hypernatraemia at 20 cases per 100,000. However, only 2 in 100,000 had documented cases of hypernatraemia.
4. In a US study of 3,718 breastfed babies[13] 71 were readmitted with hypernatraemic dehydration – a much higher rate of 1.9%.

Why are the rates so different? Data can vary slightly from study to study, but there are a number of risk factors for weight loss and dehydration.[14,15] These include:

- Caesarean section
- Birth complications and interventions
- Breast anomalies such as insufficient tissue
- Breastfeeding difficulties
- Maternal obesity
- Delayed feeding
- Fewer feeds

In countries that have good breastfeeding support and a lower level of birth interventions you would expect to see lower levels of breastfeeding complications. Just comparing the US and Dutch studies:[16,17]

- Obesity levels are lower in the Netherlands
- Healthcare is generally better for your average mother in the Netherlands
- Breastfeeding rates and therefore breastfeeding knowledge and support are higher in the Netherlands
- Birth complications and interventions are lower in the Netherlands

So it's really important to ask where a study was conducted, because it's likely your risk might be very different.

Unfortunately, this doesn't stop the press trying to pick up research from one country and drop it down in another. For example, a recent article in the *Guardian* claimed that excess weight gain during pregnancy could increase the risk of diabetes in children, with the headline: '*Midwives call for pregnancy weight targets after study highlights health risks*'.[18] First of all the study didn't actually look at diabetes, it looked at insulin resistance in children, which is a risk factor for developing diabetes. So excessive weight gain was a risk factor for developing a risk factor. But also, the study was conducted in China. Chinese women have different diets, are on average smaller and have different genetic risks compared to the UK.

This doesn't mean that the research doesn't apply – but it should certainly be interpreted with caution.[19]

3. How were people asked to take part in the research?
How people are invited to take part in research very much depends on the research question. Sometimes existing data is used, so no one has to consent to taking part. This might include anonymised hospital record data, for example. Sometimes, everyone who gives birth in a hospital at a certain time might be invited to take part in a longitudinal study.

Usually studies that have smaller numbers, such as trials, or a questionnaire or interview study, have to decide how they are going to recruit their participants. There are various sampling techniques a researcher could use to select people to invite to take part:

- *Random:* no bias or selection whatsoever. Perhaps every fifth woman on a waiting list in a clinic is approached, or every tenth person in the street. No specific characteristics are used.
- *Stratified:* this is like a random sample, but there are targets for specific inclusion of a range of participants from different age ranges, ethnic groups and so on. This is really important when researchers are trying to get a group of participants who might reflect the demographics of the general population, with for example a certain number aged over 75 or female. A few years ago we wanted to look at the general population's attitude to breastmilk. Ipsos MORI – which conducts large-scale surveys – collected answers from the general population for us. They approached people to fit the characteristics of the general population. In the UK, approximately 18% of the population are aged over 65. Therefore Ipsos MORI made sure that around 18% of the respondents were aged over 65. You can do this with whatever criteria you think are important: sex, age, education, income, voting tendencies, occupation.

- *Systematically skewed:* this is when researchers specifically want people from a certain group to take part. For example, when we collected data comparing spoon-feeding and a baby-led approach 10 years ago, we got lots of participants who were spoon-feeding and few baby-led weaners, so we had to specifically recruit to the baby-led group to get a balance in participants.

- *Purposeful:* this is when researchers specifically want participants with very specific criteria. If you want South Asian mothers who had gestational diabetes in their last pregnancy then if you stood on the street and asked everyone who came along you might be there a very long time. Unless that street just happened to be outside the weekly gestational diabetes clinic at the hospital, I guess.

- *Opportunity:* this is what usually happens. Researchers just ask whoever they can find to take part. It's particularly popular with those who have left their research to the last minute and end up asking everyone in the pub one evening. Or you only ask friendly-looking people in the street. Or you put out a Facebook request to just your local home birth group. This can lead to bias in who decides to take part. If you want to explore public attitudes to drinking and you just ask your drunk friends in the pub, you're likely to get a different result than if you asked people in a gym on a Friday evening. More samples than you'd hope are like this, because it's not always easy to get people to take part in research.

- *Snowball:* when researchers find one participant and ask them to share the study with their friends. This can introduce further bias as friends often share similar beliefs and experiences, so you get more of the same type of people taking part.

Whichever approach you take, the sample will still be biased to some extent as you (rightly) can't force people to take part, and there is never an equal chance of everyone saying yes. Even if the researchers randomly select a hospital to collect data from (and they immediately say yes) and they then had permission to randomly approach every third woman on the list for antenatal clinic, there will be a million and one reasons why some people will say yes and others will say no. Even down to things like how unwell they feel (so your sample is low on women with severe morning sickness who are too busy trying not to vomit on your shoes to think about filling in your questionnaire), or how worried they are about their complications (so you now have only women with straightforward pregnancies), to wrangling a toddler (so you're down to first-time pregnant women), and so on.

4. Check whether they tried to balance out their sample
Sometimes, when researchers realise that the people they have attracted to their research study don't represent what you would expect to find in the general population, they might place more emphasis on certain people's responses. For example, sometimes 'weighting' is used. Around 5.5% of the population in England identifies as British Asian. If a large-scale questionnaire study was conducted in the UK and the researchers looked at who responded and found that only 2.5% of the respondents were British Asian, they might 'weight' their responses to be more prominent in the sample so that it was more in line with the 5.5% level. This is done by taking the % in the population that should be there (5.5%) and dividing it by the sample that is there (2.5%). This gives a weighting of 2.2. The same is then done for the group which is oversampled. Let's say the White British group made up 95% of the sample but 85% of the population is White British: the weighting will be 85/95=0.89. Weighting is generally only done for the main outcome measure, for example if a baby is born by caesarean section or vaginally.

Then the researchers take the number of caesarean sections in the South Asian group and multiply it by 2.2. And they then take the number in the White British group and multiply it by 0.89. They then add these figures together to give a percentage rate of caesarean that is more closely reflective of the general population. This can make a real difference to 'real-life' numbers.

Weighting is common in large-scale research. For example, the UK Infant Feeding Survey in 2010[20] weighted its responses to ensure that those from Wales (lower response rate) were included at the same rate as England. They also did this for deprivation, as fewer mums from more deprived areas took part. Of course, the real issue is why fewer people from different groups take part in research, but from a statistical point of view, this helps balance the data.

5. Question whether the study attracted people with certain experiences, which might affect the study outcomes and who the findings could be generalised to

Going back to the EAT study,[21] in which allergy rates among babies introduced to solid foods at three or six months were compared, 97% of the sample was breastfed at six months compared to an average of around one-third in the UK general population. That a) tells you something about who took part, and b) means any findings can only be applied to breastfed babies. In addition to this, 82% of parents who took part had some kind of allergy themselves (eczema, asthma, hayfever) – much higher than the general population, with a quarter of the children having visible eczema at enrolment. So although the study was meant to focus on the general population, not those with an allergy risk, those with an allergy background were presumably more interested and wanting to take part, skewing the findings.

6. Has the study put the usual crowd off?

Although many a questionnaire-based study is teeming with women with degrees, sometimes, because women who are older and have a higher level of education are more likely to have a firm view on how they want to parent, those who take part in intervention or trial studies can actually end up being a lot younger, with a lower level of education. For example, in the ARRIVE trial[22] (which compared induction at 39 weeks versus waiting to see what happens) the age of women in the trial was quite young. The median age in the intervention group was 24, and it was 23 in the control group, with only around 4% of women over the age of 35. This is far younger than the average first-time mother, who is now 30 years old,[23] and most studies would find an even higher average age again due to self-selection.

Unfortunately the trial did not explore why women wanted or didn't want to take part. Overall, just 27% of those who met the eligibility criteria agreed to take part, suggesting a lot of disinterest or dislike of the idea of being induced at 39 weeks. It is likely that women who had read more widely around induction may have decided that they would prefer not to be induced.[24] Perhaps those women were more likely to be older.

One of the major findings of the trial was that it found no difference in the primary outcome (death or serious complications) between the two groups, but did find a lower risk of caesarean section and pre-eclampsia in the induction group. The problem is that the sample was so limited to younger women that we cannot confidently state that early induction does not have any impact. All we can do is cautiously state that *in women in their early 20s, in this study* there appears to be no impact. A *big* difference to the headlines.

Likewise, as mentioned previously, in the trial comparing small amounts of formula supplementation against continued exclusive breastfeeding for babies who had lost 7.5% of birth weight, 70% of those eligible to be included declined to take part, predominantly because they did not want to supplement with formula.[25] The findings stated no difference in breastfeeding rates in the short or long term, but there needs to be an addition... *among women who don't really mind whether they breastfeed exclusively or not.*

It's also important to consider who was excluded from participating, or did not have their data analysed. In the EAT study (the three months versus six months to introduce solid foods),[21] some babies were excluded from the trial, but this didn't happen equally across groups. In the group in which babies were being introduced to foods at three months, they were tested for sensitivity to any of the allergenic foods using skin-prick tests. If a baby reacted, they were given a food challenge, and if they reacted to this, they were excluded from the study. That's fine, and good practice: we don't want babies who already have an allergy to some foods being given more of them, especially not at three months. But the devil again is in the detail – the researchers did not do the same for those who were introduced to solids at six months, meaning that any babies with a pre-weaning allergy were not excluded in this group, meaning that the level of allergic babies would be higher in that group.

7. Consider whether the sample size is large enough
Sample sizes also need to be big enough to allow something to happen. Darrell Huff, in his book *How to Lie with Statistics*, gives the great example of a research study conducted to test the impact of a polio vaccine.[26] Researchers vaccinated 450 children in a community with the new vaccine and left 680 unvaccinated as controls. So the sample size was 1,130, which sounds great. However, the actual rate of infection with polio was fairly low. In that sample size of 1,130 children, only two would be expected to contract polio in a given year. Now that two wouldn't be definite, and would have been worked out on a much larger scale of say tens of thousands of children. If you wanted to be more certain of being able to predict a difference between the two groups, then more like 20 times that number of children would be needed.

What happened in the year of the study was that no cases of polio were seen at all in the unvaccinated community.

Technically the findings didn't show a protective impact of the polio vaccine, as there was nothing to protect against.

So when health outcomes are relatively rare, it affects what type of research you can actually do. For example, if researchers wanted to look at the (thankfully) relatively rare issue of maternal death during childbirth, the only way they could get a large enough sample would be to use birth record data. You couldn't set up a trial, as the numbers needed would be huge (and it also obviously wouldn't be an ethical design).

Yet sometimes very small samples are reported on, and no difference found, despite the size likely being too small to detect anything. For example, going back to the study where they compared outcomes for babies supplemented with formula or who continued breastfeeding, they also examined their microbiome (the type of bacteria in their digestive system).[25] This is because previous research has suggested that introducing formula milk could change the type of bacteria in a baby's digestive system, reducing the number of 'good' bacteria associated with breastmilk.[27]

However, even though the overall sample was of 164 infants, they only tested the microbiome of 15 (seven in the control group and eight in the early formula group). This meant that the sample was *very* small to draw conclusions from in the first place but yet the researchers concluded that formula supplementation did not affect the microbiome. Furthermore, the researchers do not mention this small microbiome sample size in their abstract. Anyone who read the abstract might very well conclude that they had measured the microbiome across the sample.

However, saying that, although a larger sample size is always going to be better than a very small one, sometimes very, very large sample sizes (containing tens or hundreds of thousands of people) can have their disadvantages. Firstly, it is less likely that the data is always completely accurate in these very large data sets as it will most likely have been taken from hospital record data which unfortunately can have a tendency to sometimes be inaccurate, missing or not be set up for the research question.[27]

But secondly, from a statistical perspective, if you have a very, very large data set you are much more likely to find that a very small difference (effect) is statistically significant when in real life the difference is not very significant to an individual at all.[28] This doesn't mean that the findings are 'wrong' but that you should be cautious and check what the actual difference to any one individual is based on the findings from the larger sample.

One example of this that is often in the news is the suggestion that eating bacon will increase your risk of cancer, with one recent study suggesting that those who ate the equivalent of one slice of bacon per day had a 20% greater chance of bowel cancer than those who ate the equivalent of about one slice a week. However, the sample size was very large – nearly 500,000 – meaning that a very, very small real-life difference was statistically significant. In reality the findings meant that eating your daily bacon sandwich was associated with a 6% risk of developing cancer... but you still had a 5% risk if you limited it to a once a week treat.[29] For some, that increase in risk will feel too big, especially perhaps if they are genetically predisposed to bowel cancer. And there are of course other reasons you might wish to avoid bacon. However, for most of us, there is no need to panic.[30]

8. Was the study conducted on humans?
'Warning to pregnant women, don't use antibacterial soap! Chemicals in the products can make children fat and disrupt their development' – Daily Mail 11/08/17 [31]

This was based on a real scientific study. Participants were fed a chemical used in antibacterial soap and the development of their children was looked at. The chemical got into the placenta and breastmilk and those babies had smaller brains and were fatter than control subjects.

Eeeek!! Don't use the soap!

Read the small print, and you find out that the study was actually conducted on mice.[32] Who were fed the chemical, rather than using it in tiny amounts on their hands (paws). The researchers said that the chemical was found in domestic waste water – well, I don't know about you, but I prefer to get my water from the tap if I'm thirsty rather than the drain outside. If you do drink drain water regularly, or eat copious amounts of soap, this study might be cause for concern.

Animal studies (ignoring the ethics for a moment) can sometimes be useful in preliminary research to start establishing a physiological mechanism. But it is a gigantic leap from mice to humans. So please wash your hands.

HOW TO KEEP INFORMED:

Always look to see who took part – or who didn't take part! This tells you a lot about who the findings can be transferred to, or who might find the interventions acceptable.

Samples need to be big enough to be sure that any difference can be detected. If samples are too small and no difference is found, then this might be because they are too small or similar, rather than there being no difference.

The location of the research really matters. What works in one country may not in another and the risks and mechanisms in one country may not apply to another.

We absolutely must work on inclusion in research – making research participation and research questions open to all. Too much research is conducted with men and White people, thinking we can simply transfer the findings to all.

16

WHAT WAS ACTUALLY MEASURED?

Unfortunately, high-quality research from a methodological perspective and useful research are not always exactly the same thing. You can conduct a study well from a methods stance: get a large enough sample, rigorously conduct your trial or large cohort study, do the correct analyses… but that all falls apart if you haven't asked the right questions.

This is increasingly common, as some researchers conduct research that they may have methods expertise in, but very little background knowledge of the topic area. So, for example, you might get economics or gender studies researchers looking at health outcomes for a birth trial… but not asking the right questions about how birth is measured or the outcomes that really matter to women because they don't quite understand the context. They don't know that they don't know, or what they don't know.

These mistakes matter. If the researcher hasn't asked the right questions, or measured things in the right way, they are not going to have data that makes sense. If they ask overly simplistic questions then their study is either not measuring what they think it is, or may lead to them missing significance because they're not looking at the right thing. At worst they can end up declaring that something doesn't matter because their research methods weren't right, rather than because there is no difference. This can have serious consequences for women and babies, because policy and practice need to be evidence-based. And if the 'evidence' says something doesn't matter, even if that evidence is wrong, then services may struggle to get the priority and funding they need.

We saw earlier how research around pregnancy, birth and babies is underfunded. On top of this, the simplicity of some of the research means that it is not measuring the right things in the right way. So here are a few things to check.

1. Have they used measures that mean anything in real life?

Sometimes research into pregnancy, birth and babies feels as though it was designed (and then interpreted by) someone who didn't really understand how to do research in this area at all. Or indeed had never been near a baby.

Research comparing outcomes for breast and formula-fed babies often falls into this category. It often measures things like:

1. Whether babies were breastfed at birth, or not. This is essentially just a measure of whether mothers intended to breastfeed, or perhaps as little as the impact of one feed of colostrum. It could include babies who pretty much just sniffed or licked a nipple.
2. Whether babies are breastfed at six weeks. Often this is set as the measuring point in research because only around half of women in the UK breastfeed until this time. Trying to measure any further down the road becomes difficult as you risk underpowering your study.
3. Whether babies were breastfed to a specific date, but not whether they were exclusively breastfed, or when formula

or solid foods were introduced.

Very few studies compare babies who were exclusively breastfed until around six months (as per the guidelines) to other feeding options. One of the main reasons for this is because so few women breastfeed exclusively until six months in the UK – just 1% or so.[1] It would be extremely difficult to measure in a trial unless you had *huge* numbers. In a cohort study, if you had a large enough sample, you could measure this, or you could use a case-control approach in which you matched women who exclusively breastfed with others. And research that has examined the impact of six months of exclusive breastfeeding in this way does find a protective effect over breastfeeding for a shorter period or breastfeeding partially. For example, one cohort study in Greece of 926 babies found that babies exclusively breastfed for six months had fewer infections than those partially breastfed or not breastfed at all.[2]

However, it seems that those in charge of the big studies, or who have the money, are not choosing to look at this. Instead, the measures described previously are used. This can mean that evidence can be majorly underpowered compared to the guidelines.

Breastfed at birth versus never breastfed – could there really be power to just one feed?

If you look at breastfed or not at birth, that one shot of colostrum would have to do pretty marvellous stuff in order to lead to improved health outcomes. It is possible that one feed of colostrum does have some effect. For example, it may help in initially populating the infant microbiome – the bacteria that reside in our digestive system.[3] Simply put, babies who are breastfed appear to have more of the 'good' bacteria in their system, which have been associated with some positive health outcomes (although much more research is needed).[4] Breastfed babies have high levels of protective bacteria known as Actinobacteria, while formula-fed babies have higher levels of pro-inflammatory bacteria called Proteobacteria. In particular, breastmilk has high levels of lactobacillus, which helps fight infections. However, we know that once formula and solid foods are introduced that the infant microbiome starts to change,[5] so large effects are probably unlikely from just one feed.

A few days of breastfeeding will also help boost an infant's immune system as colostrum, the first milk produced, is high in properties that help fight infections. For example, it is high in secretory immunoglobin A, which helps fight infections in a baby's digestive system, lungs and throat by binding itself to pathogens that come along. Although newborn babies are born with some immune protection, this is mainly a different type called immunoglobin G. They have to develop their levels of the other immunoglobins that are part of the immune system, but breastmilk passes immunoglobin A to them from the mothers own well-developed immune system. Colostrum also contains leukocytes, which are white blood cells that help fight infection, and epidermal growth factor, which helps cells to generate and regenerate if damaged by an infection. All this means that a few days of breastfeeding, or indeed partial breastfeeding, should help boost a baby's immune system.[6]

Duration of breastfeeding matters

A longer duration of breastfeeding is much more likely to have a bigger impact. But it is often not measured, or measured ineffectively. For example, one interesting systematic review and meta-analysis paper published in 2015 looked at health outcomes for women of breastfeeding, specifically breast and ovarian cancer, osteoporosis and type 2 diabetes. It searched for all papers published on these topics and looked at the outcome based on different durations of breastfeeding. It grouped studies by duration of breastfeeding including 'ever versus never', 'less than six months versus never', '6–12 months versus never' and '12 months or more versus never'.

As expected, the longer mothers breastfed, the lower their risk of breast cancer, but from a methods perspective, out of the 325 papers the researchers discovered, around a third of them (98) only looked at whether a mother ever breastfed or not. They ended up finding that ever breastfeeding reduced your risk of breast cancer by 30%, but that statement doesn't tell you anything about many real-life experiences, as women who breastfed for any length of time were included in the 'ever' group. Many of those would have breastfed for far longer than one day, but were grouped alongside these women. There is no plausible reason why breastfeeding for one day would reduce your risk of cancer that much – and indeed, when the researchers then looked at it for the other groups, there was a 17% reduction for breastfeeding for six months or less, 28% for 6–12 months and 37% for 12 months or more.

What this means in reality is that as everyone who breastfed between one day and six months was grouped in together, and we can see from the data for longer duration that more breastfeeding gives more protection, it is likely that the protection for those who breastfed for a few days is far less than 17%, while for those who breastfed for closer to six months it is more.[7]

Overall, it is likely that the longer that you breastfeed for, the greater the protection. However, I have come across very few studies that have looked at the impact of much smaller durations, to see how long you need to breastfeed for in order to see a change. One study of 6,837 babies (combined from seven different case-control studies) exploring the link between infant feeding and SIDS found that, after adjusting for other factors that could affect the relationship, breastfeeding for at least two months was associated with a significantly reduced rate of SIDS and 2–4 months gave even greater protection. Breastfeeding for less than two months did not offer any protection, while breastfeeding for longer than four months only offered slightly greater protection than up to four months.[8]

Most of the SIDS literature suggests that babies are at increased risk of SIDS during the first three months, so perhaps breastfeeding through this period helps reduce the risk through aspects such as immune transfer, a lower likelihood of sustained deeper sleep, or an increased likelihood of keeping baby in the same room at night. Given that a few weeks of breastfeeding seemed to have no impact, it suggests that it must be something about an infant *currently breastfeeding* that has an impact. However, outside of this period, breastfeeding doesn't have such an impact because the main risk period has passed.[9]

Another similar example is some research we published in 2012 looking at breastfeeding duration and 'satiety responsiveness' in toddlers (in other words, how well toddlers can control their appetite and not overeat). Rather than the usual ever breastfed or not, or breastfed at three months, we split breastfeeding duration down into very short time points, looking at whether babies were breastfed or not at birth, two weeks, four weeks, six weeks, eight weeks, 12 weeks and so on. We found no difference in how toddlers ate if they were only breastfed at birth, up to two weeks or up to four weeks – but once babies were breastfed for six weeks or more, breastfeeding promoted better appetite control.[10]

This makes sense. One of the theories for why breastfed babies are less likely to be overweight is that they have greater experience of learning to regulate their own appetite. You cannot see how much milk is in a breast, therefore the baby is more in control of deciding when they have had enough. Conversely, with a bottle, the flow of milk is faster and there can be a tendency to try to persuade a baby to consume more, meaning overall, bottle-fed babies drink a little more milk. Cues to end a feed tend to be more parent-led, meaning babies may not have so much opportunity to learn to control their own appetite. Not all babies of course – there is a lot of variation in how babies are bottle-fed, and small-scale research has shown babies drink less if bottle-fed responsively (i.e. not encouraged to keep feeding if they show any signs of being full). But it might explain the pattern on a population level.[11]

What about partially or fully breastfed?

A lot of breastfeeding research does not consider whether a baby is partially or fully breastfed. This has a number of issues. Firstly, research overall suggests that exclusive breastfeeding is more protective than partial breastfeeding. For example, research from the Generation R study in the Netherlands, a longitudinal cohort study of thousands of babies, found that exclusive breastfeeding was associated with reduced rates of gastrointestinal and respiratory tract infections compared to never breastfeeding, but no protection was seen for partial breastfeeding.[12]

Likewise, in the Millennium cohort study, analysis of data for 15,890 babies found that exclusive breastfeeding reduced the risk of hospitalisations for diarrhoeal and respiratory tract infections over no breastfeeding. Partial breastfeeding had a weaker level of protection. For example, the researchers estimated that if all babies were exclusively breastfed there would have been 53% fewer hospitalisations for diarrhoea and 27% for respiratory infections. However, if all formula-fed infants were partially breastfed the reduction would have been 31% for diarrhoea and 25% for respiratory infections.[13]

This finding is important because it shows that, in this study at least, partial breastfeeding did have a protective effect over formula feeding, especially for respiratory infections. Too often women are given the message that infant feeding is an 'either/or' situation, in which unless you can breastfeed exclusively there's no point from a health perspective. These data show otherwise – although exclusive breastfeeding gave the greatest effect, partial breastfeeding also had a positive impact. This makes sense. Partial breastfeeding will still deliver immune properties to the baby, reducing the risk of infection, but will do so in lower amounts.

However, often the difference between exclusive and partial breastfeeding is not even measured. In one study comparing growth and cognitive development of infants on two different formula milks versus a comparator breastfed group, 99% of those in the breastfed group were fully or partially breastfed at four months of age.[14] Which is it? And the average breastfeeding duration in the exclusively formula-fed groups before they were recruited into the study was just over three weeks anyway, so what were they really comparing?

Underestimating breastfeeding duration

Occasionally research has the reverse issue and babies are only counted as breastfed if breastfed for longer, which means the 'not breastfed' group could include breastfed babies. In one study that claimed there was no difference in health outcomes between breast and formula-fed babies, babies were classified as formula-fed unless they were breastfed exclusively for two months or more.[15] So babies who were breastfed for a long time but not exclusively were grouped as formula-fed. Babies who had 10 weeks of exclusive breastmilk – which is more than 80% of babies in the UK get – were classed as formula-fed. No wonder no differences in outcomes were found! This didn't stop the media claiming there was no impact of breastfeeding on health.

Another issue is that, particularly in randomised controlled trials, some babies get grouped as a particular way of feeding, even if they do not follow the guidance in that arm. For example, in the trial that looked at giving babies who had lost a lot of weight a little formula compared to encouraging exclusive breastfeeding, over one-third of the 'exclusive breastfed' group had used formula in the last 24 hours at one month old. In fact, at one week old, over a third of exclusively breastfed babies (37.3%) had received some formula by one week of age, compared to 22% of the formula top-up babies in the last 24 hours, with the exclusively breastfed babies actually receiving more formula on average per day than the formula top-up babies (13.7oz per day versus 10.2oz per day).[16] If the supposedly exclusive breastfeeding group were having on average more formula per day than the formula group, what were the researchers comparing?

No duration given at all

There is also a much-talked-about sibling pairs study, which measured outcomes for families where one baby was breastfed and the other baby formula-fed. More about the actual outcomes later, but first let's look at this concept of babies being fed a different way. The idea of a sibling study is that it may remove potential bias from outcomes because everyone grows up in the same family. This means they are likely to be exposed to the same education and income level, and so on. So if you are measuring differences for one baby who is breastfed and another who is formula-fed, you could more confidently say that the differences (or lack of them) are down to the feeding method, rather than socio-economic factors.

The problem with this design in this particular study is that there is no detail on how long babies were breastfed for. They are grouped into 'ever breastfed' versus 'never breastfed', which could mean that the ever breastfed babies received just one feed.[17] I have read the paper numerous times but cannot find any details on duration of breastfeeding. The fact that the duration details are missing is problematic. If we knew that we were comparing one baby who was breastfed for six months with one who was not breastfed at all, we would be making a more meaningful comparison.

Another study, which also found that sibling differences in outcome disappeared (apart from breastfeeding having an association with increased IQ), did give a table of the duration of breastfeeding for each sibling. 1,550 children were included in the analysis. Where the older sibling was formula-fed from birth, 1,427 of the younger siblings were too. Where the older sibling was never breastfed and the younger sibling was breastfed (n=123), 59% of the younger siblings were breastfed for 0–3 months, and 81% breastfed for less than six months.[18] Given so many were only breastfed for 0–3 months and that babies given just one feed would fall into this group, how can you be confident that the breastfed and not breastfed babies really have much difference in feeding experience at all?

In the first sibling pairs study the concept of certain infant characteristics leading to a baby being breastfed was raised. The authors argued that larger, healthier babies were more likely to be breastfed, and premature babies were more likely to be bottle-fed, so breastfed babies would have a natural additional advantage. However, that is not necessarily the case. If a baby was born sick, small or premature, it is likely that parents would be encouraged to breastfeed that baby – but those babies would be at an increased risk of illness due to their prematurity.[19]

2. Check they actually measured what they say they did

Another thing you shouldn't have to check, but you should, is that when a study states that something happens to babies at a certain age, that age is an accurate description. For example, in the EAT study,[20] the research papers and news headlines all talked about the fact that babies in the early introduction group were given solid foods from three months old. That wasn't quite true. This was the *earliest* point that babies could be introduced to solids, but many did so later. Also, parents/carers were given a timetable for when to introduce the specific allergenic foods the study was measuring. Babies were not introduced to allergenic foods for at least 5–7 days after starting weaning (they were on baby rice and fruit/veg purée before this), but actually the mean age of introduction of the allergenic foods was 20 weeks – which is very different from 12 weeks.

3. Consider whether the outcome chosen is logical

Another issue is that sometimes studies decide to use outcome measures that have nothing to do with the behaviour in question (or you would expect a weak effect) and then they use their usually non-significant finding to suggest that everything about that behaviour is overestimated and flawed.

For example, in the first sibling study discussed above, the researchers concluded that there were no differences in outcomes for children dependent on whether they were breastfed or not. However, the chosen outcomes were fairly unusual. Most studies looking at breastfeeding outcomes look at things that you could logically expect feeding to make a difference to, based on differences in milk content, such as infections or obesity. However, in the sibling study they compared outcomes such as behavioural compliance, parental attachment and hyperactivity when the babies were school children, finding no differences and concluding that breastfeeding has no long-term impact.[17] I'm not entirely sure why breastfeeding would affect the behavioural compliance of a seven-year-old, but of course the newspapers took the opportunity to declare breastfeeding pointless.

To be fair to the researchers, they did also look at some more sensible outcomes, such as obesity, asthma and intelligence, again finding no difference. Generally the research is mixed for the impact of breastfeeding on long-term asthma and intelligence, depending on the study design used. But as we have seen, we have no idea from the study just how long the breastfed babies were breastfed for. If they were only breastfed for a few days, I wouldn't expect there to be any long-term impact upon intelligence or obesity.

However, other studies that have used a sibling model (but are less well publicised because the headlines would be less sensational) have found a protective effect of breastfeeding when the outcome variables used are more suitable. For example, one study in the US looking at sibling pairs where one was breastfed and one was not found that among teens, the breastfed sibling was on average 0.39 standard deviations lower than their sibling in weight, which actually equates to 13 pounds.[21]

In terms of other outcome measures, another recent study looked at differences in bonding and attachment between babies who were breast or formula-fed, finding no difference. The authors claimed that this proved that breastfeeding did not increase maternal infant bonding.[22] This is not a conclusion that can be drawn. What the authors *can* say is that there was no difference in attachment *between the breast and formula-fed babies studied*. However, they cannot say that breastfeeding is not a form of bonding with a baby. It is, in a way that is difficult to do when you are formula feeding, for example feeding quickly for comfort or to soothe a child to sleep. The act of breastfeeding can also be bonding, through skin-to-skin contact and the impact of the hormone oxytocin being released, which promotes feelings of calm, love and bonding.[23]

This is absolutely not to say that a mother who is bottle-feeding cannot bond with her baby – just that she will bond through bottle-feeding, which is slightly different. Babies can be bottle-fed skin-to-skin. The questions used in this particular study explored things like 'I feel close to my baby'; 'I love my baby very much'; 'I feel confident when changing my baby'. I can think of no reason why mothers who do not breastfeed would not love their baby, and anyone who suggests otherwise has dubious ulterior motives.

Looking at the study, there is also the issue of relatively small sample sizes. Out of the 272 who completed the questionnaire, 87.5% had breastfed their baby at some point. Also, the vast majority (91.9%) had no bonding issues with their baby, with just 1.8% having a severe bonding issue. The study was also a cross-sectional study – a snapshot in time – meaning that even if a link between bonding issues and bottle-feeding was found, the direction could not be established. Experiencing significant bonding issues is highly correlated with mental health difficulties, which might make women more likely to bottle-feed their baby so that someone else can help support them.[24]

4. Is any outcome linked to the specific intervention studied, not just any intervention?

Thinking back to the controlled crying study discussed in the last chapter, and the poor control group who told the researchers that their baby had a sleep problem... and then no one did anything,[25] it's important to make sure that the control group experiences something that is equally detailed and valuable to them as the intervention is to the other group. Otherwise, you might unintentionally change the behaviour of the intervention group, just by involving them in something, paying attention to them, or making them think something is going to happen.

This can be explained by the *Hawthorne effect* – sometimes known as the observer effect.[26] This phenomenon was originally observed in a study that wanted to examine whether worker productivity increased in higher or lower light conditions. What it actually found was that productivity increased in both conditions, but decreased again after the study, regardless of any light given. The researchers identified that when individuals in a study are being observed, their behaviour changes. Therefore, to genuinely be able to identify any real change, you need to make sure that all participants in your study are receiving equal observation and intervention in some form. There are many ways this could occur. Just being part of something a bit new can give an improved outcome. The increased attention from researchers might reinforce this further.

The well-known placebo effect can also come into play. Originally referring to a medical study in which some participants were given an active drug and some a sugar pill, but everyone saw improvements, the effect occurs just because someone has taken part in a study and something – anything – has happened to them. A placebo can even have physiological outcomes – changes in heart rate, anxiety, pain, tiredness… all just through the power of receiving 'treatment'.[27]

Listening appointments for maternal mental health are based partly on this knowledge. Although we know that some people benefit from pharmacological intervention for mental health problems, we also know that just having someone to listen, who is spending time with you and allowing you the opportunity to offload and discuss everything that is on your mind, is an important part of mental health support. This means that studies such as the sleep training study have a major flaw: only the women in the intervention group had the opportunity to talk through their problems with a trained counsellor.[25]

Randomised controlled trials sometimes try to make sure participants are blinded, if possible, to their arm, meaning that the participants don't know whether they are in the treatment or control arm. Of course in many behavioural studies this isn't possible – a mother will know if she is baby-led weaning or spoon-feeding, for example. But in other studies, perhaps those which use medications, it is possible to at least attempt it.

However, sometimes researchers try to persuade us that treatment was blinded when it probably wasn't. For example, in one study researchers either gave babies acupuncture or the babies 'spent five minutes alone with the acupuncturist' (doing what, nobody knows). The researchers claimed that the parents didn't know which treatment their baby had, but also admitted that some babies had a spot of blood on them after the procedure… which just might have given the game away.

Funnily enough, the parents did seem to be able to spot whether needles had been stuck in their baby and at the follow-up visit 72% of parents in the acupuncture group could guess which treatment group they were in (compared to 21% in the no needles group). The researchers suggested that this was because the treatment was working, but surely those in the no needles group would know it wasn't working. And it didn't work strongly anyway.[28]

The best line in the paper, however, is '*Infants were not aware of the therapeutic relationship or possible benefits of acupuncture.*' I applaud the researchers for their audacity – they at least tried to make out that it would be the *baby* who would experience the placebo effect, but as the questions were completed by the *parent*, any placebo effect would surely operate on them. Unless, I guess, they read the questions out loud to their tiny baby and used their response to complete the questionnaire.

It's also common in research like this for whoever is doing the intervention not to be blinded. In a double-blind trial, no one knows until the end who gets what treatment – neither the participant nor the researcher. But if you are giving a baby acupuncture or not, you are going to know what you did. If you have any interaction with the parent, or even a go-between person, there is a possibility that you will give off signals about what you have done, consciously or otherwise.

Sometimes it's impossible to guarantee that you can blind participants, even if you try. Currently, there is a randomised controlled trial going on in the UK evaluating whether snipping tongue tie improves outcomes for feeding. It is trying to be blind, by not letting the parents know – but surely parents are going to look in their babies' mouths, even if they try really hard not to? And even if they don't or can't see anything, they may well feel something.[29] The pilot of the study is looking at whether blinding is possible, but in a similar trial 62% of first-time mothers, 61% of second-time mothers and 100% of third or more time mothers were able to guess whether their baby had received treatment or not. And that was mainly because they felt a difference (or no difference) afterwards.[30] This is another example of how strange things get if you insist that the only gold-standard evidence is a blinded randomised controlled trial.

5. Consider whether the participants might feel indebted to give the 'right' answer

Psychologists have also observed that people change their behaviour when they are being studied. *Demand characteristics* are ways in which participants might act because they are being studied.[31] These include:

- Being a good participant – the participant who tries to achieve what they think you want them to achieve, especially if they are grateful for your intervention.
- Being a negative participant – the one who tries to destroy the study, for fun or because they don't want the expected finding to be confirmed.
- Being an apprehensive participant – one who gets so anxious about being studied and whether they will be judged on the outcome, that their behaviour totally changes

All of these mean that without a carefully planned control group, you're never quite going to know whether an effect is accidental or not. For example, thinking about the sleep training study,[25] it is possible that being given information about how to help a baby sleep encourages you (subconsciously or otherwise) to state that your baby is sleeping better. You want to believe that the intervention has helped, or you want to give the researchers the outcome you think they are looking for – after all, they've invested a load of time helping you.

6. Consider whether the questions used led participants to give a specific answer

One more example from the sleep training study.[25] Participants were asked '*Over the last two weeks, has your baby's sleep generally been a problem for you?*' in order to define sleep problems. The response options were yes or no. They were asked the same question before the study and then after they had the intervention (or not). Now if you have just been taught about what normal sleep is, what to expect, and how to find time to care for yourself, it's possible that even if your baby's sleep pattern doesn't change in the slightest, your perception of whether it is a problem or not does.

Another example arose when we started doing some of the original work on baby-led weaning. We asked parents whether they were following a baby-led weaning approach and then the proportion of time they were spoon-feeding and using purées. We had a sizeable number in the group who identified as following baby-led weaning, but who were using spoon-feeding and purées half the time or more. We were lucky we had asked this and were able to conduct any analyses on the actual behaviour rather than the simple yes/no question.[32]

7. Beware the self-report

Related to the points discussed above, you should be wary when outcomes in a study are based on self-report. Lots of research uses self-report – because gaining researcher-observed or measured data is more expensive, time-consuming for both participant and researcher, can be invasive, and is going to lead to smaller samples. The best way to record how often a baby wakes up at night is to watch the mother and baby… but their sleep might be affected by knowing they are being observed. And it will limit the number of people who are willing and able to take part.

However, we know from studies with adults that people often under or overestimate how much sleep they get. The same is true with mothers and babies. The research team at the Baby Sleep Information Source at Durham University asked mother and baby pairs to wear actigraphs (a wearable device that can monitor sleep and activity levels) to record how much sleep they were getting. They wore them in their own homes. Participants were also given a sleep log diary, with 15-minute increments in, to fill in when their baby was awake or asleep. Data was collected for one night every two weeks from 4–18 weeks of age, giving eight samples per mother and baby pair.[33]

Incidentally this study has important implications for feeding and infant sleep. It is commonly proposed that babies who are formula-fed will sleep better than babies who are breastfed. This data is typically based on self-report. However, measurements of total sleep time and longest sleep period duration as measured by the actigraph did not differ between babies who were exclusively formula-fed and those who were exclusively breastfed at any time point from 4–16 weeks.

However, at 10, 12, 14 and 16 weeks postpartum, mothers who were exclusively formula feeding reported that their baby slept 41–58 minutes longer per night than the exclusively breastfed mothers did (although that difference was only deemed significantly different at 14 weeks). Additionally, they also reported a significantly greater longest sleep duration at each of these time points, estimating it to be between 1.64 and 2.29 hours longer than mothers who were exclusively breastfeeding. This was despite the actigraph showing no difference. And in fact, at 18 weeks, the actigraph showed breastfed babies actually had a significantly greater longest sleep duration – 55 minutes longer than for formula-fed infants, with an overall increased total sleep duration of 74 minutes (but this wasn't statistically significant).

There are many reasons why estimates of sleep might differ between mothers who are breastfeeding and those who are formula-feeding. One might be sleep location: mothers who breastfeed are more likely to co-sleep, so perhaps they are more aware of their infant waking.[34] However, in the actigraph study, when the researchers controlled for sleep location, the same findings held. Mothers who are bottle-feeding may have someone else feeding the baby, or someone else may be more involved in night-time care. There is also the possibility of bias – mothers are told that formula helps their baby to sleep, so they believe or want to report that they sleep longer. The placebo effect or desirability for a certain outcome may be at play.

Self-report for sleep duration continues to be a popular option in research. Hands up, I've done it myself [35] – although I asked for number of night-wakings rather than overall sleep duration, which is potentially slightly easier to be accurate with. However, the problem comes when these potentially inaccurate measures are used to try and change policy, or make big headlines. Just last year the news was full of articles claiming that early introduction of solids would help your baby sleep better – based on findings from the EAT study.[36] Aside from the other limitations of the study we have already discussed (low adherence rate, timing of early solids actually being closer to 20 weeks), sleep duration was based on maternal self-report and estimations were made in minutes. Can you really report with accuracy how many minutes you sleep?

8. Ensure there are before and after measures

Looking at the sleep training study one more time, a follow-up study was conducted with the babies once they were six years old. In the follow-up researchers collected cortisol samples from the children.[37] Cortisol is often used as a measure of stress. All measures were in the normal range and the researchers cited this as evidence that raised cortisol in infancy does no long-term harm. However, there were no earlier tests of cortisol to compare the results to. We have no idea about any change that occurred, or whether there were any initial differences in the group. So it is interesting that everyone seemed to be in the normal range, but it is far from the full picture. The good news is that most children who had remained in the study weren't exhibiting high stress levels.

Related to the previous point, there are essentially two types of cortisol. We have natural rises and falls in our day-to-day levels of cortisol. It peaks just after we wake, and is at its lowest around three hours after we go to sleep for our longest period. There is natural variation in cortisol peaks and troughs – and this can partly explain why some people feel more alert in the evening, and others in the morning.

We also have cortisol rises when we get stressed. It is this that indicates our reaction to anything happening. In infant sleep studies that look at the impact of any type of crying or sleep training on cortisol levels, the good ones will look at it before, during and after a crying/sleep training session. The limited work that has looked at this, shows that stress cortisol levels rise, as you would expect during crying. They remain elevated for a while before reducing again.[38] So if you measured cortisol at a far enough time point away from the event, it would be back to a lower level. Which is when a number of the other early crying studies measure it – in one case a week, a month and three months after sleep training.[39] These researchers are measuring daily cortisol levels, not stress reaction levels.

9. Check that any change isn't just due to time passing

Finally, if a headline says that something has changed after an intervention, check whether participants are being compared to a control group which has had a different experience. As noted previously, sometimes, just time passing leads to a change (for better or worse). Babies gradually cry less and wake less over time so if you don't clearly measure this you can run into problems. For example, in a study measuring the impact of probiotics on colic, babies were randomised to two groups. One group received probiotics and the other a placebo. The notable part was that over the course of the study, crying and fussing reduced in *both groups*, echoing previous research that colic symptoms generally ease over time whatever you do. So if you had been measuring the impact of the colic treatment in just one group, you might have concluded that the treatment worked, as it did reduce in the period after receiving the treatment.[40]

HOW TO KEEP INFORMED:

Always check who has conducted the research, and who is reporting on its significance. Do they have in-depth knowledge of the topic, context and influencing factors? Or do they just understand methods and think they can apply that to every question?

Always check whether the measures being used are measuring reality or what is useful.

Check the methods closely. What did interventions entail? If more than one thing, how do we know what worked and what didn't?

Check which questions were used and how data was collected. Are you comfortable that this would provide accurate answers?

Remember that all research has limitations. It's the overall pattern that matters.

17

WHAT'S THE ACTUAL
RISK TO ME?

As explained in previous chapters, much of the research conducted ends up working out what the average risk of things for an individual is based on occurrence of events across large populations. Which, if you were an average person, might give you some idea of risk. But who is? The average first-time mother is now 30.[1] The average weight and height of a UK woman is 11 stone and 5ft 5in.[2] Mean household income is £28,400.[3] And so on. And on top of that there are many more factors from genetics to luck that determine outcomes for individuals.

Overall, when thinking about risk, it's important to remember three things:

1. Our overall risk is low for most things
Thankfully, for most of us living in developed regions, the chances of anything catastrophic happening to us or our babies during pregnancy, birth and early childhood are low across populations. For example, even though the respiratory infection bronchiolitis is considered 'common', when researchers in London tracked how many babies in England developed it over a year, they found it was 2.6%.[4]

Now this is a problem for Public Health England. That 2.6% is 16,000 babies each year who all need treating, which costs money. It's also a horrible experience for you and your baby if they develop the infection. But overall the chances of your baby *not* getting it are extremely high.

2. Our risk will not be equal

For some, the risk will be far lower and for some, unfortunately, far higher. Some babies will be at greater risk because they have other risk factors which make them more likely to develop bronchiolitis (to continue our example above). For example, one study found that babies born prematurely had 1.9 times the risk of developing bronchiolitis, while babies with congenital heart disease had 3.3 times the risk. Babies with Down syndrome (2.5×) and cerebral palsy (2.4×), immunodeficiency (1.7×), cystic fibrosis (2.5×) and chronic lung disease (1.6×) were all at greater risk.[5] These are all pretty unmodifiable risk factors – you can't choose not to have them.

Genetics – something we sadly cannot change – plays a big role in many health outcomes. We are all more genetically at risk of certain illnesses than others. For example, childhood obesity has been shown to have a large genetic component. What we eat and how active we are does matter, but for those with a genetic propensity to be overweight, the battle to stay at a healthy weight will be much harder.[6] Although we know that many early experiences are associated with an increased risk of obesity (like infant feeding decisions),[7] little research has been done to look at the risk among those who have a genetic risk and those who don't.

Most people don't really know what their individual risk from a genetic perspective is. They might have patterns in their family, and some may have even been genetically tested. But most of us don't have much idea about our genetics. Research is not far enough advanced to enable us to reliably calculate what our risk might be if we take into account all of the different factors in our life and how they work together.

Another major predictor of illness risk is socioeconomic status. The very best thing you can do for your health, sadly, is to make sure you are not poor. If only that was so easy! Most illnesses are majorly socially patterned, with those living in the most deprived conditions having the worst outcomes across pregnancy, birth and infant health.[8] Globally, mothers are at a distinct health disadvantage because they are female.[9] Add in a layer of racial disparity on top and many mothers are at a further health disadvantage because they are not White.[10] Even in the UK, women of colour die in childbirth at a rate of five times that of White women – and it's not as some would like to make out just because of underlying existing health issues but rather complex, systemic prejudice.[11] Who you are and how you are perceived by others matters when it comes to your health – at a shocking level.

3. There is a major difference between relative and absolute risk

As we have seen when discussing the misuse of statistics, your *individual risk* of something is never going to be as scary as the *relative risks* that are often reported in the news. Individual risk is the chances of it happening to *you*. Relative risk is how much more frequently an illness or event occurs in certain circumstances or for some groups.

Take the example of childhood leukaemia. A few years ago there were a number of scare stories about not breastfeeding increasing your child's risk of leukaemia. That's pretty scary stuff – but not in the context of individual risk. Looking at the paper (a big meta-analysis of a number of studies) it found that ever breastfeeding reduced your child's risk of leukaemia by 9% and breastfeeding for six months or longer reduced it by 20%. It also noted that overall, if all babies were breastfed for six months or more, population rates of leukaemia would drop by 14–20%.[12] Which is excellent news for those babies, and if you're in charge of the public health budget. But what about the individual level? Thankfully, only around 900 children a year in the UK are diagnosed with leukaemia, which means an individual risk of 1 in 2,000.[13] Therefore any risk reduction is a proportion of that – 20% less than 1 in 2,000.

Taken together, these three things mean that when you hear someone saying *'But I did X and my baby was fine'*, their baby may well have been fine. But this will be based on a combination of a low overall risk – most babies not getting that illness – their own individual genetic risk, and an extra helping of good luck. It's also important to realise that many women who state this come from relatively privileged circumstances, in that education, income, ethnicity and many other factors all play a role in their baby being 'fine'. We should also be extremely careful in declaring that public health messages around babies are pointless based on the fact that you are okay.

If you are genetically at low risk of an illness, have a good education, lots of family support, are low in stress, have lots of money, are living in a good area and are White, then your risk of anything happening to your baby will be much lower than anyone who doesn't have those protective privileges. We must all be aware of our own privilege when it comes to sharing our thoughts about research findings. For some women living in the most stressful situations, being able to breastfeed their baby might be the one thing that is helping lift their baby out of the effects of at least some of that stress and disadvantage. It is a dangerous game to play to stop other women receiving the messages that just might make all the difference for them, based on what happened to you.

Our perception of risk can be skewed

As human beings, we aren't that great at recognising what is a real risk, and what is just exaggerated in our minds. Every day many of us take far greater risks with our health through our diet, lack of exercise, alcohol intake or stress levels than the things our brain chooses to worry about in the middle of the night. Everyone has irrational fears, be it spiders, snakes or sharks... but the chances of one of those creatures ever harming you is minuscule compared to the day-to-day stuff. When it comes to babies our risk misperceptions go through the roof. This is understandable. Our babies are the most precious things in the world and we will do anything to keep them safe.

However, all of this is not helped by our understanding of the word 'risk'. In scientific terms risk is used as a word that means likelihood but when we hear the word risk in reality we panic. Risk immediately sounds scary and like very bad things are going to happen. It leads easily into phrases such as 'it's not worth the risk' or labelling women's decision-making as risky. It is a favourite of news headlines as it grabs our attention and is an easy way to control and manipulate women into doing what you want them to do. It can help to swap words around. Words and phrases like 'What are the odds of?'... or 'What is the likelihood of?'... or using the word 'chance' instead of risk. Does it seem so scary?

The way in which we determine whether something is a risk or not is not usually logical. We might have hard statistics in front of us, but then we mix in a heavy dose of emotion and personal experience. Many people overestimate the risk of things like terror attacks because they are so terrifying, while slowly eating and drinking their way to heart disease. Roughly speaking, we have a 1 in 6 chance of dying of heart disease and a 1 in 7 chance of dying of cancer. But stories suggesting we eat a bit healthier and lose a bit of weight don't sell newspapers. That's mainly because we all have to die of something at some point, and modern medicine and lifestyles are keeping us alive long enough for these outcomes to happen.[14]

But then there are the strange risks. A disturbing recent study from India showed that you are now five times more likely to die from an accident while taking a selfie than from being killed by a shark.[15] (Although at this point you should also be asking, five times what? What's the real risk to me? How many people actually die in selfie-related accidents?!) Similarly, a table of risks presented in the *BMJ* finds you are more likely to die playing football than you are by murder, although I'm guessing you actually have to occasionally play football for that risk to occur.[16]

Risk experts have identified different types of things that affect whether we perceive something to be a risk or not:[17]

Who is involved?

We tend to interpret other people's behaviour as far riskier than our own when we do exactly the same thing. Most people think they are better drivers than average. If we see someone else speeding, we label them irresponsible. If we do it ourselves… well, we're good drivers, aren't we? We are more scared when we are not in control, as we perceive ourselves to be expert. Far more people are scared of planes than cars, because they're not in control.

Awareness

If something happens to a friend, even if it is a freak accident, our perception of it as a day-to-day risk is heightened. The more we see something talked about on TV and in the news, the scarier it becomes. In reality the things that are most likely to personally affect us are typically not broadcast on the news.

Trust

Do you trust who is giving you the information? If you do, you will be more worried. If you don't, you're more likely to underestimate the risk. If we have very strong fears, we may stop trusting people who give us contradictory information.

Manmade versus nature

People are more scared of terror attacks and nuclear explosions than they are of global warming or sun exposure.

Scope

We are far more worried about publicised catastrophes such as tsunamis, which kill a few hundred people in a few hours, than we are of conditions such as heart disease that kill many more over the course of a year.

Who it affects

We overestimate the risk of events if they affect children. If they look like us, or we identify with them, we worry more. That is why in the UK we panic more about a terror attack in France, where we have been on holiday, than about the many more lives that are taken by terrorists in regions of conflict every year. We also panic more if an individual is named and their photo is in the press, compared to an 'unnamed person'.

Familiarity

The more used to something we are in our day-to-day lives, the less it worries us. Whenever a rare disease pops up in headlines, people panic. Ebola? Tape up your windows and hoard food. Liver failure? Pass me another drink. For example, your lifetime risk of being killed by lightning is roughly 1 in 114,000. Yet your risk of being killed by heart disease is 1 in 5! How many people are more scared of sharks (lifetime risk of being killed by one is 1 in 3,748,067) than cows (lifetime risk of being killed by one is 1 in 173,871)?

Enjoyment

If we enjoy the risky behaviour then it's fun. How many people skydive or take drugs, yet panic at the thought of a terror attack.

What does this mean for advice about birth and babies?

Knowing what relative and absolute risks are can help you make decisions that are right for you. Unfortunately, they can never give you an exact answer, as anything to do with an outcome for your baby will be affected by lots of different things. One research study can only tell you what happened in that one research study. That's why it's important not to get too hung up on the results of any one study, but rather look at the overall pattern. I'm going to give some examples over the next pages of what different studies have found based on the reading of numerous papers (although, not all of them as that would be an almost impossible task). Given what we know about the wide range of papers out there, it's likely that you could hunt down papers with different conclusions. But remember, no one paper can be that helpful in isolation, it's the bigger picture that counts.

We can never remove all risk

Remember, when you think about the overall risk of doing something, that the default option will have its own risks too. For example, the UNICEF UK Baby Friendly Initiative publishes the risk of babies dying from Sudden Infant Death Syndrome by sleeping location.[18] We only ever hear stories in the press about babies sadly dying when sleeping on a sofa or in bed (unsafely) with a parent. We don't hear about babies who die of SIDS in their cots, because it doesn't lead to such a sensational headline (or suggest blame). The risk of SIDS is:

- 1 in 3,180 for all babies
- 1 in 174 co-sleeping on a sofa
- 1 in 174 co-sleeping after a parent has consumed alcohol or drugs
- 1 in 787 co-sleeping with a regular smoker

However, around half of all babies who die of SIDS die sleeping alone in a cot or Moses basket. And although half of these babies die while co-sleeping, 90% of those who do so will be in hazardous conditions, but 10% will be co-sleeping with no risk factors.[19] We sadly can't remove all risk, all the time. Unfortunately, as much as we would love to protect our babies from all risks forever, every choice we make carries a risk. We just need to choose the risks we are most comfortable with and remember that thankfully most of us go about our everyday lives just fine. Remember that the absolute risk for most things is very much weighted in our favour, although it may differ according to things we cannot change.

There are always two sides to every story, but not all research addresses this, or wants to, as it can ruin the 'story'. One rather strange BBC headline declared that *'Indulgent grandparents may be having an adverse impact on their grandchildren's health'*. The story came from a research review that suggested some grandparents may overindulge their grandchildren with sweets. However, the study ignored the huge swathe of research looking at the benefits of extended family and care. By all means, ban Grandma and her evil treats from the house, but overall there might be adverse consequences (which might even make your kids start comfort eating).[20] It's all about balance and careful thinking. However, if you see a headline screaming that something is a risk, always consider what the risk of *not* doing something is.

Risk elimination versus risk minimisation

This brings us to the topic of risk elimination. Some public health campaigns are renowned for taking too harsh a view of risks, assuming that if parents are simply told not to do something, everything will be okay. This doesn't work because:

1. Often the risks are only calculated for the 'natural' behaviours such as bed-sharing, vaginal birth, and not being induced, rather than taking into account the risks of clinical intervention.
2. They typically focus on the most serious risk (e.g. death)

rather than the most common risk.

3. The guidance is often unrealistic, so parents do not receive the information they need to make a decision and follow it through in the safest possible way.

4. Parents feel ashamed and guilty about going against guidance, increasing the chance they will hide this from their health professionals.

In few other areas of our lives do we take such a risk elimination approach. Take driving a car, for example. In 2017 there were 1,793 traffic-related deaths in the UK. In your lifetime you have a roughly 1 in 100 risk of dying in a car crash. Compare that to the number of babies who die during co-sleeping each year (approximately 130). We know that there are numerous things associated with traffic safety, so we improve them: we have rules about drink-driving, getting a driving licence and making cars and roads safer. We don't simply tell everyone not to drive because there is a chance they might die. Over 1,000 people each year die falling down the stairs, but at least when they're in the car they're not on those hazardous stairs many of us have in our own homes.

But in public health we often make the mistake of believing that if we just tell people not to do something, they won't do it (or at least we told them not to, so it's not our fault). What this means is that we end up actually exacerbating the issue, because rather than teaching people to reduce risks and take safety steps, you prevent them from having information. It's a bit like having staircates in your house until your children leave home, meaning they never learn to use stairs safely. An overly cautious risk elimination approach leads to issues such as:

- Unsafe co-sleeping
- Bottles of formula not being made up safely
- Inappropriate weaning foods being given
- Women birthing outside the healthcare system
- Women not telling their doctor they are taking a medication

Roughly speaking, there is about the same chance of a baby dying during co-sleeping if their mother smokes as there is a lifetime risk of dying in a motorcycle accident, or drowning (bearing in mind these are lifetime risks, and babies don't co-sleep for a lifetime, even though it seems like it). I'm not trying to compare the actual risk here, but more our attitude. We don't ban motorbikes or swimming (or going near water) because of the risks. We educate, we try to make things safer, and we hope people will act sensibly. I am betting that in the days before swimming lessons, motorcycle helmets and speed limits the death rates would have been a lot higher. So why are we not going for the education and risk reduction route for choices to do with parenting?[21]

We need to put things in the context of other risks

We take risks every single day. Getting out of bed, going down the stairs, getting in the car or walking down the street. Lying in bed is also risky. Everything has a risk. It's important to put things in the context of other health-related risks. The flipside of reassuring people that their overall risk of something is fairly low is that some people will then turn around and say that supporting women's decisions and desires when it comes to their bodies and babies doesn't matter. We live in a society where we have to continually justify with cost savings and intervention rates why we should support women to breastfeed or have a vaginal birth, when really women should receive high-quality (actually I'd accept adequate) healthcare support to enable their bodies to work if that is what they wish to do with them.

Some people argue that if 'only' a small percentage of babies are stopped from having an illness by breastfeeding, we shouldn't promote breastfeeding. But overall we have a public health system that encourages and discourages certain behaviours based on risk and population level prevention. The main issue is that even if your baby's risk of developing an illness is 3%, we don't really know who will develop it. So by taking a public health approach to try and prevent it, we can reduce the overall risk on a population level. However, luckily most babies will be fine, which is good – we want them to be fine! But there's a difference between knowing they are fine after an event and future risk.

We seem to accept health promotion for other health behaviours that also have much lower overall risks than you might expect. For example, one longitudinal study published in the *New England Journal of Medicine* following up female heavy smokers aged 30–55 found that women who smoked 25+ cigarettes a day had a 5.5 times increased risk of fatal heart disease compared to non-smokers, or triple the risk if they smoked 5–14 cigarettes a day. But out of the cohort of 119,404, just 65 died during the six-year follow-up.[22] So again, five times what risk? But we're happy to accept the public health promotion message that smoking increases the risk of heart disease.

Likewise, another study into trends in UK smoking and lung cancer found that men who smoked their entire life had a 15.9% chance of lung cancer – or an 84.1% chance of not having lung cancer.[23] That's a lot of grandfathers 'smoking all their life and being fine'. However, given all those cases of smoking-related lung cancer were, well, smoking-related, if you were in charge of public health you'd be wanting those rates to come down. Also, if you were young and deciding whether to smoke or not, you might decide a 16% chance of getting lung cancer wasn't worth it.

Another systematic review and meta-analysis looking at the lifetime risk of alcohol consumption and liver cirrhosis looked at both the risk of developing it (morbidity) and dying from it (mortality) dependent on how much alcohol was regularly drunk. Comparing drinkers to lifetime abstainers:[24]
- For women there was a 4.9× risk of dying from liver cirrhosis if you drank 24g of alcohol a day (3 units) and 12.5× risk if you drank 60g a day (7.5 units)

- For just having cirrhosis but not dying from it, there was a 3.2× risk for 24g a day and a 6.2× risk for 60g per day
- The risks were increased but less high in men

However, again it comes down to the risk of what. The study involved data from lots of different studies, so the frequency of risk of developing and dying from cirrhosis was different among the different papers. Roughly speaking, the overall risk of mortality was somewhere between 0.01 and 0.05% and the overall risk of morbidity was somewhere between 0.01 and 0.9%.

My point is not that we should all start drinking and smoking, but that we see drinking and smoking copiously as health risks. Different studies will of course give slightly different data, but these are all large meta-analysis or cohort studies. Individuals within those studies will have larger or smaller risks, and indeed the smoking or drinking may be symptomatic of other issues that might kill them, such as stress or poverty. And smoking and alcohol have far more potential negative outcomes than 'just' lung cancer or liver cirrhosis as measured in these studies. Indeed, overall estimates suggest that up to two-thirds of heavy smokers will eventually die from a smoking-related illness.[25] Alcohol is a risk factor for over 60 different illnesses, with around 1.8 million alcohol-related hospital admissions each year.[26]

But deciding on what risk is best for us is an individual decision. For some of us, any risk is simply not worth it. No matter how small the risk, we don't see any benefit of smoking or drinking so we don't do it. For others, they get pleasure or find themselves addicted or whatever reason leads them to do it. And it's the same with babies – we need to look at our overall perceived risk and preferences and how they balance together.

We also know, having looked at the previous chapters, that it is possible that some of the risks are being underestimated (or not estimated properly for different population groups).

So what is my actual risk?

Here are some real data that show you what risk looks like and puts it in real terms, for my top five 'that's risky' subjects. Remember:

1. These are just a few examples of well-conducted studies. Different studies may produce slightly different data. It is impossible to do a thorough literature review of all different studies in each different area and squeeze it into a chapter in one book. Use them as an illustrative guide.
2. I have picked studies from a range of developed countries, but remember, from the sampling chapter, overall complication rates are different for each country so could affect the findings (I've included details on the country).
3. You get to decide what constitutes a big or small risk to you. Some things might be non-negotiable for you, but others don't see the risk as big.

1. Home birth versus hospital birth

One study conducted a systematic review looking at differences in birth outcomes from 1947–2009.[27] It searched for all studies that compared outcomes for planned home births and planned hospital births that looked at maternal and newborn outcomes. It included 12 studies overall, which together included 342,056 planned home births and 207,551 planned hospital births.

One of the main outcomes for this review was the survival rate of babies born at home or in hospital.

- Perinatal death (death between 28 weeks gestation and 7 days postpartum) – 0.07% home versus 0.08% hospital (so thankfully the vast majority of babies survived regardless of birth place).
- Neonatal death (up to 28 days postpartum) – 0.15% home versus 0.04% hospital.

The authors noted '*The absolute risk was small, reflecting the low prevalence of home birth and rarity of the outcome, despite its significantly increased odds ratio*'. They were not able to state what these babies died from. They note that around 30–50% of babies who sadly die at home do so due to respiratory failure. However, they did not have the data to report on this in the study (and no data on why babies died in hospital).

What this study also did was look at the levels of other complications. Although our absolute priority would typically be whether a baby survives birth or not, this doesn't invalidate all other complications of birth, which although less deadly, may be more common. It's a case of weighing up what you think might be the worst and most likely outcome.

Overall, planned home births had fewer interventions such as epidurals, foetal heart rate monitoring, episiotomy and assisted or caesarean delivery. Specifically:

- *Episiotomy*: 7% (home) versus 10.4% (hospital)
- *Caesarean*: 5% (home) versus 9.3% (hospital)
- *Forceps/ventouse*: 3.5% (home) versus 10.2% (hospital)
- *Third-degree tear*: 1.2% (home) versus 2.5% (hospital)
- *Newborn ventilation*: 3.6% (home) versus 4.7% (hospital)

Again, the good news is that the majority of mothers and babies did not experience these outcomes. How the risk is reported is important. Take the forceps/ventouse delivery statistics. If you use the language of relative risk, you could say that mothers are three times more likely to experience forceps/ventouse if they give birth in hospital. Which sounds scary. But if you look at the bigger picture, roughly 92% of women didn't have forceps or ventouse (this in part is because some had a caesarean section, and it's difficult to work out from the paper the stats for those who had a vaginal delivery). So a better message would be 'Most births do not involve ventouse or forceps, but they do occur at a higher rate in hospitals', rather than the quite frankly terrifying sounding 'you have three times the risk of forceps in hospital'.

Notably, the authors also recognise the importance of the bigger picture, discussing how home births can be made even more safe by knowing that respiratory issues occur in a minority of cases. They discuss how home birth midwives could be further trained in ways to monitor this risk during labour, and in resuscitation options after birth if necessary. Given that home birth appears to reduce complications that are more common, simply ruling them out because of one outcome is not sensible.

Some further points to consider:

- The study looked at planned home births. You need to take into account that in most cases, it will be the lower-risk women who plan a home birth, and this will lead to outcomes being different in the two groups, regardless of the birth environment. For example, the rate of premature babies born before 37 weeks was 0.7% in the planned home group compared to 4.7% in the planned hospital group. Conversely, going overdue (42 weeks or more) was pretty much equal in both groups (2.1% for the home group and 2.2% for the hospital group).
- Again, this is risk across a *huge* group. Individuals will have a different risk based on other factors such as genetics.
- 'Home' and 'hospital' are not two generic environments where every home is calm and birth-friendly and every hospital is more intense and less birth-friendly.
- The study only used data up until 2009 – a lot has happened in the last 10 years.

2. Timing of delivery

Another area where women often feel a lot of pressure is to be induced if they have gone 'overdue' in their pregnancy (depending on the area, this can be any time from 41.5 weeks onwards). The rationale behind induction is that after 42 weeks of pregnancy, the risk of the baby dying increases. But by how much?

One interesting study looked at this, using retrospective data of all babies born after 37 weeks (without major anomalies) in California from 1997–2006, which accounted for 3,820,826 births.[28] What is interesting about this paper is that it took into account the risk of giving birth at that time point versus waiting. It recognised that both sides had a risk – because everything in life does. In particular, the earlier a baby is born, the greater their risk of Sudden Infant Death Syndrome.

Now – it should be stressed here that we are thankfully talking about tiny numbers. The vast number of women who go over 41 weeks of pregnancy deliver their babies just fine. Likewise rates of SIDS are very low. But when you have huge numbers in a study, you can look at those figures and the extremely sad cases where something does go wrong. In this paper researchers looked at the risk of the baby dying if the pregnancy was allowed to continue versus if the mother was induced. They measured in terms of risk per 10,000 babies.

- At 38 weeks the risk of induction was the same as the risk of waiting.
- At 39 weeks the risk of waiting was 12.9 in 10,000 compared to 8.8 in 10,000 for induction.
- At 40 weeks the risk of waiting was 14.9 in 10,000 compared to 9.5 in 10,000 for induction.
- At 41 weeks the risk of waiting was 17.6 in 10,000 compared to 10.8 in 10,000 for induction.

So as you can see, in the vast majority of cases babies were fine. You don't suddenly get to 41 weeks of pregnancy and the risk of something happening to your baby becomes catastrophic. The risk increases slowly. Even at 41 weeks. This of course needs to be balanced against the other more frequent but less serious risks of induction including increased risk of intervention, complications and an often more painful experience for women.[29] Although of course an alive baby is the most important outcome, considering the impact of smaller risks that are more likely to happen needs to be taken into consideration against that very, very small risk.

3. Keeping mum and baby together in hospital

Let's look at a paper entitled, scarily, 'In-hospital neonatal falls: an unintended consequence of efforts to improve breastfeeding also cause anxiety in 2019'.[30] The first lines of the abstract read: *'In-hospital neonatal falls are increasingly recognised as a postpartum safety risk with maternal fatigue contributing to these events'.*

Anyone reading that headline would understandably worry – are there babies being dropped all over the place because mothers are breastfeeding? After all, aren't most women a bit 'fatigued' after giving birth?

Thankfully this is not the case. The article was written in the context of some professionals in the US worrying about the 'new trend' of keeping mother and baby together after birth. They argue that this makes mothers too tired and that babies should be taken to a nursery so that their mothers can sleep (despite research showing that mothers don't get any more sleep if their baby is taken to the nursery, probably because they feel anxious about the separation).

The paper states in its abstract that *'We report a cluster of in-hospital neonatal falls associated with a hospital program to improve breastfeeding, which included rooming-in practices'.* This is an over-exaggeration and contortion of the actual results.

What happened was that the researchers looked at hospital records to see how many reports there were of babies being dropped over a two-year period from September 2015–August 2017. They then looked at breastfeeding data. And rooming-in data. They found:

1. Breastfeeding rates were at around 70%, rising steadily to almost all babies by April 2016.
2. Rooming-in rates were very low – zero in fact. Then they rose considerably to around 80% of infants, although some months no infants roomed-in for some reason.

Overall in the period there were three falls. Yes, just three. They occurred in months where breastfeeding rates were at around 96%, 94% and 100%. However, there were many months when breastfeeding was at around 100% that no falls occurred. In terms of rooming-in, the falls occurred in months where there was roughly 60%, 80% or 0% rooming-in.

Are you confused yet?

Now let's look at the case studies given of the mother-baby dyads who experienced a fall.

1. Elective caesarean. Breastfeeding did not start until 15 hours after delivery. Mother reported feeling very fatigued.
2. 14-year-old mother with history of foster care and depression. Mother initially breastfed 4 hours after birth but then stopped breastfeeding. On day four, she fell asleep when holding the infant and he fell to the floor. (Not a breastfeeding mother at the time of the fall.)
3. Mother with significant traumatic experiences including domestic abuse and enslavement. Baby first breastfed after 9.5 hours. Mother reported feeling drowsy from pain medication and asked for him to be taken to the hospital nursery on day two. On day three, she fell asleep breastfeeding her baby. It was unclear from the paper whether the baby was still staying in the nursery.

The discussion raises the idea that mothers dropped their baby when they fell asleep. One could argue that remaining in hospital for several days after birth makes this more likely.

4. Maternal obesity and childbirth risk

The topic of overweight and obesity during pregnancy pops up regularly in the news headlines, but what is the actual risk?

One population cohort study looked at birth outcomes for 805,275 pregnant women in Sweden according to their weight.[31] They compared outcomes for women who were a healthy BMI (19–26) to those with a BMI of 29–35 (obese) 35–40 (morbidly obese) and more than 40 (very morbidly obese). I'm not sure what happened to the women who would have been considered overweight (BMI 27–28).

In the abstract the authors focus on comparing women with a BMI over 40 and those with a healthy BMI, using relative risks to state that those with a BMI over 40 were:

- 4.8 times more likely to have pre-eclampsia
- 2.8 times more likely to have a stillbirth
- 2.7 times more likely to have a c-section
- 3.4 times more likely to have a neonatal death

The abstract does sound scary '*Maternal morbid obesity in early pregnancy is strongly associated with a number of pregnancy complications and perinatal conditions*'. However, when you look at the *individual absolute risk* for women with a healthy BMI compared to a BMI over 40 they showed risks of:

- 1.4% versus 3.5% for pre-eclampsia
- 0.3% versus 0.8% for a stillbirth
- 10.9% versus 34% for a caesarean section
- 0.1% versus 0.4% for a neonatal death

It is interesting that they chose to use the highest BMI of over 40 for the comparisons. Approximately 5% of women in the UK have a BMI over 40. The authors note that '*The associations were similar for women with BMIs between 35.1 and 40 but to a lesser degree*'.

Looking at the specific risks:

Complication	Healthy BMI	Obese	Very obese	Morbidly obese
Pre-eclampsia	1.4%	2.8%	3.4%	3.5%
Stillbirth	0.3%	0.5%	0.6%	0.8%
C-section	10.9%	16.7%	21.5%	34%
Neonatal death	0.1%	0.1%	0.3%	0.3%

What's important is that although the individual risk does increase as BMI increases a) those with a healthy BMI can still have the complication and b) it is a small overall risk, not a definitive. The only one that particularly stands out is the c-section rate, but flip that on its head: two-thirds of women with a BMI over 40 still give birth without a c-section.

One limitation of this paper is that it was based in Sweden, with 96% of the sample of White European background, so it is difficult to draw conclusions about other ethnic groups.

These findings were echoed in another cohort study of 226,958 women, this time in British Columbia in Canada.[32] The abstract was far less scary, declaring *'These results can inform pre-pregnancy weight loss counselling by defining achievable weight loss goals for patients that may reduce their risk of poor perinatal outcomes'.*

What was interesting in this study was that they also looked at all weight categories, including underweight and overweight. They found an individual risk of:

	<18.5	18.5–25	25–30	30–35	35–40	40+
Pre-eclampsia	2.4%	3.4%	6.4%	10%	12.8%	16.3%
Gestational diabetes	7.9%	5.4%	6.1%	9.7%	13.7%	16.6%
Stillbirth	0.3%	0.3%	0.3%	0.4%	0.4%	0.6%

Again, individual risk is low. The stillbirth data is a particularly good example of how you can write that something 'doubles the risk' when individual risk is actually low.

While reading all the data I also came across an interesting study that considered the risk of obesity during pregnancy when otherwise the woman was healthy. Obesity is associated with complications such as high blood pressure, pre-eclampsia and gestational diabetes, which in turn are associated with an increased risk of negative outcomes for the baby.[33] However, although the tabloids and the entire range of magazines aimed at women would collapse if this was more widely stated – it is perfectly possible to be healthy in all other ways but be overweight or obese. It's just that there is an increased risk of these things.

So what happens when a pregnant woman has a high BMI but no other health issues? Well, her risk drops considerably. In one study of 105 patient records from women who gave birth in a hospital in New Jersey, the difference in outcomes was compared for women with a BMI over 30 who had co-morbid health issues such as high blood pressure, pre-eclampsia, and gestational diabetes.[34] Comparing women with no health issues to those with one or more health issues they found:

- C-sections: 34.6% versus 58.5%
- Induction of labour: 15.4% versus 71.7%

5. Maternal age and pregnancy outcomes

One study in the UK looked at data from over 215,344 births and compared birth outcomes for women aged 30–34, 35–39 and ≥40 years with women aged 20–29.[35] The researchers predominantly reported on how women aged over 40 at birth were at an increased risk of:

- Stillbirth – 1.8 times higher
- Pre-term birth – 1.3 times higher
- Very pre-term birth – 1.3 times higher
- Macrosomic babies – 1.3 times higher
- Extremely large for gestational age babies – 1.4 times higher
- C-section – 1.8 times higher

But if you look at the individual risk of these outcomes per age group:

	20–29	30–34	35–39	40+
Stillbirth	0.4%	0.5%	0.6%	0.7%
C-section	18.4%	25.1%	29.6%	34.2%
Pre-term birth	6.1%	6.1%	6.9%	6.9%
Very pre-term birth	1.4%	1.3%	1.6%	1.6%
Macrosomia	1.4%	2.0%	2.2%	2.3%
Extremely large for gestational age	2.7%	4.0%	4.6%	4.9%

Although the risk does increase (most notably for c-section rates), looking at individual risk puts a different complexion on things.

Another study produced similar findings using retrospective data from 6,619 birth records in Oslo.[36] This simply compared women of 'advanced maternal age' (AMA) with non-advanced maternal age: older or younger than 35. The authors found only an increased risk of caesarean section in the older group. This study was interesting as it compared first- and second-time (or more) mothers:

	First-time mothers		Second-time mothers	
	AMA	*Non-AMA*	*AMA*	*Non-AMA*
Pre-term delivery	10.4%	11.5%	9.0%	8.1%
Pre-eclampsia	7.3%	6.7%	3.9%	3.5%
Gestational diabetes	1.1%	1.4%	2.5%	2.0%
Planned c-section	18.0%	10.3%	19.3%	14.4%
Emergency c-section	15.1%	12.4%	6.4%	5.5%
Low birth weight	8.3%	8.6%	5.6%	5.3%
Stillbirth	0.5%	0.5%	0.5%	0.5%

6. Co-sleeping

You will see many a headline claiming that sharing a bed with your baby is inherently dangerous.

As discussed in Chapter 14, there are a number of issues with research in this area. These include grouping all deaths where caregiver and baby share a sleeping surface (e.g. including sofas), not considering other risk factors (e.g. drinking alcohol or smoking), and not distinguishing between planned and unplanned co-sleeping.

One study used a case-control approach, looking at data from 1,472 babies who had died of SIDS and 4,679 babies (who were of a similar age and location) who did not.[37] They looked at different behaviours that were associated with SIDS and the rates at which they occurred in the SIDS and control group babies. They adjusted the odds ratios they computed for other confounding factors. They found that for overall SIDS risk:

- Bed-sharing was associated with a 2.7 times increased risk
- Bottle-feeding was associated with a 1.5 times increased risk

When they looked at lots of different factors together they concluded that if neither parent smoked, the baby was less than three months old, breastfed and had no other risk factors, then babies who were bed-sharing were five times more likely to die of SIDS. However, the absolute risk to any individual baby was a 0.08% chance of dying of SIDS if the baby was in a cot in the parents' room compared to a 0.23% chance of a baby dying of SIDS if bed-sharing.

If parents both smoke and bed-share, the risk of SIDS was 65 times higher if bed-sharing compared to room-sharing.

If the mother had drunk at least two units of alcohol then the risk of SIDS was 89 times higher for bed sharing compared to just room-sharing. However, compared to not drinking, drinking two or more units of alcohol was also linked to a five times increased risk for babies who room-shared (but did not bed-share), suggesting a wider factor other than sleep location may be increasing the risk.

Putting this into absolute risks:

- If a baby was breastfed, neither parent smoked, no alcohol drunk and the baby room-shared – 0.08 per 1,000 babies
- If a baby was breastfed, neither parent smoked, no alcohol drunk and the baby bed-shared – 0.23 per 1,000 babies
- If a baby was bottle-fed, both parents smoked, the mother drank alcohol and the baby bed-shared – 27.5 in 1,000

Note that this study did not take into account other risk factors that we know have been associated with SIDS risk, such as whether the bed-sharing was planned, the baby was ill, or the bed set-up was safe for the baby (e.g. no big duvets, no waterbeds, not in between the parents and so on). For further details on keeping a bed safer for a baby see **www.llli.org/the-safe-sleep-seven.**

So bringing this all together, this is where informed, shared decision-making really comes into play. You should be presented with all the real potential risks to you and your baby, and counselled through making a decision based on your individual circumstances, anxieties and concerns. For some people, smaller but more common risks will feel infinitely more likely and scary and for others the larger but less likely risks will be what scares them. There will never be one right decision for everyone. But women deserve the support to make the decision that is right for them based on having the truthful picture in front of them.

HOW TO KEEP INFORMED:

Check the difference between mathematical and real-life risk. What is the actual increase?

Check the absolute risk to you rather than the relative risk. Three times the risk means very little if the risk was only 0.2% in the first place.

Remember everything has a risk, including not doing anything.

Risk is calculated across populations, not for individuals. You will never have a 0.1% occurrence of something; you will have it or not. It's just that your chances of having it are 1 in 1,000. And things like your genetics, personal circumstances and luck will all influence whether you have it or not.

A really great website for reading more about actual versus relative risk is the Understanding Uncertainty website, led by Professor David Spiegelhalter, Chair of Public Understanding of Risk at Cambridge University. **understandinguncertainty.org/about**

Another great place to go is the WRISK project and website: **www.wrisk.org**. This project, which is just getting going as I write this, is looking at how risks during pregnancy are communicated to women and how health professionals and policymakers can do it better. It is a collaboration between Dr Heather Trickey at Cardiff University and the British Pregnancy Advisory Service, and will be a great support in helping anyone understand the risk to them and make the decision that is right for them.

18

MAKING THE DECISION THAT IS RIGHT FOR YOU... AND WHAT IF YOU CAN'T?

We've come to the end of the book. Hopefully you are now much more aware of how scientific information is presented in the media, and you've seen how you can dig into the research behind the headlines. Hopefully the yoga for the rage is helping. What now?

Remember that research is there to help inform your decision. It can be useful, but you can never read it all. Get an overview of what the research is saying, and then think about how it applies to you and your family. Let it play a role in the bigger picture of what you want, but remember that your own preferences, experiences, and wider familial and cultural influences are going to matter too. Whatever you decide, and whatever happens to you, information and evidence will hopefully help you feel more empowered or at peace with your decisions and outcomes.

Making the decision that is right for you

Whatever decision you make about something, someone will decide they are within their rights to tell you their thoughts about what they think you should do or how risky your decision is. I've seen this happen from every perspective. When I was planning a home birth I had people tell me I was putting everyone's lives at risk and the world as we knew it would end (it didn't but we did need a new carpet). I've also seen women told that their decision to go to a consultant-led unit is risky. Hopefully one day people will learn to keep their thoughts to themselves unless explicitly asked, but until then, how do you deal with potential risks sensibly?

The first thing is to remember that everything has a risk. Absolutely everything. From leaving the house in the morning to staying at home (remember to avoid that cheese in bed). Your own individual risk cannot be identified through reading research – research can only show what risks look like in a much bigger group of people, and how they might differ according to some of the characteristics you have.

Ultimately you have to decide what level of risk is acceptable to you. Some people find the BRAIN tool helpful in considering the overall picture. What are the potential benefits and risks of my options? What else could be possible? What is my intuition saying? And what would happen if I just did nothing?

- Benefits
- Risks
- Alternatives
- Intuition
- Nothing

Having the information about each of these stages is a central part of informed decision-making and you should have the opportunity to discuss it openly with your healthcare providers. However, as we saw at the start of the book, you may not always be given the information that you need. Hopefully you now feel more informed about how to find, understand and critique that information.

For example, if you are considering whether to have a home birth or not you might consider:

- What are the potential benefits of giving birth at home? What are the benefits of giving birth in a hospital? Which one weighs more positively?
- What are the potential risks at home? What are the potential risks in a hospital?
- What are the alternatives? How does a birth centre feel?
- What is my intuition or gut feeling saying? This is important. Our intuition can tell us a lot about what our primitive brain (which can affect how stressed we feel and thus how our labour progresses) feels about this.
- What if I did nothing? Perhaps you'd give birth in Tesco one day.

All these factors will be affected by other things personal to you:

- What does your partner think (if relevant)?
- Is this your first baby?
- Where do you live?
- Where do you feel most comfortable or indeed safest?
- What are your prior hospital experiences?
- Which professionals do you think will be involved and how do they make you feel?

And ultimately – why is a home birth important to you?

None of these things will be found in this much detail in the research literature. Even if the overall outcome for the group is positive or negative, not everyone will have the same experience. Research might suggest that overall women who give birth in water rave about how comforting they find it. But if you can't even stand having a bath then it's not going to be for you. This may be a flippant example, but the logic can be applied across decisions about birth and caring for babies.

Remember it's okay to consider your own needs

Women are continually told, subtly and otherwise, that they should not put themselves first. Right from childhood they are given the stereotypical doll and told to care for it, while boys get to have adventures with trucks and building toys.

Sometimes people say things to try and make you feel better (or to shame you) that exacerbate this. Telling women that 'All that matters is that you have a healthy baby,' or 'Fed is best,' can rightly leave women feeling that their experience doesn't matter and they were wrong for thinking it did. Of course these things matter! No one wants harm to come to their baby, or their baby to starve. But since when did that bottom line become our expectations? It's fine to want more. It's fine to want to feel in control of these monumental experiences in your life. And it's more than fine to grieve them if it doesn't happen.

What if other people judge me?

Ah, motherhood – place of perpetual judgement. Someone, somewhere, will always think you are doing it all wrong.

People love to judge mothers, particularly when they are pregnant. One quite frankly bonkers study asked US undergraduate students to rate whether they felt it was okay to feel negatively about a range of different groups. In this they had the following delightful characters – wife beaters, racists, terrorists, members of the Ku Klux Klan, drink drivers, child abusers, rapists, neo-Nazis, drug dealers, adulterers, exam cheats, gang members and many more... including pregnant women who drink alcohol. You can guess which group were thought most appropriate to judge, can't you? Yep, out of 95 different groups it was the pregnant women students felt most justified in feeling negatively towards.[1]

But why? Remember our discussion about the right-wing media, sexism and judgement of women? Well that's one big reason. People's own insecurities and desires are another. And some people are just nasty as they don't have enough cake in their lives.

Distinguish between what you want and what you think you 'ought' to do

Sometimes guilt or unease can come from what we think we 'should' do rather than what we want to do. There are of course certain things we should do in life. Like not leave the empty carton of milk in the fridge. Or eat the last slice of cake without asking. But you absolutely do not need to justify your decisions around birth and babies to anyone. You may want to talk it through with those close to you, but there is far too much expectation of women to give a reason for every last thing they do when it comes to their babies.

Professor Fiona Woollard, a philosopher, talks about this in terms of it being a 'duty mistake' or idea that we think we must act a certain way and owe it to others to explain ourselves, or that we must have a heavy science-based proof to make a decision. You don't need this. You have no moral obligation to act in a certain way when it comes to growing, birthing and caring for babies, other than to ensure that they are loved and cared for. The rest may be very important to you, of course – but there is never any need to justify it to others.[2]

What if things don't work out as you hoped?

No matter how informed we are about research and how it might affect us and our baby, Mother Nature and other factors can sometimes get in the way of our decision-making or our outcomes. We might really want to birth a certain way, feed our babies a certain way, care for them a certain way... but things outside our control may change that. If you need a caesarean section, then you need a caesarean section and suddenly for you, in your context, a caesarean is a much better idea than pushing (pun not intended) ahead with a vaginal birth.

So many of us have been there at one time or another. None of us genuinely, no matter what our social media posts say, do everything the 'right' way the guidance tells us to all the time. It just doesn't happen. We can plan, we can hope, but at the end of the day we are lucky that medicine and technology have enabled us to worry about things other than the most basic needs of life.

As a psychologist interested in eating behaviour and nutrition during pregnancy and the early years, I suffered hyperemesis (extreme morning sickness) in each of my three pregnancies. Yes, I did it three times. Yes, I did kind of forget in between each pregnancy just how bad it was. I knew all about healthy eating in pregnancy and remember at the very start of my first pregnancy (before the sickness hit) diligently stocking the fridge and freezer with salmon (for the fatty acids). It was downhill from then on as I ended up vomiting 20+ times a day at the worst of it.

In each pregnancy my diet from roughly 6–20 weeks (after that I only vomited eight times a day and could eat a slightly more varied diet) consisted of plain rice, rich tea biscuits (fingers, not the round ones), Lucozade and Haribo sweets. I occasionally managed some satsumas. By the third pregnancy my reliance on Haribo (only the tiny jelly babies, nothing else) was so well known that someone suggested I call the baby Haribo. Of course I didn't. I went for a more conventional version, Harry.

My point is that I knew what the research said, and I knew what I 'ought' to do. My body had other ideas. So be it.

One way of looking at this is to think like a gambler. If you're pregnant and planning what you would ideally like to do with your baby, reading widely helps you make an informed decision. The 'odds' lead you to decide that feeding your baby a certain way or giving birth a certain way is the right decision for you in that context. But if things change, the odds shift and you adjust your plan accordingly.

It also helps to think of the bigger picture. We've already covered how most health outcomes are so complicated that they are affected by many, many things. Remember that model of obesity and all its influences? Remember that it's highly unlikely that any one thing you do is going to change your child from being a healthy weight to being obese. The overall pattern of events in their lives is more important.

It's okay to feel bad

It's perfectly normal to feel a whole host of negative emotions when your plans don't work out. Maybe you feel angry. Sad. Anxious. Let down. Grieving. Mourning. Frustrated. Regretful. Bitter. Jealous. And likely a whole load of other words on top of that.

It's okay to feel it. It's okay to be angry. It's okay to grieve.

Some people find it easier to focus on what they have. They might find phrases like 'Fed is best' or 'your baby is healthy' helpful, for example. For others it's the exact opposite. When someone tries to tell them that all that matters is that they have a healthy baby, or the main thing is that the baby is fed, they feel as though their emotions, experiences and desires are being ignored. That they're being told they don't matter.

If you're struggling to come to terms with your birth, or anything around caring for your baby, there are many people who can help. First of all, contact your health professional and ask what support options are available in your area. There may be a birth debrief or reflections service. If you feel the care you received at any stage was not adequate, or wish to feed back in any way, you can contact your local Patient Advice and Liaison Service **www.nhs.uk/common-health-questions/nhs-services-and-treatments/what-is-pals-patient-advice-and-liaison-service.**

Although you've had your baby, think about contacting a doula. Doulas can help talk through your experiences and put them into context. They don't just support people through birth, but with everything to do with having babies, including debriefing and talking about your experiences. I did this myself in between babies one and two – it was pretty much the only way I was ever going to give birth (Kath Harbisher, I will be forever grateful). You can search for a local doula on the Doula UK website **doula.org.uk.**

The Birth Trauma Association can also help you work through your experiences and help you find support. Remember anyone with any birth experience can feel traumatised. It doesn't have to have been a physically difficult birth for you to be left feeling overwhelmed. There is lots of information on the website **birthtraumaassociation.org.uk.**

The Positive Birth Movement also has a directory of counsellors who can help you talk through any difficult experiences **www.positivebirthmovement.org/directory/counselling-support.** Likewise, the International Caesarean Awareness Network has lots of information and options for support **www.ican-online.org/support.** You may also find birth rewind therapy useful **www.traumaticbirthrecovery.com/directories.**

If your feeding experiences have not gone to plan you can contact any of the breastfeeding charities to talk through your experiences – and yes, they will absolutely support you with formula feeding. You can find details of all the different infant feeding helplines here: **www.nhs.uk/conditions/pregnancy-and-baby/breastfeeding-help-support.**

Another new and really useful resource if you are struggling, particularly with regard to any infant feeding decisions (but really the underlying ideas can apply to anything), is the Feeling Good About How We Feed Our Babies website – **www.feelingsaboutfeedingbabies.co.uk.** It covers lots of different feelings you might have about feeding, through from not being able to breastfeed to feeling embarrassed breastfeeding in public. It uses examples of ways of thinking that might help.

If you are experiencing mental health difficulties, talk to your health professional, but there are a range of charity organisations you might get in contact with, ranging from specific postnatal depression-related sites, to broader mental health charities. These include:

- The Samaritans **www.samaritans.org**
- Mind **www.mind.org.uk**
- Pre and Postnatal Depression and Support (PANDAS) **www.pandasfoundation.org.uk**
- Tommy's **www.tommys.org/pregnancy-information/im-pregnant/**

mental-health-during-and-after-pregnancy

- Postpartum support international **www.facebook.com/groups/25960478598**
- Petals – the baby loss counselling service (who also support birth trauma) **petalscharity.org**
- Bent not Broken trauma counselling project **www.facebook.com/BentNotBrokenProject**

Of course, it's not just women who are distressed by events around pregnancy, birth and babies. Men can be too. All of the above apply to men too, but you may also find a lot of support from the charity Fathers Reaching Out, set up by Mark Williams after his own experiences with postnatal depression after his son's birth **www.reachingoutpmh.co.uk.**

Changing things for the next generation of mothers

If things work out fine for you, based on your combination of factors and a helping of good fortune, that's fantastic. But there will be others out there with different experiences, and you might be able to help push for better services to support them.

Consider for example the wide body of research showing that fathers play an important role in child health and wellbeing. Fathers who are present, engaged and good role models are more likely to have children who grow up physically, educationally and psychologically well. And when fathers are absent, things can take a long-term turn for the worse. So it's really important that we do research into understanding how fathers help and publicise the importance of fathers so we can ensure that more investment and recognition is given to ensuring all children have the best possible outcomes.

But the situation is not straightforward. Many women are no longer with the fathers of their children, perhaps because he disappeared, opted out of financially supporting his children or became the sort of man you would not want near your children. And their children are just fine. In fact they're better off than when their father was there. And they're certainly not at a disadvantage in life. However, that's mainly because they are lucky in other ways. They have a mother who supports them. Enough money. Less stress in their homes. And other children won't have that and will suffer.

Now I'm sure the gut reaction of these women when they hear about the 'importance of fathers' is to throw things. It would be so easy to play down their importance – look, my child's father disappeared and he's fine! Well yes, indeed, but it's not about individuals. It's about patterns. And if enough privileged voices shout that something isn't important, then we run the risk of governments and policymakers listening… and disinvesting. Preventing the women and families who really need support from getting it.

So if something hasn't worked out how you hoped, or if it has – and you want to make a difference for the next generation of mothers who it might really matter for, come and put your voice behind campaigning for a better future for mothers and babies and those who love them.

- Join the Association for Improvements in Maternity Services (AIMS) to get involved with making pregnancy and birth better for more mothers **www.aims.org.uk**
- Birth Rights is a UK charity dedicated to improving women's experiences of pregnancy and childbirth **www.birthrights.org.uk**
- Explore the work of the Maternity Voices Partnership, dedicated to ensuring every woman has her voice heard **nationalmaternityvoices.org.uk**
- Follow the work of the Human Milk Foundation to help more babies who need it access donor human milk in the future **humanmilkfoundation.org**

We can make sure that more women in the future get the pregnancy, birth and postnatal experiences they want and deserve.

TRUSTED SOURCES

Although you are now hopefully feeling more informed about understanding the evidence and making your own decisions, sometimes you will want to be able to read about topics without thinking quite so much. So here is a *short* list of some trusted websites and individual blogs where you can find evidence-based information (still with your critical hat on!) when you're just too tired to dive into Google Scholar. Most will have references if you want to follow them up.

Guidelines for pregnancy, birth and babies
- RCOG Green Top Guidelines **www.sgh-og.com/guidelines/rcog-green-top-guidelines**
- NICE guidelines **www.nice.org.uk/guidance**
- Cochrane Reviews **www.cochranelibrary.com**

Pregnancy and birth
- AIMS
- Birthrights
- COPE – Centre of Perinatal Excellence
- Evidence Based Birth
- Midwife Thinking
- Sara Wickham

Infant feeding
- Academy of Breastfeeding Medicine
- Association of Breastfeeding Mothers
- Australian Breastfeeding Association
- Breastfeeding Network
- Breastfeeding Network Drugs in Breastmilk
- Breastfeeding Support
- Essentialparent.com

- First Steps Nutrition
- Global Health Media
- Infantrisk.com
- Jack Newman
- KellyMom
- La Leche League
- Milk Meg
- Nancy Morhbacher
- NCT
- UNICEF

For introducing solids and feeding your older child

- First Steps Nutrition
- Child Feeding Guide www.childfeedingguide.co.uk

Caring for your baby

- BASIS
- Evolutionary Parenting
- Lullaby Trust

REFERENCES

Introduction

1. www.nice.org.uk/about/what-we-do/our-programmes/nice-guidance/nice-guidelines/shared-decision-making
2. www.rcog.org.uk/globalassets/documents/guidelines/gtg_45.pdf
3. Kolip P, Büchter R 'Involvement of first-time mothers with different levels of education in the decision-making for their delivery by a planned Caesarean section. Women's satisfaction with information given by gynaecologists and midwives.' *Journal of Public Health.* 2009 Aug 1;17(4):273-80.

1. What do you want to believe?

1. Narayan, B, Case, D O, & Edwards, S L 'The role of information avoidance in everyday life information behaviors.' In *Proceedings of the American Society for Information Science and Technology,* 2011 48 (1), 1-9.
2. Nickerson, R S 'Confirmation bias: A ubiquitous phenomenon in many guises.' *Review of General Psychology.* 1998 Jun;2(2):175-220.
3. Hertz, N. *Eyes Wide Open.* HarperCollins UK; 2014.
4. Kuhlthau, C C 'Seeking meaning: A Process Approach to Library and Information Services.' 1993 New Jersey: Ablex.
5. Anderson, C A, Lepper, M R, & Ross, L 'Perseverance of social theories: The role of explanation in the persistence of discredited information.' *Journal of Personality and Social Psychology,* 1980 39(6), 1037.
6. Brown A, Harries V. Infant sleep and night feeding patterns during later infancy: Association with breastfeeding frequency, daytime complementary food intake, and infant weight. *Breastfeeding Medicine.* 2015 Jun 1;10(5):246-52.
7. Nevarez, M. D., Rifas-Shiman, S. L., Kleinman, K. P., Gillman, M. W., & Taveras, E. M. (2010). Associations of early life risk factors with infant sleep duration. *Academic pediatrics, 10*(3), 187-193.
8. Nevarez MD, Rifas-Shiman SL, Kleinman KP, Gillman MW, Taveras EM. Associations of early life risk factors with infant sleep duration. *Academic pediatrics.* 2010 May 1;10(3):187-93.
9. Hörnell A, Aarts C, Kylberg E, Hofvander Y, Gebre-Medhin M. Breastfeeding patterns in exclusively breastfed infants: a longitudinal prospective study in Uppsala, Sweden. *Acta paediatrica.* 1999 Feb;88(2):203-11.
10. White KM, Smith JR, Terry DJ, Greenslade JH, McKimmie BM. Social influence in the theory of planned behaviour: The role of descriptive, injunctive, and in-group norms. *British Journal of Social Psychology.* 2009 Mar;48(1):135-58.
11. Halpern D. *Inside the nudge unit: How small changes can make a big difference.* Random House; 2015 Aug 27.
12. Cialdini, R B 'Crafting normative messages to protect the environment.' *Current Directions in Psychological Science.* 2003 Aug; 12(4):105-9.
13. Marsden, P 'Memetics and social contagion: Two sides of the same coin.' *Journal of Memetics–Evolutionary Models of Information Transmission.* 1998; 2(2):171-85.
14. Rodgers, J L, Rowe, D C, Buster, M 'Social contagion, adolescent sexual behavior, and pregnancy: A nonlinear dynamic EMOSA model.' *Developmental Psychology.* 1998 Sep;34(5):1096.
15. Pink, S, Leopold, T, Engelhardt, H 'Fertility and social interaction at the workplace: Does childbearing spread among colleagues?' *Advances in Life Course Research.* 2014 Sep 1;21:113-22

16. Thompson, K D, Bendell, D 'Depressive cognitions, maternal attitudes and postnatal depression.' *Journal of Reproductive and Infant Psychology*. 2014 Jan 1;32(1):70-82.

17. Scott, J A, Mostyn, T 'Women's experiences of breastfeeding in a bottle-feeding culture.' *Journal of Human Lactation*. 2003 Aug;19(3):270-7.

18. Hunt L, Thomson, G 'Pressure and judgement within a dichotomous landscape of infant feeding: a grounded theory study to explore why breastfeeding women do not access peer support provision.' *Maternal & Child Nutrition*. 2017 Apr;13(2):e12279.

19. Cruwys, T, Haslam, S A, Dingle, G A, Jetten, J, Hornsey, M J, Chong, E D, Oei, T P 'Feeling connected again: Interventions that increase social identification reduce depression symptoms in community and clinical settings.' *Journal of Affective Disorders*. 2014 Apr 20; 159:139-46.

20. Nickerson, R S 'Confirmation bias: A ubiquitous phenomenon in many guises.' *Review of General Psychology*. 1998 Jun;2(2):175-220.

21. Kahneman, D *Thinking, Fast and Slow*. Macmillan; 2011.

22. Davis, M, Whalen, P J 'The amygdala: vigilance and emotion.' *Molecular Psychiatry*. 2001 Jan; 6(1):13.

23. Casey, B J, Tottenham, N, Liston, C, Durston, S 'Imaging the developing brain: what have we learned about cognitive development?' *Trends in Cognitive Sciences*. 2005 Mar 1; 9(3):104-10.

24. Sahakian, B, LaBuzetta, J N *Bad Moves: How decision-making goes wrong, and the ethics of smart drugs*. OUP, Oxford; 2013.

25. Kahneman, D, Slovic, S P, Slovic, P, Tversky, A, (Eds) *Judgment under Uncertainty: Heuristics and Biases*. Cambridge University Press; 1982.

26. Brown A, Raynor P, Lee M 'Young mothers who choose to breast feed: the importance of being part of a supportive breast-feeding community.' *Midwifery*. 2011 Feb 1; 27(1):53-9.

27. Thomas, E V '"Why even bother; they are not going to do it?" The structural roots of racism and discrimination in lactation care.' *Qualitative Health Research*. 2018 Jun; 28(7):1050-64.

28. www.breastfeedingnetwork.org.uk/guest-blog-by-ruth-dennison-why-black-breast-feeding-wcck

29. Hooker E, Ball, H L, Kelly, P J 'Sleeping like a baby: attitudes and experiences of bed-sharing in northeast England.' *Medical Anthropology*. 2001 Jan 1; 19(3):203-22

30. www.cracked.com/article_18849_6-statistically-full-s2321t-dangers-media-loves-to-hype.html

31. Thaler, R *Misbehaving: the making of behavioural economics*. Penguin; 2015.

32. Harris C R, Pashler, H E 'Evolution and human emotions.' *Psychological Inquiry*. 1995 Jan 1; 6(1):44-6.

33. Bechara, A, Damasio, H, Damasio, A R 'Emotion, decision making and the orbitofrontal cortex.' *Cerebral Cortex*. 2000 Mar 1; 10(3):295-307.

34. Brader, T *Campaigning for hearts and minds: How emotional appeals in political ads work*. University of Chicago Press; 2006.

35. Serani, D 'If it bleeds, it leads: The clinical implications of fear-based programming in news media.' *Psychotherapy and Psychoanalysis*. 2008; 24(4):240-50.

36. nautil.us/issue/60/Searches/how-to-talk-about-vaccines-on-television

37. Ito, T A, Larsen, J T, Smith, N K, Cacioppo, J T 'Negative information weighs more heavily on the brain: the negativity bias in evaluative categorizations.' *Journal of Personality and Social Psychology*. 1998 Oct; 75(4):887.

38. Barrett LF, Lindquist KA, Gendron M. Language as context for the perception of emotion. *Trends in cognitive sciences*. 2007 Aug 1;11(8):327-32.

39. Crawley H, Westland S. *Infant milks in the UK: a practical guide for health professionals*

June 2019. First Steps Nutrition Trust

40. Wansink, B, Van Ittersum, K, Painter, J E 'How descriptive food names bias sensory perceptions in restaurants.' *Food Quality and Preference*. 2005 Jul 1; 16(5):393-400.

41. Westland, S & Crawley, H 'Fruit and vegetable based purées in pouches for infants and young children.' First Steps Nutrition Trust, 2018.

2. How the news media shapes our views

1. www.pressgazette.co.uk/the-sun-overtakes-mail-online-to-become-uks-biggest-online-newspaper-brand-latest-comscore-data-shows

2. Glassner, B *The culture of fear: Why Americans are afraid of the wrong things*. Basic Books, New York; 1999.

3. Serani, D 'If it bleeds, it leads: The clinical implications of fear-based programming in news media.' *Psychotherapy and Psychoanalysis*. 2008; 24(4):240-50.

4. Duffy, B *The Perils of Perception: Why We're Wrong About Nearly Everything*. Atlantic Books; 2018.

5. Anell, A, Glenngard, A H, Merkur, S M 'Sweden: Health system review.' *Health Systems in Transition*. 2012; 14(5):1-59.

6. www.ipsos.com/ipsos-mori/en-uk/perceptions-are-not-reality

7. www.telegraph.co.uk/news/science/science-news/10555503/Spoon-fed-babies-more-likely-to-be-overweight.html

8. www.mediareform.org.uk/wp-content/uploads/2015/10/Who_owns_the_UK_media-report_plus_appendix1.pdf

9. en.wikipedia.org/wiki/Rupert_Murdoch

10. en.wikipedia.org/wiki/Jonathan_Harmsworth,_4th_Viscount_Rothermere

11. medium.com/oxford-university/where-do-people-get-their-news-8e850a0dea03

12. www.theguardian.com/media/yougov-polling-blog/2014/nov/18/yougov-profiles-the-nations-newspaper-readers

13. yougov.co.uk/topics/politics/articles-reports/2017/03/07/how-left-or-right-wing-are-uks-newspapers

14. Sibley, C G, Wilson, M S 'Differentiating hostile and benevolent sexist attitudes toward positive and negative sexual female subtypes.' *Sex Roles*. 2004 Dec 1; 51(11-12):687-96.

15. Acker, M 'Breast is best… but not everywhere: ambivalent sexism and attitudes toward private and public breastfeeding.' *Sex Roles*. 2009 Oct 1; 61(7-8):476-90.

16. Moya, M, Glick, P, Expósito, F, De Lemus, S, Hart, J 'It's for your own good: Benevolent sexism and women's reactions to protectively justified restrictions.' *Personality and Social Psychology Bulletin*. 2007 Oct; 33(10):1421-34.

17. Sutton, R M, Douglas, K M, McClellan, L M 'Benevolent sexism, perceived health risks, and the inclination to restrict pregnant women's freedoms.' *Sex Roles*. 2011 Oct 1; 65(7-8):596-605.

18. Huang, Y, Davies, P G, Sibley, C G, Osborne, D 'Benevolent sexism, attitudes toward motherhood, and reproductive rights: A multi-study longitudinal examination of abortion attitudes.' *Personality and Social Psychology Bulletin*. 2016 Jul; 42(7):970-84.

19. Christopher, A N, Mull, M S 'Conservative ideology and ambivalent sexism.' *Psychology of Women Quarterly*. 2006 Jun; 30(2):223-30.

20. Mahalik, J, Locke, B, Ludlow, L, Diemer, M, Gottfried, M, Scott, R, et al 'Development of the conformity to masculine norms inventory.' *Psychology of Men and Masculinity*, 2003 4, 3–25.

21. Ward, L M 'Does television exposure affect emerging adults' attitudes and assumptions about sexual relationships? Correlational and experimental confirmation.' *Journal of Youth and Adolescence*, 2002 31, 1–15.

22. Rudman, L, & Borgida, E 'The afterglow of construct accessibility: The behavioral con-

sequences of priming men to view women as sexual objects.' *Journal of Experimental Social Psychology*, 1995 31, 493–517.

23. Cox, C R, Goldenberg, J L, Arndt, J, & Pyszczynski, T 'Mother's milk: an existential perspective on negative reactions to breast-feeding.' *Personality and Social Psychology Bulletin*, 2007 33, 110–122.

24. Ward, L M, Merriwether, A, & Caruthers, A 'Breasts are for men: media, masculinity ideologies, and men's beliefs about women's bodies.' *Sex Roles*, 2006 55, 703–714.

25. Brown, A, Raynor, P, Lee, M 'Young mothers who choose to breast feed: the importance of being part of a supportive breast-feeding community.' *Midwifery*. 2011 Feb 1;27(1):53-9.

26. Murphy, A O, Sutton, R M, Douglas, K M, McClellan, L M 'Ambivalent sexism and the "do" s and "don't" s of pregnancy: Examining attitudes toward proscriptions and the women who flout them.' *Personality and Individual Differences*. 2011 Nov 1; 51(7):812-6.

27. Altemeyer, B 'The other "authoritarian personality".' In *Advances in Experimental Social Psychology* 1998 Jan 1 (Vol. 30, pp. 47-92). Academic Press.

28. Conway III, L G, Houck, S C, Gornick, L J, Repke, M A 'Finding the Loch Ness monster: Left-wing authoritarianism in the United States.' *Political Psychology*. 2018 Oct; 39(5):1049-67.

29. Żuk, P, Żuk, P 'Women's health as an ideological and political issue: Restricting the right to abortion, access to in vitro fertilization procedures, and prenatal testing in Poland.' *Health Care for Women International*. 2017 Jul 3; 38(7):689-704.

30. Christopher, A N, Wojda, M R 'Social dominance orientation, right-wing authoritarianism, sexism, and prejudice toward women in the workforce.' *Psychology of Women Quarterly*. 2008 Mar; 32(1):65-73.

31. Duncan, L E, Peterson, B E, Ax, E E 'Authoritarianism as an agent of status quo maintenance: Implications for women's careers and family lives.' *Sex Roles*. 2003 Dec 1; 49(11-12):619-30.

32. Pestell, R, Ball, J R 'Authoritarianism among medicine and law students.' *Australian and New Zealand Journal of Psychiatry*. 1991 Jan 1; 25(2):265-9.

33. Onraet, E, Van Hiel, A, Dhont, K, Pattyn, S 'Internal and external threat in relationship with right-wing attitudes.' *Journal of Personality*. 2013 Jun 1; 81(3):233-48.

34. www.dailymail.co.uk/femail/article-5572649/Women-reveal-drank-alcohol-pregnant. html

35. www.dailymail.co.uk/health/article-6343633/Deaths-pregnancy-rise-obesity-rates. html

36. www.telegraph.co.uk/news/2018/09/12/mumsnet-driving-women-request-caesarean-sections-leading-midwife/

37. www.dailymail.co.uk/news/article-6791165/Scientists-blame-working-mothers-Britains-childhood-obesity-epidemic-study-20-000.html

38. www.dailymail.co.uk/health/article-3662309/Working-mothers-FATTER-children-Rise-obesity-blamed-women-going-work.html

39. www.dailymail.co.uk/health/article-5020779/Working-mothers-LIKELY-obese-children.html

40. www.dailymail.co.uk/news/article-6897311/Women-help-prevent-children-obese-exercising-pregnancy-study-says.html

41. www.dailymail.co.uk/health/article-6695067/Single-mothers-likely-obese-children. html

42. www.dailymail.co.uk/health/article-6976361/Parenting-classes-reverse-UKs-obesity-crisis.html

43. www.dailymail.co.uk/health/article-1353521/Children-working-mothers-6-times-

likely-fat.html

3. The role of the internet

1. www.ons.gov.uk/businessindustryandtrade/itandinternetindustry/bulletins/interne-tusers/2019
2. www.statista.com/statistics/271851/smartphone-owners-in-the-united-kingdom-uk-by-age/
3. medium.com/oxford-university/where-do-people-get-their-news-8e850a0dea03
4. www.pewinternet.org/2011/02/28/peer-to-peer-health-care-2/
5. Usborne, S 'Cyberchondria: the perils of internet self-diagnosis.' *Independent.* 17 Feb, 2009.
6. Wong, D K, Cheung, M K 'Online Health Information Seeking and eHealth Literacy Among Patients Attending a Primary Care Clinic in Hong Kong: A Cross-Sectional Survey.' *Journal of Medical Internet Research.* 2019; 21(3):e10831.
7. Chu, J T, Wang, M P, Shen, C, Viswanath, K, Lam, T H, & Chan, S S C 'How, when and why people seek health information online: qualitative study in Hong Kong.' *Interactive Journal of Medical Research*, 2017 6(2), e24.
8. Fox, S, & Duggan, M 'Health online 2013.' *Health, 2013,* 1-55.
9. Rains, S A 'Perceptions of traditional information sources and use of the world wide web to seek health information: findings from the health information national trends survey.' *Journal of Health Communication.* 2007 Oct 11; 12(7):667-80.
10. www.ofcom.org.uk/research-and-data/media-literacy-research/adults/adults-media-use-and-attitudes
11. Lagan, B M, Sinclair, M, George Kernohan, W 'Internet use in pregnancy informs women's decision making: a web-based survey.' *Birth.* 2010 Jun; 37(2):106-15.
12. Tan, S S, Goonawardene, N 'Internet health information seeking and the patient-physician relationship: a systematic review.' *Journal of Medical Internet Research.* 2017; 19(1):e9.
13. www.nhs.uk/conditions/pregnancy-and-baby/getting-baby-to-sleep/
14. Brown A, Harries V. Infant sleep and night feeding patterns during later infancy: Association with breastfeeding frequency, daytime complementary food intake, and infant weight. Breastfeeding Medicine. 2015 Jun 1;10(5):246-52.
15. www.healthline.com/nutrition/7-health-benefits-dark-chocolate#section1
16. www.businessinsider.com/7-surprising-health-benefits-of-drinking-gin-2017-10?r=US&IR=T
17. www.theguardian.com/food/2019/jun/02/up-to-25-cups-of-coffee-a-day-safe-for-heart-health-study-finds
18. Ahmad, F, Hudak, P L, Bercovitz, K, Hollenberg, E, Levinson, W 'Are physicians ready for patients with Internet-based health information?' *Journal of Medical Internet Research.* 2006; 8(3):e22.
19. Dhillon, A S, Albersheim, S G, Alsaad, S, Pargass, N S, Zupancic, J A 'Internet use and perceptions of information reliability by parents in a neonatal intensive care unit.' *Journal of Perinatology.* 2003 Jul; 23(5):420.
20. Chang, T, Verma, B A, Shull, T, Moniz, M H, Kohatsu, L, Plegue, M A, Collins-Thompson, K 'Crowdsourcing and the accuracy of online information regarding weight gain in pregnancy: a descriptive study.' *Journal of Medical Internet Research.* 2016; 18(4):e81.
21. De Santis, M, De Luca, C, Quattrocchi, T, Visconti, D, Cesari, E, Mappa, I, Nobili, E, Spagnuolo, T, Caruso, A 'Use of the Internet by women seeking information about potentially teratogenic agents.' *European Journal of Obstetrics & Gynecology and Reproductive Biology.* 2010 Aug 1; 151(2):154-7.

22. www.dailymail.co.uk/health/article-1165972/Concerns-raised-milk-helps-babies-sleep-longer.html
23. www.iflscience.com/health-and-medicine/you-can-buy-intervaginal-speakers-so-your-baby-can-listen-to-tunes/
24. www.alexa.com/topsites/category/Health
25. www.healthcareglobal.com/top-10/top-10-healthcare-websites
26. Bryant, A G, Narasimhan, S, Bryant-Comstock, K, Levi, E E 'Crisis pregnancy center websites: information, misinformation and disinformation.' *Contraception*. 2014 Dec 1; 90(6):601-5.
27. www.thetimes.co.uk/article/fake-abortion-website-faces-legal-action-kmbmrl8f0
28. www.nestlenutrition-institute.org
29. Semigran, H L, Linder, J A, Gidengil, C, Mehrotra, A 'Evaluation of symptom checkers for self-diagnosis and triage: audit study.' *BMJ*. 2015 Jul 8; 351:h3480.
30. Comer, B 'Docs look to Wikipedia for condition info' Manhattan Research [Internet] New York: *Medical Marketing and Media*; 21 Apr 2009 [cited 4 Nov 2010].
31. Hughes, B, Joshi, I, Lemonde, H, Wareham, J 'Junior physicians' use of Web 2.0 for information seeking and medical education: a qualitative study.' *International Journal of Medical Information*. 2009 Oct; 78(10):645–55
32. Brokowski, L, Sheehan, A H 'Evaluation of pharmacist use and perception of Wikipedia as a drug information resource.' *Annals of Pharmacotherapy*. 2009 Nov; 43(11):1912–3
33. Kupferberg, N, Protus, B M 'Accuracy and completeness of drug information in Wikipedia: an assessment.' *Journal of the Medical Library Association*. 2011 Oct; 99(4):310.
34. Syed-Abdul, S, Fernandez-Luque, L, Jian, W S, Li, Y C, Crain, S, Hsu, M H, Wang, Y C, Khandregzen, D, Chuluunbaatar, E, Nguyen, P A, Liou, D M 'Misleading health-related information promoted through video-based social media: anorexia on YouTube.' *Journal of Medical Internet Research*. 2013;15(2):e30.
35. Pant, S, Deshmukh, A, Murugiah, K, Kumar, G, Sachdeva, R, Mehta, J L 'Assessing the credibility of the "YouTube approach" to health information on acute myocardial infarction.' *Clinical Cardiology*. 2012 May; 35(5):281-5.
36. www.healthline.com/health-news/fake-blogs-warning-about-medical-advice-from-online-experts#1
37. www.businessinsider.com/gwyneth-platrows-goop-lawsuit-vaginal-egg-claims-2018-9?r=US&IR=T
38. Archer, C 'Social media influencers, post-feminism and neoliberalism: How mum bloggers'playbour' is reshaping public relations.' *Public Relations Inquiry*. 2019 May; 8(2):149-66.
39. services.nhslothian.scot/feedingyourbaby/Documents/Statement_on_formula_preparation_machines_Nov%202016.pdf
40. www.expressandstar.com/entertainment/showbiz/2018/12/03/ferne-mccanns-tv-show-breached-broadcasting-rules/
41. www.unicef.org.uk/babyfriendly/baby-friendly-resources/international-code-marketing-breastmilk-substitutes-resources/the-code/
42. static1.squarespace.com/static/59f75004f09ca48694070f3b/t/5d131024a4f6110001954423/1561530417559/Infant_Milks_June_2019.pdf
43. Bell, S 'The infodiet: how libraries can offer an appetizing alternative to Google.' *The Chronicle of Higher Education*. 2004 50(24) Available at: chronicle.com/prm/weekly/v50/i24/24b01501.htm
44. Hertz N. Eyes wide open. HarperCollins; 2013.
45. Levitin DJ. The organized mind: Thinking straight in the age of information overload. Penguin; 2014 Aug 19.

46. US Preventative Services Task Force. 'Folic acid for the prevention of neural tube defects: US Preventative Services Task Force recommendation statement.' *Annals of Internal Medicine*, 150, 626-631

47. Kirsch, D 'A few thoughts on cognitive overload.' *Intellectica*. 2000 30 19–51.

48. Bawden, D 'Information Overload' (Library and Information Briefing Series, Library and Information Technology Centre, South Bank University, London, 2001).

49. Adamic LA, Huberman BA. Zipf's law and the Internet. Glottometrics. 2002 Jun;3(1):143-50.

50. Granka, L A, Joachims, T, Gay, G 'Eye-tracking analysis of user behavior in WWW search.' In *Proceedings of the 27th annual international ACM SIGIR conference on Research and Development in Information Retrieval*. 2004 Jul 25 (pp. 478-479). ACM.

51. McCoy BR. Digital distractions in the classroom phase II: Student classroom use of digital devices for non-class related purposes.

52. www.theguardian.com/commentisfree/2018/aug/25/skim-reading-new-normal-mary-anne-wolf

53. Liu, Z 'Reading behavior in the digital environment: Changes in reading behavior over the past ten years.' *Journal of Documentation*. 2005 Dec 1;61(6):700-12.

54. Carr N. Is Google making us stupid? What the internet is doing to our brains. The Atlantic July/August 2010

55. Hooper, V, Herath, C 'Is Google Making Us Stupid? The Impact of the Internet on Reading Behaviour.' InBled eConference 2014 (p1).

56. Fitzsimmons, G, Weal, M, Drieghe, D 'Skim reading: An adaptive strategy for reading on the Web.' 6th ACM Web Science Conference, WebSci 2014.

57. CIBER, *Information Behaviour of the Researcher of the Future (2008)*.

58. Miall, D S & Dobson, T 'Reading hypertext and the experience of literature.' *Journal of Digital Information*. 2006 2(1).

59. Mangen, A, Walgermo, B R, & Brønnick, K 'Reading linear texts on paper versus computer screen: Effects on reading comprehension.' *International Journal of Educational Research*, 2013 *58*, 61-68.

4. Social media tricks

1. wearesocial.com/blog/2019/01/digital-2019-global-internet-use-accelerates

2. www.journalism.org/2015/06/01/millennials-political-news/

3. Lupton, D 'The use and value of digital media for information about pregnancy and early motherhood: a focus group study.' *BMC Pregnancy and Childbirth*. 2016 Dec; 16(1):171.

4. Holtz, B, Smock, A, Reyes-Gastelum, D 'Connected motherhood: Social support for moms and moms-to-be on Facebook.' *Telemedicine and e-Health*. 2015 May 1; 21(5):415-21.

5. Shaw, L H, Gant, L M 'In defense of the Internet: The relationship between Internet communication and depression, loneliness, self-esteem, and perceived social support.' *Internet Research*. 2004 Jul 5; 28(3).

6. Barclay, L, Everitt, L, Rogan, F, Shmied, V, and Wyllie, A '"Becoming a mother" – an analysis of women's experience of early motherhood.' *Journal of Advanced Nursing*. 1997 25, 719-728.

7. Meadows, S 'The association between perceptions of social support and maternal mental health: A cumulative perspective.' *Journal of Family Issues*. 2011, 32, 181-208.

8. Gibson, L, Hanson, V L 'Digital motherhood: How does technology help new mothers?' In *Proceedings of the SIGCHI conference on human factors in computing systems*. 2013 Apr 27 (pp. 313-322). ACM.

9. Bartholomew, M K, Schoppe-Sullivan, S J, Glassman, M, et al 'New parents' Facebook

use at the transition to parenthood.' *Family Relations.* 2012 61(3): 455–469.

10. Moore, S, Kawachi, I 'Twenty years of social capital and health research: a glossary.' *Journal of Epidemiology and Community Health.* 2017 May 1; 71(5):513-7.

11. Holtz, B, Smock, A, Reyes-Gastelum, D 'Connected motherhood: Social support for moms and moms-to-be on Facebook.' *Telemedicine and e-Health.* 2015 May 1; 21(5):415-21.

12. BabyCenter 'BabyCentre's "2011 21st century Mum Report".' 22 September 2011. www. investegate.co.uk/article.aspx?id=20110922 11000571560

13. Madge, C, & O'Connor, H 'Parenting gone wired: empowerment of new mothers on the internet?' *Social & Cultural Geography.* 2006 7:02, 199-220.

14. Brady, E, & Guerin, S '"Not the Romantic, All Happy, Coochy Coo Experience": A Qualitative Analysis of Interactions on an Irish Parenting Web Site.' *Family Relations: Interdisciplinary Journal of Applied Family Studies.* 2010; 15, 14-27.

15. Skelton, K R, Evans, R, LaChenaye, J, Amsbary, J, Wingate, M, Talbott, L 'Exploring Social Media Group Use Among Breastfeeding Mothers: Qualitative Analysis.' *JMIR Pediatrics and Parenting.* 2018; 1(2):e11344.

16. Everett, F 'Facebook's motherhood challenge makes me want to punch my computer screen.' *The Guardian,* 3 February 2016. Available at: www.theguardian.com/comment-isfree/2016/feb/02/face-book-motherhood-challenge

17. Tandoc, E C, Ferrucci, P and Duffy, M 'Facebook use, envy, and depression among college students: is facebooking depressing?' *Computers in Human Behavior.* 2015 43: 139-146.

18. Schoppe-Sullivan SJ, Yavorsky JE, Bartholomew MK, Sullivan JM, Lee MA, Dush CM, Glassman M. Doing gender online: New mothers' psychological characteristics, Facebook use, and depressive symptoms. Sex roles. 2017 Mar 1;76(5-6):276-89.

19. Price, S L, Aston, M, Monaghan, J, Sim, M, Tomblin Murphy, G, Etowa, J, Pickles, M, Hunter, A, Little, V 'Maternal knowing and social networks: Understanding first-time mothers' search for information and support through online and offline social networks.' *Qualitative Health Research.* 2018 Aug;28(10):1552-63.

20. Centola D. An experimental study of homophily in the adoption of health behavior. Science. 2011 Dec 2;334(6060):1269-72.

21. Johnson, T J & Kaye, B K 'The dark side of the boon? Credibility, selective exposure and the proliferation of online sources of political information.' *Computers in Human Behavior.* 2013 29(4), 1862-1871.

22. www.bbc.co.uk/news/uk-41838386

23. Pennycook G, Rand DG. Lazy, not biased: Susceptibility to partisan fake news is better explained by lack of reasoning than by motivated reasoning. Cognition. 2019 Jul 1;188:39-50.

24. whyy.org/articles/poll-most-americans-believe-traditional-media-outlets-dispense-fake-news/

25. www.vox.com/the-goods/2018/12/28/18158968/facebook-microphone-tapping-recording-instagram-ads

26. twitter.com/scarlet_xroads/status/1119253342478307328

27. Bessi, A, Coletto, M, Davidescu, G A, Scala, A, Caldarelli, G, & Quattrociocchi, W 'Science vs conspiracy: Collective narratives in the age of misinformation.' *Plos One.* 2015.

28. Broniatowski, D A, Jamison, A M, Qi, S, AlKulaib, L, Chen, T, Benton, A, Quinn, S C, Dredze, M 'Weaponized health communication: Twitter bots and Russian trolls amplify the vaccine debate.' *American Journal of Public Health.* 2018 Oct; 108(10):1378-84.

29. Conover, M, Ratkiewicz, J, Francisco, M, Gonçalves, B, Menczer, F and Flammini, A 'Political polarization on Twitter.' In *Proceedings of the 5th International AAAI Conference on Weblogs and Social Media.* 2011, 89–96.

30. Edwards, C, Edwards, A, Spence, P R and Shelton, A K 'Is that a bot running the so-cial media feed? Testing the differences in perceptions of communication quality for a human agent and a bot agent on Twitter.' *Computers in Human Behavior.* 2014 *33,* 372–376.

31. Lee, K, Eoff, B D, and Caverlee, J 'Seven months with the devils: A long-term study of content polluters on Twitter.' In *Proceedings of the 5th International AAAI Conference on Weblogs and Social Media.* 2011, 185–192.

32. Aiello, L M, Deplano, M, Schifanella, R and Ruffo, G 'People are strange when you're a stranger: Impact and influence of bots on social networks.' In *Proceedings of the 6th AAAI International Conference on Weblogs and Social Media.* 2012. AAAI, 10–17.

33. Freitas, C A et al 'Reverse engineering social bot infiltration strategies in Twitter.' In *Proceedings of the 2015 IEEE/ACM International Conference on Advances in Social Networks Analysis and Mining.* ACM 2015.

34. Boshmaf, Y, Muslukhov, I, Beznosov, K and Ripeanu, M 'Design and analysis of a so-cial botnet.' *Computer Networks.* 2013 *57,* 2 (2013), 556–578.

35. Ferrara, O, Varol, C, Davis, F, Menczer, and Flammini, A. 'The rise of social bots.' Comm. ACM, 59(7):96–104, 2016.

36. Shao, C, Ciampaglia, G L, Varol, O, Flammini, A, Menczer, F 'The spread of fake news by social bots.' arXiv preprint arXiv:1707.07592. 2017 Jul 24:96-104.

37. Edwards, C, Edwards, A, Spence, P R, Shelton, A K 'Is that a bot running the social media feed? Testing the differences in perceptions of communication quality for a human agent and a bot agent on Twitter.' *Computers in Human Behavior.* 2014 Apr 1; 33:372-6.

38. Short, J, William, E, Christie, B *The social psychology of telecommunications.* New York: Wiley, 1976.

39. Neubaum G, Krämer NC. My friends right next to me: A laboratory investigation on predictors and consequences of experiencing social closeness on social networking sites. *Cyberpsychology, Behavior, and Social Networking.* 2015 Aug 1;18(8):443-9.

40. Thoits, P 'Social support as coping assistance.' *Journal of Consulting and Clinical Psychology.* 1986, volume 54, number 4, pp. 416–423.

41. www.americanpressinstitute.org/publications/reports/survey-research/news-trust-digital-social-media/

42. ifballiance.org/about#vic-widget-27-container-anchor

43. Morris, M R, Counts, S, Roseway, A, Hoff, A & Schwarz, J 'Tweeting is believing? Understanding microblog credibility perceptions.' In S Poltrock & C Simone (Eds), *Proceedings of the ACM 2012 Conference on Computer Supported Cooperative Work* (pp.441-450). Seattle, WA: ACM Press, 2012.

44. Goldacre, Ben (30 September 2004). 'Dr Gillian McKeith (PhD) continued.' *The Guardian.* London. Retrieved 31 March 2010.

45. de Almeida Brites, J 'The language of psychopaths: A systematic review.' *Aggression and Violent Behavior.* 2016 Mar 1; 27:50-4.

46. Stadtler, M, Bromme, R 'The Content–Source Integration Model: A taxonomic description of how readers comprehend conflicting scientific information.' In: Rapp, D N, Braasch, J (Eds) *Processing Inaccurate Information: Theoretical and Applied Perspectives from Cognitive Science and the Educational Sciences.* Cambridge, MA: MIT Press; 2014. p. 379–402

47. Flanagin, A J & Metzger, M J 'The role of site features, user attributes, and information verification behaviors on the perceived credibility of web-based information.' *New Media & Society,* 2007 9(2), 319-342.

48. Bossaller, J S 'Evidence, Not Authority: Reconsidering Presentation of Science for Difficult Decisions.' *Reference and User Services Quarterly.* 2014 53(3), 232-241.

49. Frey, D, Shulz-Hardt, S, & Stahlberg, D 'Information seeking among individuals and groups and possible consequences for decision making in business and politics.' In Witte, E H, & Davis, J H, (Eds), *Understanding Group Behavior, Volume 1: Consensual Action By Small Groups*. 2013 1, 211-225.

50. Goertzel, T 'Belief in conspiracy theories.' *Political Psychology*. 1994 15, 731-42.

51. Shachaf, P and Hara, N, 'Beyond vandalism: Wikipedia trolls.' *Journal of Information Science*. 2010 *36*(3), pp.357-370.

52. Buckels, E E, Trapnell, P D and Paulhus, D L, 'Trolls just want to have fun.' *Personality and Individual Differences*. 2014 *67*, pp.97-102.

53. www.forbes.com/sites/marshallshepherd/2019/03/07/sealioning-is-a-common-trolling-tactic-on-social-media-what-is-it/#30cf12ac7a41

54. cyber.harvard.edu/sites/cyber.harvard.edu/files/2017-08_harmfulspeech.pdf

55. Dunning, D 'The Dunning–Kruger effect: On being ignorant of one's own ignorance.' In *Advances in Experimental Social Psychology*. 2011 Jan 1 (Vol. 44, pp. 247-296). Academic Press.

56. Tavris, C, Aronson, E. *Mistakes were made (but not by me): Why we justify foolish beliefs, bad decisions, and hurtful acts*. Pinter & Martin, London, 2016.

57. Bode, L, Vraga, E K 'In related news, that was wrong: The correction of misinformation through related stories functionality in social media.' *Journal of Communication*. 2015 Jun 23; 65(4):619-38.

58. Jerit, J, Barabas, J 'Partisan perceptual bias and the information environment.' *The Journal of Politics*. 2012 Jul; 74(3):672-84.

59. Fernbach, P M, Rogers, T, Fox, C R, Sloman, S A 'Political extremism is supported by an illusion of understanding.' *Psychological Science*. 2013 Jun; 24(6):939-46.

60. Lewandowsky, S, Ecker, U K, Seifert, C M, Schwarz, N, Cook, J 'Misinformation and its correction: Continued influence and successful debiasing.' *Psychological Science in the Public Interest*. 2012 Dec;13(3):106-31.

61. DiFonzo, N, Robinson, N M, Suls, J M, Rini, C 'Rumors about cancer: Content, sources, coping, transmission, and belief.' *Journal of Health Communication*. 2012 Oct 1; 17(9):1099-115.

62. Nyhan, B, Reifler, J. 'When corrections fail: The persistence of political misperceptions.' *Political Behavior*. 2010 Jun 1; 32(2):303-30.

63. www.theguardian.com/science/2019/jun/30/the-science-of-influencing-people-six-ways-to-win-an-argument

64. Barrett, L F, Bliss-Moreau, E 'She's emotional. He's having a bad day: Attributional explanations for emotion stereotypes.' *Emotion*. 2009 Oct;9(5):649.

65. Omerod, K *Why Social Media is Ruining your Life*. Cassell, 2018.

66. Hicks, S, Brown, A 'Higher Facebook use predicts greater body image dissatisfaction during pregnancy: the role of self-comparison.' *Midwifery*. 2016 Sep 1; 40:132-40.

67. Padoa T, Berle D, Roberts L. Comparative social media use and the mental health of mothers with high levels of perfectionism. *Journal of Social and Clinical Psychology*. 2018 Sep;37(7):514-35.

5. Who is the messenger?

1. Wilson, P *Second-hand knowledge: an inquiry into cognitive authority*. Westport, CT: Greenwood Press, 1983.

2. Harries V, Brown A. The association between use of infant parenting books that promote strict routines, and maternal depression, self-efficacy, and parenting confidence. *Early Child Development and Care*. 2019 Jul 3;189(8):1339-50.

3. Harries V, Brown A. The association between baby care books that promote strict care routines and infant feeding, night-time care, and maternal–infant interactions. *Mater-*

nal & Child Nutrition. 2019 Jun 19:e12858.

4. Metzger, M J, Flanagin, A J & Medders, R B 'Social and heuristic approaches to credibility evaluation online.' *Journal of Communication.* 2010 *60*(3), 413-439.

5. www.slideshare.net/EdelmanInsights/2017-edelman-trust-barometer-global-results-71035413

6. www.pewresearch.org/fact-tank/2017/07/20/republicans-skeptical-of-colleges-impact-on-u-s-but-most-see-benefits-for-workforce-preparation/

7. blogs.lse.ac.uk/usappblog/2017/08/30/had-enough-of-experts-anti-intellectualism-is-linked-to-voters-support-for-movements-that-are-skeptical-of-expertise/

8. blogs.scientificamerican.com/observations/trump-to-cdc-these-7-words-are-now-forbidden/

9. d25d2506sfb94s.cloudfront.net/cumulus_uploads/document/x4iynd1mn7/TodayResults_160614_EUReferendum_W.pdf

10. Collini S. *What are universities for?* Penguin UK; 2012 Feb 23.

11. www.nytimes.com/2017/03/21/books/the-death-of-expertise-explores-how-ignorance-became-a-virtue.html

12. Anderson, A A, Scheufele, D A, Brossard, D, Corley, E A 'The role of media and deference to scientific authority in cultivating trust in sources of information about emerging technologies.' *International Journal of Public Opinion Research.* 2011 Aug 25;24(2):225-37.

13. Kahan, D M, Jenkins-Smith, H, Braman, D 'Cultural cognition of scientific consensus.' *Journal of Risk Research.* 2011 Feb 1; 14(2):147-74.

14. Weibel, D, Wissmath, B, Groner, R 'How gender and age affect newscasters' credibility—an investigation in Switzerland.' *Journal of Broadcasting & Electronic Media.* 2008 Aug 8; 52(3):466-84.

15. Vedantam, S 'Male Scientist Writes of Life as Female Scientist.' *Washington Post*: www.washingtonpost.com/wp-dyn/content/article/2006/07/12/AR2006071201883.html

16. cdn.agilitycms.com/who-makes-the-news/Imported/reports_2010/national/UK.pdf

17. Hancock, A B, & Rubin, B A 'Influence of Communication Partner's Gender on Language.' *Journal of Language and Social Psychology.* 2014 *34*(1), 46-64.

18. Solnit R. Men explain things to me. Haymarket Books; 2014 Apr 14.

19. Laserna, C M, Seih, Y, & Pennebaker, J W 'Um... Who Like Says You Know: Filler Word Use as a Function of Age, Gender, and Personality.' *Journal of Language and Social Psychology.* 2014 *33*(3), 328-338

20. www.inc.com/deborah-grayson-riegel/how-to-get-rid-of-filler-words-sound-more-professional-in-4-weeks.html

21. Salerno, J M, Peter-Hagene, L C 'One angry woman: Anger expression increases influence for men, but decreases influence for women, during group deliberation.' *Law and Human Behavior.* 2015 Dec; 39(6):581

22. Barrett, L F, Bliss-Moreau, E 'She's emotional. He's having a bad day: Attributional explanations for emotion stereotypes.' *Emotion.* 2009 Oct; 9(5):649.

23. Steinpreis, R E, Anders, K A, Ritzke, D 'The impact of gender on the review of the curricula vitae of job applicants and tenure candidates: A national empirical study.' *Sex Roles.* 1999 Oct 1;41(7-8):509-28.

24. Eaton, A A, Saunders, J F, Jacobson, R K, West, K 'How Gender and Race Stereotypes Impact the Advancement of Scholars in STEM: Professors' Biased Evaluations of Physics and Biology Post-Doctoral Candidates.' *Sex Roles.* 2019:1-5.

25. Okimoto, T G, & Brescoll, V L 'The price of power: Power seeking and backlash against female politicians.' *Personality and Social Psychology Bulletin.* 2010, 36, 923–936.

26. Brescoll, V L, Okimoto, T G, Vial, A C 'You've come a long way... maybe: How moral

emotions trigger backlash against women leaders.' *Journal of Social Issues*. 2018 Mar; 74(1):144-64.

27. Williams, M J, & Tiedens, L T 'The subtle suspension of backlash: A meta-analysis of penalties for women's implicit and explicit dominance behavior.' *Psychological Bulletin*. 2016, 57, 675–688.

28. Haidt, J 'The moral emotions.' In R J Davidson, K R Scherer, & H H Goldsmith (Eds), *Handbook of Affective Sciences* (pp.852–870). Oxford University Press, 2003.

29. Moore, M M, Williams, G I 'No jacket required: Academic women and the problem of the blazer.' *Fashion, Style & Popular Culture*. 2014 Aug 1;1(3):359-76.

30. Gray, S 'To Curl Up or Relax? That is the Question: Tenured Black Female Faculty Navigation of Black Hair Expression in Academia.' Southern Illinois University at Carbondale; 2017.

31. Muzzatti SL, Samarco CV, editors. *Reflections from the wrong side of the tracks: Class, identity, and the working class experience in academe*. Rowman & Littlefield; 2006.

32. Salway S, Chowbey P, Such E, Ferguson B. Researching health inequalities with community researchers: practical, methodological and ethical challenges of an 'inclusive'research approach. *Research Involvement and Engagement*. 2015 Dec;1(1):9.

33. www.hesa.ac.uk/news/18-01-2018/sfr248-higher-education-staff-statistics

34. www.theguardian.com/education/2019/feb/04/black-female-professors-report

35. Head, M G, Fitchett, J R, Cooke, M K, Wurie, F B, Atun, R 'Differences in research funding for women scientists: a systematic comparison of UK investments in global infectious disease research during 1997–2010.' *BMJ Open*. 2013 Dec 1; 3(12):e003362.

36. Zhou, C D, Head, M G, Marshall, D C, Gilbert, B J, El-Harasis, M A, Raine, R, O'Connor, H, Atun, R, Maruthappu, M 'A systematic analysis of UK cancer research funding by gender of primary investigator.' *BMJ Open*. 2018 Apr 1; 8(4):e018625.

37. Barrett, L, Barrett, P 'Women and academic workloads: career slow lane or Cul-de-Sac?' *Higher Education*. 2011 Feb 1;61(2):141-55.

38. www.nature.com/news/gender-balance-women-are-funded-more-fairly-in-social-science-1.18310

39. Filardo, G, da Graca, B, Sass, D M, Pollock, B D, Smith, E B, Martinez, M A. 'Trends and comparison of female first authorship in high impact medical journals: observational study (1994-2014).' *BMJ*. 2016 Mar 2; 352:i847.

40. Renn, O, Levine, D 'Credibility and trust in risk communication.' In *Communicating Risks to the Public*. 1991 (pp. 175-217). Springer, Dordrecht.

41. Hendriks, F, Kienhues, D, Bromme, R 'Measuring laypeople's trust in experts in a digital age: The Muenster Epistemic Trustworthiness Inventory (METI).' *PloS One*. 2015 Oct 16; 10(10):e0139309.

42. Eiser, J R, Stafford, T, Henneberry, J, Catney, P '"Trust me, I'm a scientist (not a developer)": Perceived expertise and motives as predictors of trust in assessment of risk from contaminated land.' *Risk Analysis: An International Journal*. 2009 Feb;29(2):288-97.

43. Bica OC, Giugliani ER. Influence of counseling sessions on the prevalence of breastfeeding in the first year of life: a randomized clinical trial with adolescent mothers and grandmothers. Birth. 2014 Mar;41(1):39-45.

44. archive.defense.gov/Transcripts/Transcript.aspx?TranscriptID=2636

45. Kuklinski, J H, Quirk, P J, Jerit, J, Schwieder, D, Rich, R F 'Misinformation and the currency of democratic citizenship.' *Journal of Politics*. 2000 Aug; 62(3):790-816.

46. www.theguardian.com/uk-news/2016/jun/26/cornwall-fears-loss-of-funding-after-backing-brexit

47. Fischhoff, B, Slovic, P, Lichtenstein, S 'Knowing with certainty: The appropriateness of extreme confidence.' *Journal of Experimental Psychology: Human Perception and Performance*. 1977 Nov; 3(4):552.

48. Paulhus, D L, Harms, P D, Bruce, M N, & Lysy, D C 'The over-claiming technique: Measuring self-enhancement independent of ability.' *Journal of Personality and Social Psychology*. 2003 84, 890–904

49. Bishop, G F, Tuchfarber, A J, & Oldendick, R W 'Opinions on fictitious issues: The pressure to answer survey questions.' *Public Opinion Quarterly*. 1986 50, 240–250

50. Barnsley, L, Lyon, P, Ralson, S, Hibbert, E, Cunningham, I, Gordon, F, et al 'Clinical skills in junior medical officers: A comparison of self-reported confidence and observed competence.' *Medical Education*. 2004 38, 358–367.

51. Brocas I, Carrillo JD. Are we all better drivers than average? Self-perception and biased behaviour.

52. theconversation.com/distrust-of-experts-happens-when-we-forget-they-are-human-beings-76219

53. www.businessinsider.com/what-is-the-eu-is-top-google-search-in-uk-after-brexit-2016-6

54. Von Wagner C, Knight K, Steptoe A, Wardle J. Functional health literacy and health-promoting behaviour in a national sample of British adults. *Journal of Epidemiology & Community Health*. 2007 Dec 1;61(12):1086-90.

55. Motta, M, Callaghan, T, Sylvester, S 'Knowing less but presuming more: Dunning-Kruger effects and the endorsement of anti-vaccine policy attitudes.' *Social Science & Medicine*. 2018 Aug 1; 211:274-81.

56. Dunning, D 'The Dunning–Kruger effect: On being ignorant of one's own ignorance.' In *Advances in Experimental Social Psychology*. 2011 Jan 1 (Vol. 44, pp. 247-296). Academic Press.

57. Dunning, D, Johnson, K, Ehrlinger, J, & Kruger, J 'Why people fail to recognize their own incompetence.' *Current Directions in Psychological Science*. 2003 12, 83–87.

58. Ehrlinger, J, Johnson, K, Banner, M, Dunning, D, & Kruger, J 'Why the unskilled are unaware? Further explorations of (lack of) self-insight among the incompetent.' *Organizational Behavior and Human Decision Processes*. 2008 105, 98–121.

59. Dunning, D, & Stern, L B 'Distinguishing accurate from inaccurate eyewitness identifications via inquiries about decision processes.' *Journal of Personality and Social Psychology*. 1994 67, 818–835

60. Ehrlinger, J, & Dunning, D 'How chronic self-views influence (and potentially mislead) assessments of performance.' *Journal of Personality and Social Psychology*. 2003 84, 5–17

6. Research funding, financial gains and conflict of interest

1. www.ukri.org

2. wellcome.ac.uk/news/new-funding-model-replace-public-engagement-fund

3. www.nytimes.com/2019/03/19/health/postpartum-depression-drug.html

4. www.theguardian.com/us-news/2018/jan/16/why-does-it-cost-32093-just-to-give-birth-in-america

5. Nestle, M 'Food industry funding of nutrition research: the relevance of history for current debates.' *JAMA Internal Medicine*. 2016 Nov 1;176(11):1685-6.

6. Lesser, L I, Ebbeling, C B, Goozner, M, Wypij, D, Ludwig, D S 'Relationship between funding source and conclusion among nutrition-related scientific articles.' *PLoS Medicine*. 2007 Jan 9; 4(1):e5.

7. Vartanian, L R, Schwartz, M B, Brownell, K D 'Effects of Soft Drink Consumption on Nutrition and Health: A Systematic Review and Meta-Analysis.' *American Journal of Public Health*. 2007;97(4):667-75.

8. PrescQIPP. 'Appropriate prescribing of specialist infant formulae (foods for special medical purposes).' 2016. www.prescqipp.info/media/1346/b146-infant-feeds-21.pdf

9. NHS Digital. Prescription cost analysis—England, 2017. digital.nhs.uk/data-and-information/publications/statistical/prescription-cost-analysis/prescription-cost-analysis-england-2017

10. Venter, C, Patil, V, Grundy, J, et al 'Prevalence and cumulative incidence of food hypersensitivity in the first 10 years of life.' *Pediatric Allergy and Immunology*. 2016; 27:452-8.10.1111/pai.12564 26999747

11. van Tulleken, C 'Overdiagnosis and industry influence: how cow's milk protein allergy is extending the reach of infant formula manufacturers.' *BMJ*. 2018 *363*, k5056.

12. well.blogs.nytimes.com/2015/08/09/coca-cola-funds-scientists-who-shift-blame-for-obesity-away-from-bad-diets/?_r=0

13. Kearns CE, Schmidt LA, Glantz SA. Sugar industry and coronary heart disease research: a historical analysis of internal industry documents. JAMA internal medicine. 2016 Nov 1;176(11):1680-5.

14. Lundh, A, Lexchin, J, Mintzes, B, Schroll, J B, Bero, L 'Industry sponsorship and research outcome.' *Cochrane Database Systematic Review* 2017(2):MR000033.

15. Critchley, C R 'Public opinion and trust in scientists: The role of the research context, and the perceived motivation of stem cell researchers.' *Public Understanding of Science*. 2008 Jul; 17(3):309-27.

16. www.eatdrinkpolitics.com/wp-content/uploads/AND_Corporate_Sponsorship_Report.pdf

17. www.firststepsnutrition.org/websites-organisations

18. World Health Organization. *International Code of Marketing of Breastmilk Substitutes.* Geneva: World Health Organization; 1981

19. Berry NJ, Jones S, Iverson D. It's all formula to me: women's understandings of toddler milk ads. Breastfeeding Review. 2010 Mar;18(1):21.

20. Alden DL, Steenkamp JB, Batra R. Brand positioning through advertising in Asia, North America, and Europe: The role of global consumer culture. *Journal of marketing*. 1999 Jan;63(1):75-87.

21. www.savethechildren.org.uk/content/dam/gb/reports/health/dont-push-it.pdf

22. Palmer G. The politics of breastfeeding: When breasts are bad for business. Pinter & Martin Publishers; 2009.

23. Godlee F, Cook S, Coombes R, El-Omar E, Brown N. Calling time on formula milk adverts. BMJ 2019;364:l1200

24. www.rcpch.ac.uk/news-events/news/rcpch-statement-relationship-formula-milk-companies

25. www.barnardos.ie/news/2018/june/danone-early-life-nutrition-celebrates-15-years-of-support-of-barnardos-childrens-charity

26. www.irishexaminer.com/breakingnews/business/barnardos-defends-danone-deal-930683.html

27. www.babymilkaction.org/wp-content/uploads/2016/08/monitoringuk070916.pdf

28. www.babymilkaction.org/archives/18478

29. Lam A. From 'ivory tower traditionalists' to 'entrepreneurial scientists'? Academic scientists in fuzzy university—industry boundaries. Social studies of science. 2010 Apr;40(2):307-40.

30. www.nutritioncoalition.us/news/2019/6/10/first-ever-birth-24-month-dietary-guidelines-deliberations-and-complications

31. www.nytimes.com/2018/12/08/health/medical-journals-conflicts-of-interest.html

32. cjasn.asnjournals.org/content/13/1/26.long

33. www.nejm.org/doi/full/10.1056/NEJMoa1609709

34. Ziai, K, Pigazzi, A, Smith, B R, Nouri-Nikbakht, R, Nepomuceno, H, Carmichael, J C, Mills, S, Stamos, M J, Jafari, M D 'Association of compensation from the surgical

and medical device industry to physicians and self-declared conflict of interest.' *JAMA Surgery*. 2018 Nov 1; 153(11):997-1002.

35. Koletzko, B, Bhutta, Z A, Cai, W, Cruchet, S, Guindi, M E, Fuchs, G J, et al 'Compositional requirements of follow-up formula for use in infancy: Recommendations of an international expert group coordinated by the Early Nutrition Academy.' *Annals of Nutrition Metabolism*. 2013;62(1):44-54.

36. Laving, A R, Hussain, S R, Atieno, D O 'Overnutrition: Does complementary feeding play a role?' *Annals of Nutrition Metabolism*. 2018; 73:15-8.

37. Laving AR, Hussain SR, Atieno DO: Overnutrition: Does Complementary Feeding Play a Role? *Ann Nutr Metab*. 2018; 73 Suppl 1: 15–8

38. Hennessy M, Cullerton K, Baker P, Brown A, Crawley H, Hayes C, Kearney PM, Kelly C, McKee M, Mialon M, Petticrew M. Time for complete transparency about conflicts of interest in public health nutrition research [version 2; referees: 2 approved]. HRB Open Research. 2019 Mar 4.

39. Haivas, I, Schroter, S, Waechter, F, Smith, R 'Editors' declaration of their own conflicts of interest.' *CMAJ*. 2004;171(5):475-6.

40. womensenews.org/2018/12/exclusive-investigative-report-harvards-pediatric-nutrition-star-comes-under-scrutiny-for-conflicts-of-interest/

41. Bass JL, Gartley T, Kleinman R. Unintended consequences of current breastfeeding initiatives. JAMA pediatrics. 2016 Oct 1;170(10):923-4.

42. www.infactcanada.ca/Chandra_Jan30_2006.htm

43. retractionwatch.com/2016/07/26/who-is-ranjit-kumar-chandra-a-timeline-of-notoriety/

44. Chandra, R K, Puri, S, Hamed, A 'Influence of maternal diet during lactation and use of formula feeds on development of atopic eczema in high risk infants.' *BMJ*. 1989 Jul 22; 299(6693):228.

45. Chandra, R K, Singh, G U, Shridhara, B E 'Effect of feeding whey hydrolysate, soy and conventional cow milk formulas on incidence of atopic disease in high risk infants.' *Annals of Allergy*. 1989 Aug; 63(2):102-6.

7. How do you know which research to trust?

1. Greenhalgh, T *How to Read a Paper: The basics of evidence-based medicine*. John Wiley & Sons; 2010.

8. Research methods 101

1. Greenhalgh, T *How to Read a Paper: The basics of evidence-based medicine*. John Wiley & Sons; 2010.

2. Bryman, A *Social Research Methods*. Oxford University Press. 2016.

3. Bowling, A *Research methods in health: investigating health and health services*. McGraw Hill. 2014.

4. Coolican, H *Research Methods and Statistics in Psychology*. Psychology Press. 2017.

5. Carneiro I, Howard, N *Introduction to Epidemiology*. McGraw Hill. 2011.

6. Liamputtong, P *Research methods in health: foundations for evidence-based practice*. 2010.

7. Smith, G C, Pell, J P 'Parachute use to prevent death and major trauma related to gravitational challenge: systematic review of randomised controlled trials.' *BMJ* 2003; 327:1459-61. doi:10.1136/bmj.327.7429.1459 pmid:14684649

8. www.bristol.ac.uk/alspac/researchers/publications/

9. cls.ucl.ac.uk/cls-studies/millennium-cohort-study/

10. cls.ucl.ac.uk/cls-studies/1958-national-child-development-study/

11. McAndrew, F, Thompson, J, Fellows, L, Large, A, Speed, M, Renfrew, M J 'Infant Feed-

ing Survey 2010.' *Leeds: Health and Social Care Information Centre.* 2012 Nov 20.

12. www.who.int/csr/disease/ebola/one-year-report/factors/en/

13. Lincoln, Y S, Guba, E G 'But is it rigorous? Trustworthiness and authenticity in naturalistic evaluation.' *New Directions for Program Evaluation.* 1986 Jun; 1986(30):73-84.

14. Evans, D 'Hierarchy of evidence: a framework for ranking evidence evaluating healthcare interventions.' *Journal of Clinical Nursing.* 2003 Jan;12(1):77-84.

15. Daniels, K, Loewenson, R, George, A, Howard, N, Koleva, G, Lewin, S, Marchal, B, Nambiar, D, Paina, L, Sacks, E, Sheikh, K 'Fair publication of qualitative research in health systems: a call by health policy and systems researchers.' *International Journal for Equity in Health.* 2016 Dec; 15(1):98.

16. Konner, M 'Nursing frequency and birth spacing in Kung hunter-gatherers.' *IPPF Medical Bulletin.* 1978 Apr 1;15(2):1-3.

17. Ghosh, R, Mascie-Taylor, C N and Rosetta, L 'Longitudinal study of the frequency and duration of breastfeeding in rural Bangladeshi women.' *American Journal of Human Biology: The Official Journal of the Human Biology Association,* 2006 *18*(5), pp.630-638.

18. Zeitlin, M F, Ahmed, N U 'Nutritional correlates of frequency and length of breastfeeds in rural Bangladesh.' *Early Human Development.* 1995 Apr 14; 41(2):97-110.

9. Lies, damned lies, and statistics

1. Marriott, N 'The future of statistical thinking.' *Significance.* 2014 Dec 1; 11(5):78-80.

2. Huff, D *How to Lie with Statistics.* WW Norton & Company. 1993.

3. Levitin, D. *A Field Guide to Lies and Statistics: A Neuroscientist on how to Make Sense of a Complex World.* Penguin UK; 2016.

4. Spiegelhalter, D *The Art of Statistics.* Pelican

5. Rumsey, D J *U Can: Statistics for Dummies.* John Wiley & Sons; 2015.

6. Wheelan, C *Naked statistics: Stripping the dread from the data.* WW Norton & Company; 2013.

7. theconversation.com/giving-your-baby-solid-food-early-wont-help-them-sleep-better-99645

8. Grieger, J A, Grzeskowiak, L E, Bianco-Miotto, T, Jankovic-Karasoulos, T, Moran, L J, Wilson, R L, Leemaqz, S Y, Poston, L, McCowan, L, Kenny, L C, Myers, J 'Pre-pregnancy fast food and fruit intake is associated with time to pregnancy.' *Human Reproduction.* 2018 May 4; 33(6):1063-70.

9. McAndrew, F, Thompson, J, Fellows, L, Large, A, Speed, M, Renfrew, M J 'Infant Feeding Survey 2010.' *Leeds: Health and Social Care Information Centre.* 2012.

10. www.statisticssolutions.com/transforming-data-for-normality/

11. publications.parliament.uk/pa/cm201719/cmselect/cmenvaud/1805/180505.htm#_id-TextAnchor021

12. Simons SS, Beijers R, Cillessen AH, de Weerth C. Development of the cortisol circadian rhythm in the light of stress early in life. *Psychoneuroendocrinology.* 2015 Dec 1;62:292-300.

13. www.thesun.co.uk/news/7168515/ivf-babies-children-blood-pressure/

14. Meister TA, Rimoldi SF, Soria R, von Arx R, Messerli FH, Sartori C, Scherrer U, Rexhaj E. Association of assisted reproductive technologies with arterial hypertension during adolescence. *Journal of the American College of Cardiology.* 2018 Sep 11;72(11):1267-74.

15. Schünemann, H, Hill, S, Guyatt, G, Akl, E A, Ahmed, F 'The GRADE approach and Bradford Hill's criteria for causation.' *Journal of Epidemiology & Community Health.* 2011 May 1; 65(5):392-5.

10. How to understand a research paper

1. www.ndr.de/der_ndr/presse/More-than-5000-German-scientists-have-published-papers-in-pseudo-scientific-journals,fakescience178.html
2. Lukić, T, Blešić, I, Basarin, B, Ivanović, B, Milošević, D, Sakulski, D 'Predatory and fake scientific journals/publishers – a global outbreak with rising trend: a review.' *Geographica Pannonica.* 2014; 18:69–81.
3. Oermann, M H, Conklin, J L, Nicoll, L H, Chinn, P L, Ashton, K S, Edie, A H, Amarasekara, S, Budinger, S C 'Study of predatory open access nursing journals.' *Journal of Nursing Scholarship.* 2016 Nov; 48(6):624-32.
4. Davis, P 'Open access publisher accepts nonsense manuscript for dollars.' *The Scholarly Kitchen;* 2009.
5. Bohannon, J 'Who's afraid of peer review?' *Science.* 2013;342:60–5.
6. Stromberg, J '"Get Me Off Your Fucking Mailing List" is an Actual Science Paper Accepted by a Journal.' *Vox.* 2014 Nov; 21:10-1.

11. What about other types of writing?

1. www.dailymail.co.uk/health/article-1347006/Breast-feeding-6-months-causes-allergies-warn-British-researchers.html
2. Fewtrell, M, Wilson, D C, Booth, I, Lucas, A 'Six months of exclusive breast feeding: how good is the evidence?' *BMJ* (Online). 2011 Jan 13; 342.
3. Pérez-Escamilla, R, Buccini, G S, Segura-Pérez, S, Piwoz, E 'Perspective: Should Exclusive Breastfeeding Still Be Recommended for 6 Months?' *Advances in Nutrition.* 2019 May 31.
4. www.gov.uk/government/publications/feeding-in-the-first-year-of-life-sacn-report
5. Bass, J, Gartley, Y, & Kleinman, R 'Unintended Consequences of Current Breastfeeding Initiatives.' *JAMA*, doi:1001/jamapediatrics.2016.1529
6. www.who.int/nutrition/bfhi/ten-steps/en/
7. Pérez-Escamilla, R, Martinez, J L, Segura-Pérez, S 'Impact of the Baby-friendly Hospital Initiative on breastfeeding and child health outcomes: a systematic review.' *Maternal & Child Nutrition.* 2016 Jul; 12(3):402-17.
8. Charpak, N, Gabriel Ruiz, J, Zupan, J, Cattaneo, A, Figueroa, Z, Tessier, R, & Mokhachane, M 'Kangaroo mother care: 25 years after.' *Acta Paediatrica.* 2005 94(5), 514-522.
9. Bystrova, K, Ivanova, V, Edhborg, M, Matthiesen, A S, Ransjö-Arvidson, A B, Mukhamedrakhimov, R, & Widström, A M 'Early contact versus separation: effects on mother–infant interaction one year later.' *Birth.* 2009 36(2), 97-109.
10. Buccini, G D, Pérez-Escamilla, R, Venancio, S I 'Pacifier use and exclusive breastfeeding in Brazil.' *Journal of Human Lactation.* 2016 Aug; 32(3):NP52-60.
11. Jaafar, S H, Ho, J J, Jahanfar, S, Angolkar, M 'Effect of restricted pacifier use in breastfeeding term infants for increasing duration of breastfeeding.' *Cochrane Database of Systematic Reviews.* 2016(8).
12. Herlenius, E, & Kuhn, P 'Sudden unexpected postnatal collapse of newborn infants: a review of cases, definitions, risks, and preventive measures.' *Translational Stroke Research.* 2013 4(2), 236-247.
13. Helsley, L, McDonald, J V, & Stewart, V T 'Addressing In-Hospital.' *The Joint Commission Journal on Quality and Patient Safety.* 2010 36(7), 327-333.
14. Ball, H L, Ward-Platt, M P, Heslop, E, Leech, S J, & Brown, K A 'Randomised trial of infant sleep location on the postnatal ward.' *Archives of Disease in Childhood.* 2006 91(12), 1005-1010.
15. www.nct.org.uk/professional/research/maternity%20statistics/maternity-statistics-england

16. www.cdc.gov/nchs/data/nvsr/nvsr59/nvsr59_05.pdf
17. www.rcm.org.uk/learning-and-career/learning-and-research/ebm-articles/pain-and-epidural-use-in-normal-childbirth
18. Brown, A, & Jordan, S 'Impact of birth complications on breastfeeding duration: an internet survey.' *Journal of Advanced Nursing.* 2013 69(4), 828-839.
19. Hookway L. *Holistic sleep coaching: gentle alternatives to sleep training for health and childcare professionals.* Praeclarus Press. 2018.
20. Tomori C. *Nighttime breastfeeding: An American cultural dilemma.* Berghahn Books; 2014 Oct 1.
21. www.badscience.net/2007/02/ms-gillian-mckeith-banned-from-calling-herself-a-doctor
22. www.telegraph.co.uk/news/health/news/8580454/Ignore-official-weaning-guidelines-says-Annabel-Karmel.html
23. www.youtube.com/watch?v=JvroKVBY-CM
24. Bernhardt, J M, Felter, E M 'Online pediatric information seeking among mothers of young children: results from a qualitative study using focus groups.' *Journal of Medical Internet Research.* 2004;6(1):e7.
25. theconversation.com/taking-paracetamol-during-pregnancy-may-affect-the-childs-behaviour-in-early-years-123392
26. 26. Golding J, Gregory S, Clark R, Ellis G, Iles-Caven Y, Northstone K. Associations between paracetamol (acetaminophen) intake between 18 and 32 weeks gestation and neurocognitive outcomes in the child: A longitudinal cohort study. *Paediatric and perinatal epidemiology.* 2019 Sep 15.

12. Randomised controlled trials

1. Sung, V, Hiscock, H, Tang, M L, Mensah, F K, Nation, M L, Satzke, C, Heine, R G, Stock, A, Barr, R G, Wake, M 'Treating infant colic with the probiotic Lactobacillus reuteri: double blind, placebo controlled randomised trial.' *BMJ.* 2014 Apr 1; 348:g2107.
2. Knight, M, Chiocchia, V, Partlett, C, Rivero-Arias, O, Hua, X, Hinshaw, K, Tuffnell, D, Linsell, L, Juszczak, E, Enderby, H, Thakar, R 'Prophylactic antibiotics in the prevention of infection after operative vaginal delivery (ANODE): a multicentre randomised controlled trial.' *The Lancet.* 2019 May 13.
3. Yeh, R W, Valsdottir, L R, Yeh, M W, Shen, C, Kramer, D B, Strom, J B, Secemsky, E A, Healy, J L, Domeier, R M, Kazi, D S, Nallamothu, B K 'Parachute use to prevent death and major trauma when jumping from aircraft: randomized controlled trial.' *BMJ.* 2018 Dec 13; 363:k5094.
4. www.visualcomplexity.com/vc/project.cfm?id=622
5. www.youtube.com/watch?v=inTkvx5m0es
6. Wahlqvist, M L, Krawetz, S A, Rizzo, N S, Dominguez-Bello, M G, Szymanski, L M, Barkin, S, Yatkine, A, Waterland, R A, Mennella, J A, Desai, M, Ross, M G 'Early-life influences on obesity: from preconception to adolescence.' *Annals of the New York Academy of Sciences.* 2015 Jul 1; 1347(1):1-28.
7. Rauschert, S, Mori, T A, Beilin, L J, Jacoby, P, Uhl, O, Koletzko, B, Oddy, W H, Hellmuth, C 'Early life factors, obesity risk, and the metabolome of young adults.' *Obesity.* 2017 Sep; 25(9):1549-55.
8. Snethen, J A, Hewitt, J B, Goretzke, M 'Childhood obesity: the infancy connection.' *Journal of Obstetric, Gynecologic & Neonatal Nursing.* 2007 Sep 1; 36(5):501-10.
9. Shiovitz, T M, Bain, E E, McCann, D J, Skolnick, P, Laughren, T, Hanina, A, Burch, D 'Mitigating the effects of nonadherence in clinical trials.' *The Journal of Clinical Pharmacology.* 2016 Sep 1; 56(9):1151-64.
10. Murali, K M, Mullan, J, Chen, J H, Roodenrys, S, Lonergan, M 'Medication adherence

in randomized controlled trials evaluating cardiovascular or mortality outcomes in dialysis patients: A systematic review.' *BMC Nephrology.* 2017 Dec; 18(1):42.

11. Perkin, M R, Logan, K, Marrs, T, Radulovic, S, Craven, J, Flohr, C, Lack, G, Young, L, Offord, V, DeSousa, M, Cullen, J 'Enquiring About Tolerance (EAT) study: feasibility of an early allergenic food introduction regimen.' *Journal of Allergy and Clinical Immunology.* 2016 May 1; 137(5):1477-86.

12. Williams Erickson L, Taylor R, Haszard J, Fleming E, Daniels L, Morison B, Leong C, Fangupo L, Wheeler B, Taylor B, Te Morenga L. Impact of a modified version of baby-led weaning on infant food and nutrient intakes: the BLISS Randomized Controlled Trial. *Nutrients.* 2018 Jun;10(6):740.

13. Taylor, R W, Williams, S M, Fangupo, L J, Wheeler, B J, Taylor, B J, Daniels, L, Fleming, E A, McArthur, J, Morison, B, Erickson, L W, Davies, R S 'Effect of a baby-led approach to complementary feeding on infant growth and overweight: a randomized clinical trial.' *JAMA Pediatrics.* 2017 Sep 1; 171(9):838-46.

14. Brown, A, Lee, M D 'Early influences on child satiety-responsiveness: the role of weaning style.' *Pediatric Obesity.* 2015 Feb; 10(1):57-66.

15. Townsend, E, Pitchford, N J 'Baby knows best? The impact of weaning style on food preferences and body mass index in early childhood in a case–controlled sample.' *BMJ Open.* 2012 Jan 1; 2(1):e000298.

16. McAndrew, F, Thompson, J, Fellows, L, Large, A, Speed, M, Renfrew, M J 'Infant Feeding Survey 2010.' *Leeds: Health and Social Care Information Centre.* 2012.

17. Patel, R, Oken, E, Bogdanovich, N, Matush, L, Sevkovskaya, Z, Chalmers, B, Hodnett, E D, Vilchuck, K, Kramer, M S, Martin, R M 'Cohort profile: the promotion of breastfeeding intervention trial (PROBIT).' *International Journal of Epidemiology.* 2013 Mar 7; 43(3):679-90.

18. 18 Duijts L, Jaddoe VW, Hofman A, Moll HA. Prolonged and exclusive breastfeeding reduces the risk of infectious diseases in infancy. Pediatrics. 2010 Jul 1;126(1):e18-25.

19. Kramer, M S, Chalmers, B, Hodnett, E D, Sevkovskaya, Z, Dzikovich, I, Shapiro, S, Collet, J P, Vanilovich, I, Mezen, I, Ducruet, T, Shishko, G 'Promotion of Breastfeeding Intervention Trial (PROBIT): a randomized trial in the Republic of Belarus.' *JAMA.* 2001 Jan 24; 285(4):413-20.

20. Flaherman, V J, Narayan, N R, Hartigan-O'Connor, D, Cabana, M D, McCulloch, C E, Paul, I M 'The effect of early limited formula on breastfeeding, readmission, and intestinal microbiota: a randomized clinical trial.' *The Journal of Pediatrics.* 2018 May 1; 196:84-90.

21. Grobman WA, Rice MM, Reddy UM, Tita AT, Silver RM, Mallett G, Hill K, Thom EA, El-Sayed YY, Perez-Delboy A, Rouse DJ. Labor induction versus expectant management in low-risk nulliparous women. New England Journal of Medicine. 2018 Aug 9;379(6):513-23.

22. McGrath, S K, Kennell, J H 'A randomized controlled trial of continuous labor support for middle-class couples: Effect on cesarean delivery rates.' *Birth.* 2008 Jun; 35(2):92-7.

13. More about ethics

1. Israel, M, Hay, I 'Research ethics for social scientists.' *Sage*; 2006 Jun 15.

2. The Nuremberg Code history.nih.gov/research/downloads/nuremberg.pdf

3. www.wma.net/policies-post/wma-declaration-of-helsinki-ethical-principles-for-medical-research-involving-human-subjects/

4. Beck, H P, Levinson, S, Irons, G 'Finding little Albert: A journey to John B. Watson's infant laboratory.' *American Psychologist.* 2009 Oct; 64(7):605.

5. Bandura, A, Ross, D, Ross, S A 'Imitation of film-mediated aggressive models.' *The Journal of Abnormal and Social Psychology.* 1963 Jan;66(1):3.

6. www.spring.org.uk/2007/06/monster-study.php

7. nypost.com/2018/06/23/these-triplets-were-separated-at-birth-for-a-twisted-psych-study/

8. Kramer, M S, Chalmers, B, Hodnett, E D, Sevkovskaya, Z, Dzikovich, I, Shapiro, S, Collet, J P, Vanilovich, I, Mezen, I, Ducruet, T, Shishko, G 'Promotion of Breastfeeding Intervention Trial (PROBIT): a randomized trial in the Republic of Belarus.' *JAMA*. 2001 Jan 24; 285(4):413-20.

9. Pourhoseingholi MA, Baghestani AR, Vahedi M. How to control confounding effects by statistical analysis. Gastroenterology and Hepatology from bed to bench. 2012;5(2):79.

14. Channel your inner five-year-old and always ask 'Why?'

1. www.reuters.com/article/us-health-pregnancy-fish-diet/eating-lots-of-fish-in-pregnancy-linked-to-obesity-risk-for-kids-idUSKCN0VO226

2. Stratakis N, Roumeliotaki T, Oken E, Barros H, Basterrechea M, Charles MA, Eggesbø M, Forastiere F, Gaillard R, Gehring U, Govarts E. Fish intake in pregnancy and child growth: a pooled analysis of 15 European and US birth cohorts. JAMA pediatrics. 2016 Apr 1;170(4):381-90.

3. Ladomenou, F, Moschandreas, J, Kafatos, A, Tselentis, Y, Galanakis, E 'Protective effect of exclusive breastfeeding against infections during infancy: a prospective study.' *Archives of Disease in Childhood*. 2010 Dec 1; 95(12):1004-8.

4. Mueller, N T, Bakacs, E, Combellick, J, Grigoryan, Z, Dominguez-Bello, M G 'The infant microbiome development: mom matters.' *Trends in Molecular Medicine*. 2015 Feb 1; 21(2):109-17.

5. Yang, I, Corwin, E J, Brennan, P A, Jordan, S, Murphy, J R, Dunlop, A 'The infant microbiome: implications for infant health and neurocognitive development.' *Nursing Research*. 2016 Jan; 65(1):76.

6. Andreas, N J, Kampmann, B, Le-Doare, K M 'Human breast milk: A review on its composition and bioactivity.' *Early Human Development*. 2015 Nov 1;91(11):629-35.

7. Moore ER, Bergman N, Anderson GC, Medley N. Early skin-to-skin contact for mothers and their healthy newborn infants. *Cochrane database of systematic Reviews*. 2016(11).

8. Gregson S, Blacker J. Kangaroo care in pre-term or low birth weight babies in a postnatal ward. *British journal of midwifery*. 2011 Sep;19(9):568-77.

9. Feldman R, Rosenthal Z, Eidelman AI. Maternal-preterm skin-to-skin contact enhances child physiologic organization and cognitive control across the first 10 years of life. *Biological psychiatry*. 2014 Jan 1;75(1):56-64.

10. Blomqvist YT, Frölund L, Rubertsson C, Nyqvist KH. Provision of Kangaroo Mother Care: supportive factors and barriers perceived by parents. Scandinavian Journal of Caring Sciences. 2013 Jun;27(2):345-53.

11. Kostandy RR, Ludington-Hoe SM, Cong X, Abouelfettoh A, Bronson C, Stankus A, Jarrell JR. Kangaroo Care (skin contact) reduces crying response to pain in preterm neonates: pilot results. Pain management nursing. 2008 Jun 1;9(2):55-65.

12. Bramson L, Lee JW, Moore E, Montgomery S, Neish C, Bahjri K, Melcher CL. Effect of early skin-to-skin mother—Infant contact during the first 3 hours following birth on exclusive breastfeeding during the maternity hospital stay. Journal of Human Lactation. 2010 May;26(2):130-7.

13. Cong X, Cusson RM, Walsh S, Hussain N, Ludington-Hoe SM, Zhang D. Effects of skin-to-skin contact on autonomic pain responses in preterm infants. The Journal of Pain. 2012 Jul 1;13(7):636-45.

14. Cong X, Ludington-Hoe SM, Hussain N, Cusson RM, Walsh S, Vazquez V, Briere CE,

Vittner D. Parental oxytocin responses during skin-to-skin contact in pre-term infants. *Early human development*. 2015 Jul 1;91(7):401-6.

15. Bigelow A, Power M, MacLellan-Peters J, Alex M, McDonald C. Effect of mother/ infant skin-to-skin contact on postpartum depressive symptoms and maternal physiological stress. *Journal of Obstetric, Gynecologic & Neonatal Nursing*. 2012 May 1;41(3):369-82.

16. McKenna JJ, McDade T. Why babies should never sleep alone: a review of the co-sleeping controversy in relation to SIDS, bedsharing and breast feeding. *Paediatric respiratory reviews*. 2005 Jun 1;6(2):134-52.

17. Blair PS, Sidebotham P, Pease A, Fleming PJ. Bed-sharing in the absence of hazardous circumstances: is there a risk of sudden infant death syndrome? An analysis from two case-control studies conducted in the UK. *PLoS One*. 2014 Sep 19;9(9):e107799.

18. Ward TC. Reasons for mother–infant bed-sharing: A systematic narrative synthesis of the literature and implications for future research. *Maternal and child health journal*. 2015 Mar 1;19(3):675-90.

19. www.telegraph.co.uk/news/health/news/12193136/Half-of-new-mothers-lie-about-sharing-bed-with-their-baby.html

20. www.lullabytrust.org.uk/new-survey-shows-40-of-parents-are-not-co-sleeping-safely

21. Flaherman VJ, Narayan NR, Hartigan-O'Connor D, Cabana MD, McCulloch CE, Paul IM. The effect of early limited formula on breastfeeding, readmission, and intestinal microbiota: a randomized clinical trial. *The Journal of pediatrics*. 2018 May 1;196:84-90.

22. Chantry CJ, Dewey KG, Peerson JM, Wagner EA, Nommsen-Rivers LA. In-hospital formula use increases early breastfeeding cessation among first-time mothers intending to exclusively breastfeed. *The Journal of pediatrics*. 2014 Jun 1;164(6):1339-45.

23. www.cdc.gov/nchs/fastats/delivery.htm

24. Brown A, Jordan S. Impact of birth complications on breastfeeding duration: an internet survey. *Journal of advanced nursing*. 2013 Apr;69(4):828-39.

25. www.cdc.gov/breastfeeding/data/reportcard.htm

26. Coomarasamy A, Devall AJ, Cheed V, Harb H, Middleton LJ, Gallos ID, Williams H, Eapen AK, Roberts T, Ogwulu CC, Goranitis I. A randomized trial of progesterone in women with bleeding in early pregnancy. *New England Journal of Medicine*. 2019 May 9;380(19):1815-24.

27. Bernardo H, Cesar V, World Health Organization. Long-term effects of breastfeeding: a systematic review.

28. Koletzko B, Broekaert I, Demmelmair H, Franke J, Hannibal I, Oberle D, Schiess S, Baumann BT, Verwied-Jorky S. Protein intake in the first year of life: a risk factor for later obesity?. InEarly nutrition and its later consequences: new opportunities 2005 (pp. 69-79). Springer, Dordrecht.

29. European Child Obesity Trial Study group. Lower protein in infant formula is associated with lower weight up to age 2 y: a randomized clinical trial. *The American journal of clinical nutrition* 89, no. 6 (2009): 1836-1845.

30. Weber M, Grote V, Closa-Monasterolo R, Escribano J, Langhendries JP, Dain E, Giovannini M, Verduci E, Gruszfeld D, Socha P, Koletzko B. Lower protein content in infant formula reduces BMI and obesity risk at school age: follow-up of a randomized trial. *The American journal of clinical nutrition*. 2014 Mar 12;99(5):1041-51.

31. 34 Brown A, Raynor P, Lee M. Maternal control of child-feeding during breast and formula feeding in the first 6 months post-partum. *Journal of Human Nutrition and Dietetics*. 2011 Apr;24(2):177-86.

32. Rapley GA. Baby-led weaning: Where are we now? *Nutrition Bulletin*. 2018 Sep;43(3):262-8.

33. Brown A, Jones SW, Rowan H. Baby-led weaning: the evidence to date. *Current nutri-*

tion reports. 2017 Jun 1;6(2):148-56.

34. Larkin P, Begley CM, Devane D. Women's experiences of labour and birth: an evolutionary concept analysis. *Midwifery.* 2009 Apr 1;25(2):e49-59.

35. Smith J, Plaat F, Fisk NM. The natural caesarean: a woman-centred technique. *BJOG: An International Journal of Obstetrics & Gynaecology.* 2008 Jul;115(8):1037-42.

36. Hiscock H, Bayer J, Gold L, Hampton A, Ukoumunne OC, Wake M. Improving infant sleep and maternal mental health: a cluster randomised trial. *Archives of disease in childhood.* 2007 Nov 1;92(11):952-8.

37. Shi H, Enriquez A, Rapadas M, Martin EM, Wang R, Moreau J, Lim CK, Szot JO, Ip E, Hughes JN, Sugimoto K. NAD deficiency, congenital malformations, and niacin supplementation. *New England Journal of Medicine.* 2017 Aug 10;377(6):544-52.

15. Who took part?

1. Pawson, R, Tilley, N, Tilley, N 'Realistic evaluation.' *Sage*; 1997 Jun 23.

2. Rowe RE, Garcia JO. Social class, ethnicity and attendance for antenatal care in the United Kingdom: a systematic review. *Journal of Public Health.* 2003 Jun 1;25(2):113-9.

3. Pizzi C, De Stavola BL, Pearce N, Lazzarato F, Ghiotti P, Merletti F, Richiardi L. Selection bias and patterns of confounding in cohort studies: the case of the NINFEA web-based birth cohort. J *Epidemiol Community Health.* 2012 Nov 1;66(11):976-81.

4. Zuberi T, Bonilla-Silva E, editors. *White logic, white methods: Racism and methodology.* Rowman & Littlefield Publishers; 2008 May 2.

5. Perez CC. *Invisible Women: Exposing Data Bias in a World Designed for Men.* Random House; 2019 Mar 7.

6. www.bbc.co.uk/news/uk-england-47115305

7. Declercq ER, Sakala C, Corry MP, Applebaum S. Listening to mothers II: report of the second national US survey of women's childbearing experiences: conducted January–February 2006 for childbirth connection by Harris Interactive* in partnership with Lamaze International. *The Journal of perinatal education.* 2007;16(4):9.

8. www.health.gov.au/internet/publications/publishing.nsf/Content/int-comp-whocode-bf-init~int-comp-whocode-bf-init-ico~int-comp-whocode-bf-init-ico-norway

9. Laing IA. Hypernatremic dehydration in newborn infants. *Acta Pharmacol Sin.* 2002;23(suppl):48-51.

10. Manganaro R, Mami C, Marrone T, Marseglia L, Gemelli M. Incidence of dehydration and hypernatremia in exclusively breast-fed infants. *J Pediatr.* 2001;139(5):673-675.

11. Oddie SJ, Craven V, Deakin K, Westman J, Scally A. Severe neonatal hypernatraemia: a population based study. *Arch Dis Child Fetal Neonatal Ed.* 2013;98(5):F384-F387.

12. Pelleboer RA, Bontemps ST, Verkerk PH, Van Dommelen P, Pereira RR, Van Wouwe JP. A nationwide study on hospital admissions due to dehydration in exclusively breastfed infants in the Netherlands: its incidence, clinical characteristics, treat- ment and outcome. *Acta Paediatr.* 2009;98(5):807-811.

13. Moritz ML, Manole MD, Bogen DL, Ayus JC. Breastfeeding-associated hypernatremia: are we missing the diagnosis? *Pediatrics.* 2005 Sep 1;116(3):e343-7.

14. Dewey KG, Nommsen-Rivers LA, Heinig MJ, Cohen RJ. Risk factors for suboptimal infant breastfeeding behavior, delayed onset of lactation, and excess neonatal weight loss. *Pediatrics.* 2003;112(3):607-619.

15. Boskabadi H, Maamouri G, Ebrahimi M, Ghayour-Mobarhan M, Esmaeily H, Sahebkar A, Ferns GA. Neonatal hypernatremia and dehydration in infants receiving inadequate breastfeeding. *Asia Pacific journal of clinical nutrition.* 2010 Sep 1;19(3):301-7.

16. www.cbs.nl/en-gb/news/2011/47/obesity-rate-in-the-netherlands-lower-than-in-other-oecd-countries

17. Wammes JO, Jeurissen PA, Westert GE. The Dutch Health System, 2014. Utrecht:

NVAG. www. nvag. nl/afbeeldingen/2015/nscholing/Netherlands% 20Health% 20Care% 20System. 2014;202014:20.

18. www.theguardian.com/lifeandstyle/2018/sep/18/gaining-too-much-or-too-little-weight-in-pregnancy-could-affect-babys-health

19. Tam CH, Ma RC, Yuen LY, Ozaki R, Li AM, Hou Y, Chan MH, Ho CS, Yang X, Chan JC, Tam WH. The impact of maternal gestational weight gain on cardiometabolic risk factors in children. *Diabetologia*. 2018 Dec 1;61(12):2539-48.

20. McAndrew F, Thompson J, Fellows L, Large A, Speed M, Renfrew MJ. Infant feeding survey 2010. Leeds: Health and Social Care Information Centre. 2012 Nov 20.

21. Perkin MR, Logan K, Marrs T, Radulovic S, Craven J, Flohr C, Lack G, Young L, Offord V, DeSousa M, Cullen J. Enquiring About Tolerance (EAT) study: feasibility of an early allergenic food introduction regimen. *Journal of Allergy and Clinical Immunology*. 2016 May 1;137(5):1477-86.

22. Grobman WA, Rice MM, Reddy UM, Tita AT, Silver RM, Mallett G, Hill K, Thom EA, El-Sayed YY, Perez-Delboy A, Rouse DJ. Labor induction versus expectant management in low-risk nulliparous women. *New England Journal of Medicine*. 2018 Aug 9;379(6):513-23.

23. www.ons.gov.uk/peoplepopulationandcommunity/birthsdeathsandmarriages/livebirths/bulletins/birthsbyparentscharacteristicsinenglandandwales/2015

24. Schwarz C, Gross MM, Heusser P, Berger B. Women's perceptions of induction of labour outcomes: Results of an online-survey in Germany. *Midwifery*. 2016 Apr 1;35:3-10.

25. Flaherman VJ, Narayan NR, Hartigan-O'Connor D, Cabana MD, McCulloch CE, Paul IM. The effect of early limited formula on breastfeeding, readmission, and intestinal microbiota: a randomized clinical trial. *The Journal of Pediatrics*. 2018 May 1;196:84-90.

26. Huff D. *How to lie with statistics*. WW Norton & Company; 1993 Oct 17.

27. Abdelrahman W, Abdelmageed A. Medical record keeping: clarity, accuracy, and timeliness are essential. BMJ: *British Medical Journal*. 2014 Jan 9;348:f7716.

28. Kühberger A, Fritz A, Lermer E, Scherndl T. The significance fallacy in inferential statistics. *BMC research notes*. 2015 Dec;8(1):84.

29. Bradbury KE, Murphy N, Key TJ. Diet and colorectal cancer in UK Biobank: a prospective study. *International journal of epidemiology*. 2019 Apr 17.

30. www.newscientist.com/article/dn20104-how-to-understand-the-risk-of-a-bacon-sandwich-giving-you-bowel-cancer/

31. Mueller NT, Bakacs E, Combellick J, Grigoryan Z, Dominguez-Bello MG. The infant microbiome development: mom matters. *Trends in molecular medicine*. 2015 Feb 1;21(2):109-17.

32. www.dailymail.co.uk/health/article-4781934/Why-pregnant-women-shouldn-t-use-antibacterial-soap.html

33. Enright HA, Falso MJ, Malfatti MA, Lao V, Kuhn EA, Hum N, Shi Y, Sales AP, Haack KW, Kulp KS, Buchholz BA. Maternal exposure to an environmentally relevant dose of triclocarban results in perinatal exposure and potential alterations in offspring development in the mouse model. *PloS one*. 2017 Aug 9;12(8):e0181996.

16. What was actually measured?

1. McAndrew F, Thompson J, Fellows L, Large A, Speed M, Renfrew MJ. Infant feeding survey 2010. Leeds: Health and Social Care Information Centre. 2012 Nov 20.

2. Ladomenou F, Moschandreas J, Kafatos A, Tselentis Y, Galanakis E. Protective effect of exclusive breastfeeding against infections during infancy: a prospective study. *Archives of disease in childhood*. 2010 Dec 1;95(12):1004-8.

3. Mueller NT, Bakacs E, Combellick J, Grigoryan Z, Dominguez-Bello MG. The infant microbiome development: mom matters. *Trends in molecular medicine*. 2015 Feb 1;21(2):109-17.

4. Yang I, Corwin EJ, Brennan PA, Jordan S, Murphy JR, Dunlop A. The infant microbiome: implications for infant health and neurocognitive development. *Nursing research*. 2016 Jan;65(1):76.

5. Fallani M, Amarri S, Uusijarvi A, Adam R, Khanna S, Aguilera M, Gil A, Vieites JM, Norin E, Young D, Scott JA. Determinants of the human infant intestinal microbiota after the introduction of first complementary foods in infant samples from five European centres. *Microbiology*. 2011 May 1;157(5):1385-92.

6. Andreas NJ, Kampmann B, Le-Doare KM. Human breast milk: A review on its composition and bioactivity. *Early human development*. 2015 Nov 1;91(11):629-35.

7. Chowdhury, R., Sinha, B., Sankar, M. J., Taneja, S., Bhandari, N., Rollins, N., ... & Martines, J. (2015). Breastfeeding and maternal health outcomes: a systematic review and meta-analysis. *Acta Paediatrica*, 104, 96-113.

8. Thompson JM, Tanabe K, Moon RY, Mitchell EA, McGarvey C, Tappin D, Blair PS, Hauck FR. Duration of breastfeeding and risk of SIDS: an individual participant data meta-analysis. *Pediatrics*. 2017 Nov 1;140(5):e20171324.

9. Ball HL, Volpe LE. Sudden Infant Death Syndrome (SIDS) risk reduction and infant sleep location–Moving the discussion forward. *Social science & medicine*. 2013 Feb 1;79:84-91.

10. Brown, A., & Lee, M. (2012). Breastfeeding during the first year promotes satiety responsiveness in children aged 18–24 months. *Pediatric obesity*, 7(5), 382-390.

11. Bartok CJ, Ventura AK. Mechanisms underlying the association between breastfeeding and obesity. *International Journal of Pediatric Obesity*. 2009 Jan 1;4(4):196-204.

12. Duijts L, Jaddoe VW, Hofman A, Moll HA. Prolonged and exclusive breastfeeding reduces the risk of infectious diseases in infancy. *Pediatrics*. 2010 Jul 1;126(1):e18-25.

13. Quigley MA, Kelly YJ, Sacker A. Breastfeeding and hospitalization for diarrheal and respiratory infection in the United Kingdom Millennium Cohort Study. *Pediatrics*. 2007 Apr 1;119(4):e837-42.

14. Timby N, Domellöf E, Hernell O, Lönnerdal B, Domellöf M. Neurodevelopment, nutrition, and growth until 12 mo of age in infants fed a low-energy, low-protein formula supplemented with bovine milk fat globule membranes: a randomized controlled trial. *The American journal of clinical nutrition*. 2014 Feb 5;99(4):860-8.

15. Raissian KM, Su JH. The best of intentions: Prenatal breastfeeding intentions and infant health. *SSM-Population Health*. 2018 Aug 31;5:86-100.

16. Flaherman VJ, Narayan NR, Hartigan-O'Connor D, Cabana MD, McCulloch CE, Paul IM. The effect of early limited formula on breastfeeding, readmission, and intestinal microbiota: a randomized clinical trial. *The Journal of pediatrics*. 2018 May 1;196:84-90.

17. Colen CG, Ramey DM. Is breast truly best? Estimating the effects of breastfeeding on long-term child health and wellbeing in the United States using sibling comparisons. *Social Science & Medicine*. 2014 May 1;109:55-65.

18. Evenhouse E, Reilly S. Improved estimates of the benefits of breastfeeding using sibling comparisons to reduce selection bias. *Health services research*. 2005 Dec;40(6p1):1781-802.

19. Lewis ED, Richard C, Larsen BM, Field CJ. The importance of human milk for immunity in preterm infants. *Clinics in perinatology*. 2017 Mar 1;44(1):23-47.

20. Perkin MR, Logan K, Marrs T, Radulovic S, Craven J, Flohr C, Lack G, Young L, Offord V, DeSousa M, Cullen J. Enquiring About Tolerance (EAT) study: feasibility of an early allergenic food introduction regimen. *Journal of Allergy and Clinical Immunology*.

2016 May 1;137(5):1477-86.

21. Metzger MW, McDade TW. Breastfeeding as obesity prevention in the United States: a sibling difference model. *American journal of human biology*. 2010 May;22(3):291-6.

22. Hairston IS, Handelzalts JE, Lehman-Inbar T, Kovo M. Mother-infant bonding is not associated with feeding type: a community study sample. *BMC pregnancy and childbirth*. 2019 Dec;19(1):125.

23. Uvnäs-Moberg K, Handlin L, Petersson M. Self-soothing behaviors with particular reference to oxytocin release induced by non-noxious sensory stimulation. *Frontiers in psychology*. 2015 Jan 12;5:1529.

24. Gonidakis F, Rabavilas AD, Varsou E, Kreatsas G, Christodoulou GN. A 6-month study of postpartum depression and related factors in Athens Greece. *Comprehensive psychiatry*. 2008 Jun 30;49(3):275-82.

25. Hiscock H, Bayer J, Gold L, Hampton A, Ukoumunne OC, Wake M. Improving infant sleep and maternal mental health: a cluster randomised trial. *Archives of disease in childhood*. 2007 Nov 1;92(11):952-8.

26. Landsberger H. *Hawthorne Revisited*, Ithaca, 1958.

27. Benedetti F, Mayberg HS, Wager TD, Stohler CS, Zubieta JK. Neurobiological mechanisms of the placebo effect. *Journal of Neuroscience*. 2005 Nov 9;25(45):10390-402.

28. Landgren K, Hallström I. Effect of minimal acupuncture for infantile colic: a multicentre, three-armed, single-blind, randomised controlled trial (ACU-COL). *Acupuncture in Medicine*. 2017 Jun;35(3):171-9.

29. www.npeu.ox.ac.uk/frosttie

30. Berry J, Griffiths M, Westcott C. A double-blind, randomized, controlled trial of tongue-tie division and its immediate effect on breastfeeding. *Breastfeeding Medicine*. 2012 Jun 1;7(3):189-93.

31. Orne, Martin T. Demand Characteristics and the concept of Quasi-Controls. in Artifacts in Behavioral Research: Robert Rosenthal and Ralph L. Rosnow's Classic Books, beginning with page 110

32. Brown A, Lee M. A descriptive study investigating the use and nature of baby-led weaning in a UK sample of mothers. *Maternal & child nutrition*. 2011 Jan;7(1):34-47.

33. Rudzik AE, Robinson-Smith L, Ball HL. Discrepancies in maternal reports of infant sleep vs. actigraphy by mode of feeding. *Sleep medicine*. 2018 Sep 1;49:90-8.

34. Ball HL, Howel D, Bryant A, Best E, Russell C, Ward-Platt M. Bed-sharing by breastfeeding mothers: who bed-shares and what is the relationship with breastfeeding duration? *Acta Paediatrica*. 2016 Jun;105(6):628-34.

35. Brown A, Harries V. Infant sleep and night feeding patterns during later infancy: Association with breastfeeding frequency, daytime complementary food intake, and infant weight. *Breastfeeding Medicine*. 2015 Jun 1;10(5):246-52.

36. Perkin MR, Bahnson HT, Logan K, Marrs T, Radulovic S, Craven J, Flohr C, Lack G. Association of early introduction of solids with infant sleep: a secondary analysis of a randomized clinical trial. *JAMA pediatrics*. 2018 Aug 1;172(8):e180739-.

37. Price AM, Wake M, Ukoumunne OC, Hiscock H. Five-year follow-up of harms and benefits of behavioral infant sleep intervention: randomized trial. *Pediatrics*. 2012 Oct 1;130(4):643-51.

38. Middlemiss, W., Granger, D. A., Goldberg, W. A., & Nathans, L. (2012). Asynchrony of mother–infant hypothalamic–pituitary–adrenal axis activity following extinction of infant crying responses induced during the transition to sleep. *Early human development*, 88(4), 227-232.

39. Gradisar, M., Jackson, K., Spurrier, N. J., Gibson, J., Whitham, J., Williams, A. S., … & Kennaway, D. J. (2016). Behavioral interventions for infant sleep problems: a randomized controlled trial. *Pediatrics*, 137(6), e20151486.

40. Sung V, Hiscock H, Tang ML, Mensah FK, Nation ML, Satzke C, Heine RG, Stock A, Barr RG, Wake M. Treating infant colic with the probiotic Lactobacillus reuteri: double blind, placebo controlled randomised trial. *BMJ*. 2014 Apr 1;348:g2107.

17. What's the actual risk to me?

1. www.independent.co.uk/life-style/health-and-families/womens-body-changes-since-1957-self-image-fashion-weight-health-sizes-positive-a7633036.html
2. www.independent.co.uk/news/health/pregnancy-baby-thirties-live-longer-life-expectancy-coimbra-fertility-a7867901.html
3. www.ons.gov.uk/peoplepopulationandcommunity/personalandhouseholdfinances/incomeandwealth/bulletins/householddisposableincomeandinequality/yearending2018
4. www.imperial.ac.uk/news/190428/common-chest-infection-puts-babies-risk/
5. Murray, J, Bottle, A, Sharland, M, Modi, N, Aylin, P, Majeed, A, Saxena, S, Medicines for Neonates Investigator Group 'Risk factors for hospital admission with RSV bronchiolitis in England: a population-based birth cohort study.' *PloS One*. 2014 Feb 26; 9(2):e89186.
6. Wardle, J, Carnell, S, Haworth, C M, Plomin, R 'Evidence for a strong genetic influence on childhood adiposity despite the force of the obesogenic environment.' *The American Journal of Clinical Nutrition*. 2008 Feb 1; 87(2):398-404.
7. Snethen, J A, Hewitt, J B, Goretzke, M 'Childhood obesity: the infancy connection.' *Journal of Obstetric, Gynecologic & Neonatal Nursing*. 2007 Sep 1; 36(5):501-10.
8. Lindquist, A, Kurinczuk, J J, Redshaw, M, Knight, M 'Experiences, utilisation and outcomes of maternity care in England among women from different socio-economic groups: findings from the 2010 National Maternity Survey.' *BJOG: An International Journal of Obstetrics & Gynaecology*. 2015 Nov 1;122(12):1610-7.
9. Barros, A J, Victora, C G 'Measuring coverage in MNCH: determining and interpreting inequalities in coverage of maternal, newborn, and child health interventions.' *PLoS Medicine*. 2013 May 7;10(5):e1001390.
10. Kimbro, R T, Bzostek, S, Goldman, N, Rodríguez, G 'Race, ethnicity, and the education gradient in health.' *Health Affairs*. 2008 Mar; 27(2):361-72.
11. www.ndph.ox.ac.uk/news/new-report-on-uk-deaths-during-and-after-pregnancy
12. Amitay, E L, Keinan-Boker, L 'Breastfeeding and childhood leukemia incidence: a meta-analysis and systematic review.' *JAMA Pediatrics*. 2015 Jun 1; 169(6):e151025
13. www.childrenwithcancer.org.uk/childhood-cancer-info/childhood-cancer-facts-figures
14. injuryfacts.nsc.org/all-injuries/preventable-death-overview/odds-of-dying/
15. Bansal, A, Garg, C, Pakhare, A, Gupta, S 'Selfies: A boon or bane?' *Journal of Family Medicine and Primary Care*. 2018 Jul; 7(4):828.
16. www.bmj.com/content/suppl/2003/09/25/327.7417.694.DC1
17. niemanreports.org/articles/understanding-factors-of-risk-perception/
18. www.unicef.org.uk/babyfriendly/wp-content/uploads/sites/2/2016/07/Co-sleeping-and-SIDS-A-Guide-for-Health-Professionals.pdf
19. Blair, P S, Sidebotham, P, Evason-Coombe, C, Edmonds, M, Heckstall-Smith, E M & Fleming, P 'Hazardous co-sleeping environments and risk factors amenable to change: case-control study of SIDS in south west England.' *BMJ*. 2009 339:b3666
20. www.bbc.co.uk/news/health-41981549
21. injuryfacts.nsc.org/all-injuries/preventable-death-overview/odds-of-dying/
22. Willett, W C, Green, A, Stampfer, M J, Speizer, F E, Colditz, G A, Rosner, B, Monson, R R, Stason, W, Hennekens, C H 'Relative and absolute excess risks of coronary heart disease among women who smoke cigarettes.' *New England Journal of Medicine*. 1987 Nov 19; 317(21):1303-9.

23. Peto, R, Darby, S, Deo, H, Silcocks, P, Whitley, E, Doll, R 'Smoking, smoking cessation, and lung cancer in the UK since 1950: combination of national statistics with two case-control studies.' *BMJ.* 2000 Aug 5; 321(7257):323-9.

24. Rehm, J, Taylor, B, Mohapatra, S, Irving, H, Baliunas, D, Patra, J, Roerecke, M 'Alcohol as a risk factor for liver cirrhosis: a systematic review and meta-analysis.' *Drug and Alcohol Review.* 2010 Jul; 29(4):437-45.

25. www.washingtonpost.com/news/wonk/wp/2015/02/26/the-terrifying-rate-at-which-smokers-die-from-smoking/?utm_term=.b929d8d2927f

26. www.gov.uk/government/publications/the-public-health-burden-of-alcohol-evidence-review

27. Wax, J R, Lucas, F L, Lamont, M, Pinette, M G, Cartin, A and Blackstone, J 'Maternal and newborn outcomes in planned home birth vs planned hospital births: a metaanalysis.' *American Journal of Obstetrics and Gynecology.* 2010 203(3), pp.243-e1.

28. Rosenstein MG, Cheng YW, Snowden JM, Nicholson JM, Caughey AB. Risk of stillbirth and infant death stratified by gestational age. *Obstetrics and gynecology.* 2012 Jul;120(1):76.

29. Seijmonsbergen-Schermers, A. E., Scherjon, S. and Jonge, A. (2019), Induction of labour should be offered to all women at term. *BJOG: Int J Obstet Gy.* doi:10.1111/1471-0528.15887

30. Driscoll, C A, Pereira, N, Lichenstein, R 'In-hospital neonatal falls: an unintended consequence of efforts to improve breastfeeding.' *Pediatrics.* 2019 Jan 1;143(1):e20182488.

31. Cedergren, M I 'Maternal morbid obesity and the risk of adverse pregnancy outcome.' *Obstetrics & Gynecology.* 2004 Feb 1; 103(2):219-24.

32. Schummers, L, Hutcheon, J A, Bodnar, L M, Lieberman, E, Himes, K P 'Risk of adverse pregnancy outcomes by prepregnancy body mass index: a population-based study to inform prepregnancy weight loss counseling.' *Obstetrics and Gynecology.* 2015 Jan; 125(1):133.

33. Ramachenderan J, Bradford J, Mclean M. Maternal obesity and pregnancy complications: a review. *Australian and New Zealand Journal of Obstetrics and Gynaecology.* 2008 Jun;48(3):228-35.

34. Suidan, R S, Apuzzio, J J, Williams, S F 'Obesity, comorbidities, and the cesarean delivery rate.' *American Journal of Perinatology.* 2012 Sep; 29(08):623-8.

35. Kenny, L C, Lavender, T, McNamee, R, O'Neill, S M, Mills, T, Khashan, A S 'Advanced maternal age and adverse pregnancy outcome: evidence from a large contemporary cohort.' *PloS One.* 2013 Feb 20; 8(2):e56583.

36. Wang, Y, Tanbo, T, Åbyholm, T, Henriksen, T 'The impact of advanced maternal age and parity on obstetric and perinatal outcomes in singleton gestations.' *Archives of Gynecology and Obstetrics.* 2011 Jul 1; 284(1):31-7.

37. Carpenter, R, McGarvey, C, Mitchell, E A, Tappin, D M, Vennemann, M M, Smuk, M, Carpenter, J R 'Bed sharing when parents do not smoke: is there a risk of SIDS? An individual level analysis of five major case–control studies.' *BMJ Open.* 2013 May 1; 3(5):e002299.

18. Making the decision that is right for you... and what if you can't?

1. Crandall CS, Eshleman A, O'brien L. Social norms and the expression and suppression of prejudice: the struggle for internalization. *Journal of personality and social psychology.* 2002 Mar;82(3):359.

INDEX